Fashion Spreads

Dress, Body, Culture

Series Editor **Joanne B. Eicher,** *Regents' Professor, University of Minnesota*

Books in this provocative series seek to articulate the connections between culture and dress which is defined here in its broadest possible sense as any modification or supplement to the body. Interdisciplinary in approach, the series highlights the dialogue between identity and dress, cosmetics, coiffure, and body alternations as manifested in practices as varied as plastic surgery, tattooing, and ritual scarification. The series aims, in particular, to analyze the meaning of dress in relation to popular culture and gender issues and will include works grounded in anthropology, sociology, history, art history, literature, and folklore.

ISSN: 1360-466X

Previously published titles in the Series

Helen Bradley Foster, *"New Raiments of Self": African American Clothing in the Antebellum South*
Claudine Griggs, *"S/he: Changing Sex and Changing Clothes"*
Michaele Thurgood Haynes, *Dressing Up Debutantes: Pageantry and Glitz in Texas*
Dani Cavallaro and Alexandra Warwick, *Fashioning the Frame: Boundaries, Dress and the Body*

DRESS, BODY, CULTURE

Fashion Spreads

Word and Image in Fashion Photography Since 1980

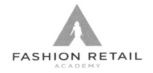

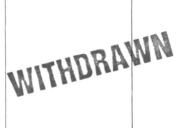

FASHION RETAIL
ACADEMY

Library

Renewals: 020 7307 2365

Email: library@fra.ac.uk

15 Gresse Street, London W1T

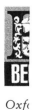

BE

Oxf

Contents

Acknowledgements   ix

List of Figures   xi

Introduction   1

Part 1: Back to the Future: Fashion Publishing Since 1980

Introduction to Part 1   17

1   *Vogue*   19

2   *The Face*   35

3   *Arena*   49

Conclusion to Part 1   59

Part 2: Written Clothing and Image Clothing: Roland Barthes' 'The Fashion System' in Perspective

Introduction to Part 2   65

4   *The Fashion System*: A Synopsis   69

5   Going Beyond *The Fashion System*: A Critique   83

Conclusion to Part 2   101

Part 3: Bodylines: Identity and Otherness in Fashion Photography

Introduction to Part 3   107

6   Who's That Girl? Alex and Kate: A Tale of Two
        Bodies in Contemporary Fashion Photography   111

7   *Statue Men:* The Phallic Body, Identity and
        Ambiguity in Fashion Photography   143

**Appendix 1: Directory of Fashion Photographers, Stylists
and Magazine Features 1980–1996**   189

**Appendix 2: Photographers for British *Vogue*
1980–1995**   211

Bibliography   215

Index   235

Acknowledgements

I should like to thank the following people for their invaluable involvement and endless support in the preparation of this book: Kevan Rose, Marsha Meskimmon, David Crowley, Tracy Fowler, Jane O'Connor, and my Ph.D. supervisor at the University of Warwick, Dr Joanne Collie, for her illuminating comments on French translation. Also many thanks to SURI (Staffordshire University Research Initiative), which awarded me sabbatical leave during the Autumn/Winter Semester of 1996–7 so that I could convert my Ph.D. thesis into the present study. A final debt of gratitude is due to Kathryn Earle for having the faith to commission this book, to Nick Logan at Wagadon for his extremely generous permission to reproduce numerous fashion spreads from *The Face*, *Arena* and *Arena Homme Plus*, to Bruce Weber likewise for the permission to reproduce Figures 4–6 and 42, and to Anna Sherbany for her help in preparing the plates.

List of Figures

1–3   'Guys N Dolls', photographer Mark Lewis, stylist Finbar at Max Presents, *The Face* July/August 1988, courtesy of *The Face*/Wagadon Ltd.

4   Bruce Weber, 'New Morning Nebraska – Pioneers of 82 Wear Plains Clothes', British *Vogue* January 1982, courtesy of Bruce Weber.

5 and 6   Bruce Weber, 'Under Weston Eyes – Bruce Weber in a Romantic Encounter With Edward Weston', British *Vogue* December 1982, courtesy of Bruce Weber.

7   Sheila Rock, 'Style: A West Side Story', *The Face* October 1981, courtesy of *The Face*/Wagadon Ltd.

8   'The Last Daze of the Raj', photographer Sheila Rock, stylist Stephen Linard, *The Face* May 1983, courtesy of *The Face*/Wagadon Ltd.

9   'Heavy Metal', photographers Buffalo (Jamie Morgan and Ray Petri), *The Face* April 1986, courtesy of *The Face*/Wagadon Ltd.

10   'Flesh', model Nick Moss, photographer Mario Sorrenti, stylist Cathy Dixon, *The Face* April 1993, courtesy of *The Face*/Wagadon Ltd.

11   'Cuba Libre', photographer Juergen Teller, stylist Venetia Scott, *The Face* February 1992, courtesy of *The Face*/Wagadon Ltd.

12   'Leisure Lounge', photographer Andrea Giacobbe, stylist Maida, *The Face* October 1994, courtesy of *The Face*/Wagadon Ltd.

13   'England's Dreaming', photographer Corinne Day, stylist Melanie Ward, *The Face* August 1993, courtesy of *The Face*/Wagadon Ltd.

14   'London March 88', photographer Andrew Bettles, stylist Paul Frecker, *The Face* May 1988, courtesy of The Face/Wagadon Ltd.

15   'Head Hunters – Back To The No Future', photographer Jean Baptiste Mondino, stylist Judy Blame, *The Face* August 1993, courtesy of *The Face*/Wagadon Ltd.

16 and 17   'Throwback', photographer Michel Haddi, *Arena* January/February 1988, courtesy of *Arena*/Wagadon Ltd.

18   'Who's Shooting Who?', photographer Oliver Maxwell, stylist Elaine Jones, *The Face* July 1986, courtesy of *The Face*/Wagadon Ltd.

19   'Malcolm X', photographer Norman Watson, stylists Karl and Derick (UTO), *The Face* November 1992, courtesy of *The Face*/Wagadon Ltd.

20   'Apparitions', photographer Andrew Macpherson, stylist Amanda Grieve, *The Face* December 1984, courtesy of *The Face*/Wagadon Ltd.

21   'Veiled Threats', photographer Andrew Macpherson, stylist Amanda Grieve, *The Face* January 1985, courtesy of *The Face*/Wagadon Ltd.

22   'Simplex Concordia – Jason with Ketuta's head, Ketuta with Jason's head', photographer Andrea Giacobbe, stylist Maida, *The Face* July 1996, courtesy of *The Face*/Wagadon Ltd.

23   'fin de siècle', photographer Michel Haddi, stylist Debra Berkin, *Arena* January/February 1988, courtesy of *Arena*/Wagadon Ltd.

24   'once upon a time' , photographer Randall Mesdon, stylist, David Bradshaw, *Arena* November 1992, courtesy of *Arena*/Wagadon Ltd.

25   'borneo', photographer Corinne Day, stylist Melanie Ward, The Face August 1991, courtesy of *The Face*/Wagadon Ltd.

26   'Hotel Motel, Holiday In', photographer Enrique Badulescu, stylist Mitzi Lorenz, *The Face* April 1991, courtesy of *The Face*/Wagadon Ltd.

27–31   'Alex Eats', photographer Anthony Gordon, stylist Katy Lush, *The Face* April 1988, courtesy of *The Face*/Wagadon Ltd.

32   'The Baby Sitter', photographer Bertrand Marignac, *The Face* March 1994, courtesy of *The Face*/Wagadon Ltd.

33   'Idle Kitsch', photographer Ellen Von Unwerth, *Arena* March/April 1993, courtesy of *Arena*/Wagadon Ltd.

34   'Mashed', photographer Terry Richardson, stylist Karl Templer, *The Face* June 1995, courtesy of *The Face*/Wagadon Ltd.

35   'Grease Monkeys', photographer Herb Ritts, The Face October 1984, courtesy of *The Face*/Wagadon Ltd.

36   'High Noon', photographer Johnny Rosza, *Unique* October/November 1986, private collection.

37   Advertising billboards for Marlboro and RSVP Gay Cruises, Greenwich Village, New York City, 1991, photography P. Jobling.

38–41   'Close Encounters', photographer Nick Knight, stylist Simon Foxton, *Arena Homme Plus* Spring/Summer 1995, courtesy of *Arena*/Wagadon Ltd.

42   'Hollywood', photographer Bruce Weber, *Per Lui* July/August 1985, courtesy of Bruce Weber.

43   'On and Off the Road', photographer Michel Haddi, stylist Debra Berkin, *Arena* December 1986/January 1987, courtesy of *Arena*/Wagadon Ltd.

44   'Punk', photographer Nick Knight, stylist Simon Foxton, *The Face* February 1986, courtesy of *The Face*/Wagadon Ltd.

45   Advertisement for Van Gils, Strictly for Men, 1989, courtesy of the Advertising Archives.

46   'Forever Leather', photographer Marc Lebon, stylist Debbi Mason, *The Face* November 1991, courtesy of *The Face*/Wagadon Ltd.

47   'Fairground Attraction', photographer Ellen Von Unwerth, stylist Corinne Nocella, Arena July/August 1988, courtesy of *Arena*/Wagadon Ltd.

48   'Wet', photographer Kate Garner, stylists Karl and Derick (UTO), *The Face* August 1991, courtesy of *The Face*/Wagadon Ltd.

49   'Have a nice day', photographer Christopher Griffith, stylist David Bradshaw, *Arena* July/August 1994, courtesy of *Arena*/Wagadon Ltd.

50   'Trade', photographer Steve Callaghan, stylist Karl Templer, *The Face* June 1996, courtesy of *The Face*/Wagadon Ltd.

Introduction

The Fashion photograph is not just any photograph, it bears little relation to the news photograph or to the snapshot, for example; it has its own units and rules; within photographic communication, it forms a specific language which no doubt has its own lexicon and syntax, its own banned or approved 'turns of phrase'.

Roland Barthes, The Fashion System, 1990.

In 10 years' time people will look back on a series of pictures titled 'Under-Exposure' and wonder what on earth we thought we were up to.

Marion Hume, The Independent, 26 May 1993.

Fashion photography is traditionally regarded as the lightweight end of photographic practice. Its close relationship to the economic imperatives of turnover makes the fashion photograph the transitory image *par excellence*.

Rosetta Brookes, 'Double-Page spread – fashion and
advertising photography', Camerawork, 1980.

The fashion magazine and the fashion photograph tend to be regarded by many historians and critics as ephemeral and exiguous forms of cultural production. Hence, in 1979 Nancy Hall-Duncan commented that, 'Fashion photographs are ostensibly as transitory as last year's style or this month's magazine issue.'[1] While in 1991 Eamonn McCabe, picture editor of *The Guardian*, declared in somewhat parallel terms: 'Fashion photography is like its models, nobody wants it for very long.'[2] However, such statements tend to sound overly reductive, and although we all wear clothing or fashion on our bodies, as Roland Barthes has also argued, there are significant differences between how actual garments and representations of them are both produced and consumed. Indeed, the magazine is a prime motivator in helping us to assess the meaning of clothing, of determining what is in fashion and what is out. But more often than not, it does so by persuading us to overlook the mundane materiality and utility of the garments portrayed, and to ruminate instead on the symbolism of fashion:

1

The study of the garment 'represented' (by image and text), i.e. the garment dealt with by the Fashion magazine, affords an immediate methodological advantage over the analysis of real clothing . . . 'Real' clothing is burdened with practical considerations (protection, modesty, adornment); these finalities disappear from 'represented' clothing, which no longer serves to protect, to cover, or to adorn, but at most to signify protection, modesty or adornment.[3]

The role of fashion publishing can be seen to be an instrumental factor, therefore, in promoting seasonal changes in styles of clothing. Yet at the same time, it seeks to authorise certain looks and body shapes, predominantly a svelte, ectomorphic ideal for women and a muscle-bound, mesomorphic one for men, and in this way it can appear to be more conservative and predictable. As Grace Mirabella, the former editor of American *Vogue* maintains: 'fi-nally, fi-nally the magazines dictate what's at the top. We don't design clothes, but we can be very selective in our reporting. The insistence by us on a certain ease and modernity has been decisive, and we try to resist moving away from that.'[4]

In short, it can be argued that fashion photography is not necessarily for people who want to know what clothes really look like, for example the fashion buyers of large stores and their customers. The catwalk, designer's studio and changing room perform this function, affording the opportunity for scrutinising garments on bodies in movement, or for trying them on, while simultaneously enhancing their appeal with atmospheric music and lighting. Certainly the fashion spread can be seen to share similar concerns to the display of garments in arenas such as these in so far as it also trades on ideas of fantasy and masquerade. But the representation of clothing does not offer exactly the same point of identification as clothing demonstrated on the catwalk, or displayed on a mannequin or model in the studio. Rather, much fashion photography beckons us into a world of unbridled fantasies by placing fashion and the body in any number of discursive contexts. Thus it would be myopic to argue that such imagery is innocent or without deeper ideological signification. Indeed, on many occasions fashion photography has either little or nothing to do with clothing, or else clothing itself seems to become an alibi for the representation of other contemporaneous issues and ideas. The shift to a neo-realist style of representation in 1993 by photographers like Corinne Day and Davide Sorrenti and the concomitant debate concerning their imputed celebration of heroin chic is an illuminating case in point. For such photographers the most important thing has been to portray the streetwise attitude of young people and the contempt many of them have for high fashion (Figure 13). Sorrenti, for example, preferred to work with his own friends rather than with professional models, to represent them in their own milieux rather than in the studio, and to leave every blemish they may have had untouched. In 1996 an image of his girlfriend James King, taken in her apartment and showing her cutting holes into her tights, caused a furore, earning him a reputation as the champion of drug addiction and sleaze. Although there are no real signs in the picture that King had been doing drugs, the battle lines nonetheless had been drawn. Following the untimely death of Sorrenti of a heroin overdose in February 1997, for example, President Clinton threw his weight behind those who claimed a correlation between recent developments in fashion photography and the incidence of drug abuse, expatiating: 'Glorifying death is not good for any society.'[5]

Clearly, the expression of an attitude such as this bears witness to the fact that fashion photography can both make a profound impact on the social and cultural scene, and have the potential to make a lasting rather than fleeting impression on the consciousness of any individual. Moreover, as the arguments surrounding heroin chic demonstrate, nor does it always offer up an idealised or a desirable 'image' of who we want to be, or even of who we are. If we look beneath the surface of the fashion magazine, therefore, a whole cluster of more complex and serious issues emerge concerning the objectification of sex, gender, race and class, as well as the politics of consumption and pleasure. Nowhere is this more apparent than in the way bodies are represented in various narrative contexts and situations. We need to ask, therefore, who are these images for? To what extent do they either offer self-contained, sexual or identificatory fantasies or are they symptomatic of the wider cultural issues of the society and time for which and in which they are produced? These points will be unpacked in more detail in the course of this study. But for the moment it is worth sketching in how they are crystallised in a pivotal spread called 'Guys N Dolls', photographed by Mark Lewis and styled by Finbar for the July/August (1988) issue of *The Face*. As we turn the pages we encounter an elaborate masquerade, based on an eclectic range of cinematic reference points and in which various typologies of femininity and masculinity unfold.

The piece opens with a photograph captioned 'Blue Movie', depicting a young girl lying on a hospital bed and sucking her thumb (Figure 1). The textual reference here appears to be the transgressive paedophilia of Nabokov's *Lolita*, which became the focus of an eponymous film by Stanley Kubrik in 1961. Accordingly, the juvenile age of the model, who bears more than a passing resemblance to her cinematic counterpart Sue Lyon, is connoted by the 'Lovehearts' candies at the bottom right of the picture and the giant red lollipop on the right – in this context surely a symbol of phallic mastery as well? Next, we encounter two images of macho, black males

(Figure 2). The first, entitled 'Ship Ahoy, Lifeboy', features an image of a muscular sailor-figure lying supine on a bed with his legs apart, on to which a phallic flick-knife, naval emblem and bottle of rum have been montaged. The pose of the model, the knife, and the word 'Narcissus' embroidered on the rim of his hat appear to connote the murderous and sexually deviant anti-hero of Jean Genet's novel *Querelle de Brest*, which Fassbinder turned into a movie in 1982. The picaresque exploits of Querelle were similarly used in 1995 as the basis of the fashion spread 'Close Encounters', photographed by Nick Knight and styled by Simon Foxton (Figures 38–41), which is discussed more fully in Part III of this study. The second montage, 'He's Sharp? The King of Clubs', comprises a model posing as a dandyish gangster, a cigarette packet, a bottle of whiskey, a set of dice, some playing cards, and another phallic signifier – this time in the form of a handgun. The tropes of this composition appear to trade more closely on the title of the entire spread, which is ostensibly named after Joseph Mankiewicz's *Guys and Dolls* (1955), a film musical based loosely on 'The Idyll of Miss Sarah Brown', one of Damon Runyon's Broadway stories dealing with bootleggers, gamblers, and gang warfare in New York City during the Prohibition era.

The last opening of the spread comprises two more images of women (Figure 3). The first, 'Watch Those Birdies!', with its besieged model who looks like the actress Tippi Hedren, and silhouetted profile of a male figure at bottom left, is a somewhat self-conscious parody of Hitchcock's suspense thriller *The Birds* (1963). But the way that the model's head is entrapped in a cage also seems to reference a common motif in Surrealist art – André Masson's representation for the Surrealist Exhibition in 1938 of a mannequin with her head imprisoned in a bird cage, for example, or Man Ray's 1930 photograph of Lee Miller with her face and head screened by a wire mesh hat. The final image, 'There's A Tiger On That Tank', similarly seems to trade on a double signification. On the one hand, the caption puns the tagline of many Esso petrol advertising campaigns, while on the other, along with the motif of the Jane character stroking an aggressive lion included at top right, and the female model who straddles the motorbike, it also signifies an idea of female sexuality as primitive or animal. In contrast to the image of the caged woman on the facing page, however, what we seem to confront here is a more subversive and active femininity. The model adopts a pose and wears clothing that evoke the part played by Marianne Faithfull in *Girl on A Motorcycle* (1968), for example, and as such, she upsets the usual association of motorbiking with rebellious, male protagonists like Marlon Brando in *The Wild One* (1954).

Taken as a totality, then, 'Guys N Dolls' can be regarded as an entropically incongruous and typically simulacral, postmodern pastiche in which the past is replayed as if it were nothing more than a stylistic option or series of masks. Moreover, in the way that it constructs a narrative based on other media texts, the spread enables us to take refuge in what Baudrillard calls hyperreality. Now, as he argues: 'It is no longer a question of imitation, nor duplication, nor even parody. It is a question of substituting signs of the real for the real.'[6] Yet, at the same time, it would be erroneous to think that the impact of postmodern aesthetics on the iconography of fashion automatically divests it of any deeper signification whatsoever. For what 'Guys N Dolls' also illuminates is the way that both fashion and the fashion magazine are central institutions for the discursive production and circulation of sexualities, vehicles for 'putting sex in the picture', to paraphrase Foucault:

> The central issue then . . . is not to determine whether one says yes or no to sex . . . but to account for the fact that it is spoken about, to discover who does the speaking, the positions and viewpoints from which they speak, the institutions which prompt people to speak about it and which store and distribute the things which are said. What is at issue, briefly, is . . . the way in which sex is 'put into discourse'.[7]

It is with such an idea of fashion as discourse, and more particularly with the representation of the body in the fashion spread between 1980 and 1996, that this study is concerned. There are, of course, other authors who have dealt with fashion photography from various worthwhile and productive perspectives. Chief among these is Nancy Hall-Duncan's pioneering volume *The History of Fashion Photography* (1979). This covers the chronological development of various styles in fashion imagery in *Vogue* and *Harper's Bazaar*, and the contribution of photographers as diverse as Steichen, Horst, Man Ray, Avedon, Penn and Newton during the twentieth century. It was not until 1991–2, however, with the centenary of American *Vogue* and the seventy-fifth anniversary of British *Vogue* very much on the horizon, that the history of fashion photography began to be consolidated in several major exhibitions and related publications. These included Martin Harrison's *Appearances* (1991), which compares and contrasts images produced by photographers in Britain, Europe and America after 1945; *The Idealizing Vision*, a diverse collection of essays by William Ewing, Richard Martin, Valerie Steele and Anna Wintour among others, published by Aperture in 1991; and *On the Edge* (1992), a decade-by-decade survey of the most iconic photographs published in American *Vogue* since its inception in 1892, edited by Kennedy Fraser.[8] My own project has much in common with all these works in so far as it attempts to account for the production and consumption of fashion photography in the light of prevailing period styles, sexual politics and social values. It does, however, differ from them in two significant and interdependent respects. The images discussed and/or reproduced in the works I have just cited tend to be original artwork, for example, removed from the commercial context of the magazines in which they subsequently appeared. Whereas, without exception, it has been my intention to analyse and/or reproduce fashion photographs as they appeared on the printed page. Consequently, rather than concentrating exclusively on isolated images, the avowed aim of this study has been to elaborate the relationship of parts to the whole in the fashion spread. By this, I mean to convey two things. First an idea of intratextuality, that is the way that captions, descriptions and photographs are laid out as a composite entity within any given fashion spread, and the meanings that accrue from the relationship of one picture to another and of words to images. And second, an idea of intertextuality, that is the ways in which such spreads appear either to evoke or quote other media – be they works of literature, advertisements, films, or pop videos.

The current study is also deliberately selective, and I do not make any claim to furnishing an exhaustive chronological survey or history of fashion photography between 1980 and 1996. I have included for analysis here images by several producers who have gained an international reputation in the field – Bruce Weber, Herb Ritts, Nick Knight, Norman Watson, Corinne Day and Ellen von Unwerth among them (Figures 4–6, 13, 19, 33, 35 and 38–41). Yet in so doing, it has not been my conscious intention to compound any notion of the canon by unfolding an apostolic succession of the great and good who have been involved in the production of fashion photographs. Instead, my task has been to elaborate a number of the identifiable themes and chief ideas that have emerged in fashion photography since 1980 and to analyse them in the context of a series of case studies. This has entailed making certain strategic choices – which kinds of fashion magazines to include, for instance, and how many of each type. For the purpose of comparison and as a matter of methodological expediency, I decided to concentrate predominantly on British titles, and to examine three distinct categories of publication, destined principally for diverse consumers – traditional or high-fashion magazines whose readership is predominantly female, style periodicals for youth culture and, finally, magazines designated for men who are interested in fashion. Thus, by process of elimination, my elected paradigm became British *Vogue*, founded in 1916 and one of the longest-running fashion publications; *The Face*, founded in 1980 and one of the most internationally renowned and influential style magazines; and *Arena*, founded in 1986 and the first British periodical to have successfully pioneered a more thoughtful approach to the male consumer. In addition, sporadic issues of other titles were also consulted to achieve a sense of international perspective. These include *Unique*, the British and American editions of *GQ*, and certain copies of European periodicals.

Indeed, the launch date of *The Face* in May 1980 also served to determine the chronological starting-point of this study. However, it is not my intention to endorse a crude idea of decadeism, nor to claim that in 1980 suddenly everything in fashion spreads began to look different. For, as I argue in my assessment of *The Face*, much of its early iconography bears more than a passing stylistic resemblance to the 1960s pop magazine *Fabulous*, and in analysing the representation of male and female bodies, for instance, I reassess longstanding debates on pornography and censorship, and pleasure and spectatorship. Moreover, in carving out three different categories of magazine, I do not mean to imply that such boundaries are always so watertight, nor that the readers of one are entirely unaware of or do not consume the others. Rather, in the absence of any conclusive statistical data, I feel it would be safer to assert that the *typical* reader of *The Face* is probably not the same person who typically reads either its stablemate Wagadon publication *Arena* or *Vogue*, an idea that I address in my comparison of 'Alex Eats' and 'Under Exposure' in Part III (Figures 27–31). It must also be realised that while *The Face* is designated a youth culture magazine, its aesthetic, if not directional, appeal is wider than this; in 1987, for example, the age range of *The Face*'s readership was between 15 and 34 years old.[9] At the same time, although both it and *Arena* belong to Wagadon publishing, were originally conceived and edited by Nick Logan, and designed by Neville Brody, they have not necessarily developed along parallel lines: only a handful of the photographers who have contributed to *The Face* have also worked for *Arena*, for example, and the latter, along with its offshoot *Arena Homme Plus*, has clearly tended to foreground both men's fashion and men in fashion photography to a more marked degree.

On another level, the three titles elected for concentrated analysis in this study may be regarded as similar in so far as they are not exclusively fashion periodicals, and to a certain extent we can find some overlap in the themes represented in the spreads of each of them – most notably, nostalgia, travel, surrealism, sex and gender (see Appendix I). But while *Vogue*, *The Face* (particularly since 1986), and *Arena* may be considered to be aesthetically close with regard to production values, in many respects their treatment of such themes is not always the same. Under the respective editorships of Beatrix Miller (1964–June 1986), Anna Wintour (July 1986–November 1987), and Liz Tilberis (December 1987–January 1992), for example, British *Vogue* tended to employ big name photographers like Bruce Weber or Herb Ritts, to dwell on exclusive, designer fashions, mostly for women, and to photograph supermodels like Linda Evangelista and Christy Turlington wearing them, and to include many more straightforward studio-based spreads. Occasionally, more imaginative narrative spreads shot on location by Bruce Weber were featured (Figures 4–6), or sometimes more sexually daring work appeared, such as John Stember's provocative 'Soft Under-statements' (British *Vogue*, November 1980), which seemed to harp on the notoriety of earlier shoots by Helmut Newton like 'The Story of Ohhh!' for American *Vogue* in May 1975.[10] It was not until Alexandra Shulman became editor in 1992 that the fashion spreads in British *Vogue* began to incorporate the type of street or grunge style iconography more usually associated with magazines like *The Face* and *i-D*, witness 'Under Exposure' (May 1993). By 1993, we also find the names of several of the photographers who had already carved out their reputations with *The Face* and *Arena*, most notably Corinne Day and Nick Knight, cropping up in the credits of *Vogue*.

Both *The Face* and *Arena* have likewise undergone several changes of editor since their inception; the former was edited successively by Nick Logan (May 1980–October 1990), Sheryl Garratt (October 1990–October 1995), and Richard Benson (since November 1995); and the latter by Logan (November 1986–December 1989), Dylan Jones (December 1989–Autumn 1992), Kathryn Flett (Autumn 1992–October 1995), Peter Howarth (November 1995–February 1997), and Ekow Eshun (since March 1997). Notwithstanding such comings and goings, however, in contrast to *Vogue* both magazines have been consistently more adventurous in giving work to young, aspiring photographers and in their predilection for a narrative or discursive approach to subject-matter, as is evidenced in my comparative analysis of the fashion spreads included in the following chapters.

In turn, every fashion spread published in these magazines between 1980 and 1996 has been listed in Appendix I. The latter constitutes a classified directory of the major identifiable themes and ideas to be found in fashion spreads during the period, attributed alphabetically to the photographers and stylists involved in their production. It was on the basis of such empirical data that it was possible to determine the final selection of images included for analysis in each of the subsequent chapters. The directory itself, however, has also proved an invaluable source of information for establishing some general points and, it is hoped, will act as a catalyst for further research.

As things stand, therefore, the material under discussion in this study has been organised into three separate parts. Each one has its own discursive framework and diverse methodological perspective, yet is also dialectically related to the others in a wider argument concerning the construction of the body in word and image in contemporary fashion photography. Part I, 'Back to the Future' serves to provide an overview of the genesis and evolution of the three chief titles consulted, and consists of successive chapters on *Vogue*,

The Face and *Arena*. It takes as its starting-point Barthes' idea of the magazine as a 'machine for making Fashion' while examining the social, economic and aesthetic factors that have been instrumental in forging an identity for fashion photography since 1980.[11] As it is the longest-standing of the three periodicals it has, however, been necessary to sketch in some of the earlier developments in the history of *Vogue* in order better to understand and compare its relationships to the other two periodicals. In assessing the iconography of British *Vogue* after 1980, I have concentrated particularly on the interdependence of word and image in two spreads with photographs by Bruce Weber. The first, 'New Morning Nebraska – Pioneers of 82 Wear Plains Clothes', references fragments from the novels of American lesbian author Willa Cather (Figure 4), while the second, 'Under Weston Eyes', pays homage to the American photographer Edward Weston by including entries from his daybooks and commentary on his work by others (Figures 5 and 6). In each case, an interesting isology is elaborated between the form and content of the photographs and the pieces of writing cited that has implications for the meaning of authorship and originality. In addition, with their nostalgic emphasis, Weber's contemporary photographs evince a kind of fake, hyperreal vision of American history in which the past and present paradoxically seem to collapse into each other.

This postmodern treatment of time and history is pursued further in the chapters on *The Face* and *Arena*. With regard to *The Face*, I have used Dick Hebdige's incisive critique of the magazine as a central platform from which to argue the shift towards the image in postmodern culture and the death of the word that this implies. Hebdige cogently argues that: 'Truth – in so far as it exists at all – is first and foremost pictured: embodied in images which have their own power and effects.'[12] But when it comes to examining the way that fashion is represented in the magazine, this iconocentrism is not always so much in evidence. As I argue it, therefore, we can only gain a fuller understanding of the symbolism in spreads like 'Apparitions' and 'Veiled Threats' by considering text and image in tandem (Figures 20–1). Finally, in discussing *Arena*, I have focused on the image of new man, the principal masculine stereotype of the 1980s. I have endeavoured to reveal how in many instances the image of 1980s new man took its authority from an idea of masculinity that can be traced back to the early twentieth century, and that in forging together the past and the present, it constructs a mythical representation of masculinity.

Part 2, 'Written Clothing and Image Clothing', is a detailed exploration of Roland Barthes' text *The Fashion System*, first published in French in 1967 and still the only work that has attempted to evaluate the relationship of words and images in fashion publishing. For Barthes it is not so much the actual garments themselves that create the meaning of fashion, but the ways in which they can be articulated in verbal and iconic forms of representation. Accordingly, his central thesis concerns the distinction between verbal accounts of fashion and photographs or illustrations, what he refers to respectively as written clothing (*le vêtement écrit*) and image-clothing (*le vêtement-image*). But he affords priority to the first of these two terms, maintaining that words seem to proffer a purer reading of the fashion text than pictures. To be sure, Barthes' analysis of fashion publishing is extremely dense and complex. Yet for all that, it is also an indispensable work for anyone who is interested in the correspondence between words and images and the idea of repetitive performativity in the fashion spread. Thus, in examining what he has to say, my argument has been arranged into two chapters. Given the structural complexity of *The Fashion System*, Chapter 4 aims to give an overview of the chief ideas and terminology deployed in the work, while Chapter 5 builds on this and attempts to unravel some of the textual knots and ambiguities contained in it by drawing on 'Amoureuse', one of the typical fashion spreads from the late 1950s that Barthes would have encountered in researching the iconography of *Elle*. In particular, my intention has been to locate Barthes' writing into a broader philosophical context concerning logocentrism, and the way that his thesis appears to invert the iconocentric emphasis of postmodern culture. With reference to 'Amoureuse' and material from the 1980s, I have also assessed the way that Barthes treats fashion as an exclusively female pursuit and his failure to address both the representation of men in fashion texts and the role of the male consumer. Part 2 of this study, therefore, forms a methodological bridge between Part 1, inasmuch as Parts 1 and 2 are both concerned with the tension between words and images in fashion publishing, and Part 3, inasmuch as Parts 2 and 3 both deal with the nexus between fashion and the performative reiteration of gender identities.

Certainly gender and sexuality have been implicated in fashion photography since the early twentieth century. But during the 1970s there was a marked shift of emphasis in the way that the female body was represented as a fetishistic object of desire in the work of photographers like Helmut Newton, Guy Bourdin, Chris von Wangenheim and Deborah Turbeville. Nudity became more common, and fashion photography also took on connotations of lesbianism, as in Newton's infamous image of two models smoking a cigarette in a hotel lobby for French *Vogue* (March 1979), or of paedophilia, as in von Wangenheim's image of a young boy in naval costume lying on a carpet with a seductive, female model for American *Vogue* (April 1974). This more ingenuous, and often shocking, depiction of sex and gender was compounded during the 1980s when men's bodies as well as women's became objects of desire in the spectacle of fashion photography and advertising. In this respect, it is hardly surprising to note that all 455 fashion spreads listed in Appendix I include images of bodies of one type or another: masculine and feminine, straight and gay, and white and non-white. Consequently, Part III explores the intense interest in sex and the body that has subtended much fashion imagery between 1980 and 1996, and the relationship that such representations have to issues concerning identity formation and otherness, power, and visual pleasure. Thus I mean to interrogate the nexus between the body and fashion in terms of production and consumption, and the investment that different photographers and spectators might have in the fashion text. Who is it exactly that does the constructing and does the looking? Men *or* women, or men *and* women? White *or* non-white, or white *and* non-white? Straight *or* gay or straight *and* gay? Young *or* old or young *and* old? In coming to terms with these questions my argument is inextricably linked to certain aspects of psychoanalytical theory. Accordingly, I have referenced both Freudian and Lacanian ideas on identity and otherness, as well as more recent developments in feminist and queer theory by writers such as Julia Kristeva, Luce Irigaray, Judith Butler and Diana Fuss.

More particularly, Chapter 6 concentrates on the objectification of female sexualities by mobilising the central trope of the 'girl', or to put it more precisely, the woman-child. I have used two chief case studies in this context: 'Alex Eats' from *The Face*, photographed by Anthony Gordon, and 'Under Exposure' from *Vogue*, photographed by Corinne Day (Figures 27–31). In grafting the two features together for analysis, there is a whole cluster of interconnecting concerns that I want to address and questions that I want to raise. Are there any significant differences between male and female photographers in their objectification of the female body? Do the readers of the two magazines in question have different perspectives on what is acceptable photographic practice and what is not? Why should 'Under Exposure' have been implicated in debates concerning child pornography? Why does 'Alex Eats' stray into the territory of anorexia and bulimia, and what are the psychosexual implications of such a portrayal? Here, I have drawn extensively on the rich legacy of *écriture féminine*, chiefly ideas concerning abjection by Julia Kristeva, and the essential or homosexual maternal propounded by both Kristeva and Luce Irigaray. In contrast, Chapter 7 deals with the representation of masculinities, and more especially it focuses on the ideal of the phallic, muscle-bound body. With reference to a diverse range of fashion spreads, therefore, I have attempted to elaborate many of the ambiguities in the objectification of gender, sexuality and ethnicity that the phallic body implies – see, for example, Figures 38–41. But, as Bob Connell has argued: 'To recognize diversity in masculinities is not enough. We must also recognize the *relations* between different kinds of masculinity: relations of alliance, dominance and subordination.'[13] Hence this chapter includes examination of body fascism, the part played by Surrealism in the representation of the phallic woman, and, in particular, the border-crossing between straight and gay sexualities that is connoted in many contemporary fashion spreads. In assessing the latter, I have dealt with sex and gender as liminal or fluid entities, and have analysed the provisional status of the phallic body in the context of Judith Butler's compelling and penetrating theory of identity as performativity.

As a totality, this study embraces a broad spectrum of issues and ideas, and given the nature of the material under discussion, it is also based on a diverse range of sources – from theoretical texts to articles and letters in specialist and popular magazines and newspapers. The latter form a particularly fertile hunting-ground for anyone intent on keeping abreast of recent debates concerning the role of fashion photography, and on gleaning the attitudes of both producers and consumers to the subject-matter, and I have exploited them as much as possible in constructing my own argument. In the final analysis, therefore, if this study has any value at all, it is to encourage us not to dismiss the fashion texts that we encounter in magazines as the superficial products of a throwaway culture; something that we mindlessly flick through in the hairdressing salon or dental surgery, and that has no demonstrable relevance to our lives or effect on our consciousness. As Mike Featherstone contends: 'Images invite comparisons: they are constant reminders of what we are and might with effort yet become.'[14] In common with any other form of cultural production, then, the fashion spread not only emanates from the society in which it was produced but also comments on it, and to lose sight of this fact alone has repercussions far beyond the representation of fashion.

Notes

1. N. Hall-Duncan, *The History of Fashion Photography* (New York, 1979), p. 10.
2. E. McCabe, 'A ray of light in a phoney world', *The Guardian* (25 February 1991), p. 33.
3. Roland Barthes, *The Fashion System*, trans. M. Ward and R. Howard (Berkeley, 1990), p. 8.
4. Cited in N. Coleridge, *The Fashion Conspiracy* (London, 1989), p. 250.
5. Cited in 'Fatal Exposure', *The Works*, BBC 2 (25 October 1997).
6. J. Baudrillard, 'The Precession of Simulacra' in *Simulacra and Simulation*, trans. S. F. Glaser (Ann Arbor, 1994), p. 2.

7. M. Foucault, *The History of Sexuality: Vol. 1, An Introduction*, trans. R. Hurley (Harmondsworth, 1976), p. 11.

8. *Appearances* was published to tie in with a major exhibition held at the Victoria and Albert Museum, London in 1991, while *On the Edge* commemorated an exhibition at the New York Public Library in 1992.

9. D. O'Donaghue, *Lifestyles and Psychographics* (London, 1989), p. 64.

10. In 'Soft Understatements' the model has been photographed lying face down on a bed wearing see-through pants. Her body is stiff, as if a mannequin's, her legs trail on the floor, and her buttocks are visible and slightly raised.

11. Barthes, *The Fashion System*, p. 51.

12. D. Hebdige, 'The bottom line on Planet One – Squaring up to THE FACE', Ten.8, No. 19 (1985), p. 41.

13. R. W. Connell, *Masculinities* (Oxford, 1995), p. 37.

14. M. Featherstone, 'The Body in Consumer Culture', in M. Featherstone, M. Hepworth and B. S. Turner (eds), *The Body: Social Process and Cultural Theory* (London, 1991), p. 178.

Part 1

Back to the Future: Fashion Publishing Since 1980

Introduction to Part 1

Fashion photography provokes viewers and consumers into confirming their own identity through structures of desire . . . constituting a nexus between fashion and selfhood.

Jennifer Craik, *The Face* of Fashion.

Since 1980 fashion publishing in Britain has become more diverse and diffuse than it has ever been. By the end of the decade, the market position of established and popular titles in the women's press such as *Woman's Own*, *19* and *Cosmopolitan* began to be challenged by more daring prototypes such as the English editions of *Elle* and *Marie Claire*, launched in 1985 and 1988 respectively.[1] More significantly, a triad of youth culture magazines, *The Face*, *i-D* and *Blitz*, all launched in 1980, had taken the initiative of giving work to inventive young photographers, many of them recent graduates from art and design school. By 1985 their contribution to the fashion shoot had begun to make much of the iconography in traditional magazines such as *Vogue* (British edition founded 1916) and *Harper's and Queen* (founded 1970) appear staid and lacking in imagination. At the same time, a revolution in the men's magazine market had been set into chain with the appearance of new titles such as *Unique* (founded 1985), *Arena* (founded 1986), *For Him* (founded 1987 and latterly known as *FHM*), and the British edition of *GQ* (founded 1988). This trend has continued into the 1990s, when avant-garde fashion photography also became the province of independently produced titles like *Dazed and Confused* (founded 1994) and *Don't Tell It* (1995–7).

All these new titles prioritised an ideal of conspicuous consumption, and the delectable fashion photographs they contained had a huge part to play in transforming attitudes towards both style culture and gender and sexuality. A more detailed analysis of particular examples of the latter and the work of many of the photographers included in the following chapters can be found in Part 3, which evaluates the construction of gender, sexuality and ethnicity in fashion photography and the representation of the body in terms of production and consumption. But at this stage of my discussion I feel it is necessary and useful to sketch in some of the more general developments in fashion photography with reference to my representative sample of titles: British *Vogue*, *The Face* and *Arena*. Here, I wish to trace the evolution of the different photographic styles and narrative themes that were generated in these magazines, taking into account their ideological aims and objectives in terms of editorial policy, and locating them into a broader socio-economic framework. For the purpose of establishing a consistent analysis of the interdependence between word and image, I have also chosen to compare and contrast a handful of fashion spreads that represent the body in the context of history and nostalgia. Accordingly, in assessing the narrative structure of such spreads and both their historicist and historical connotations, I have drawn on ideas concerning postmodernism and hyperreality as expressed by Jean Baudrillard and Dick Hebdige, as well as Roland Barthes' essay 'Myth Today'. This Part, therefore, picks up on Barthes' central idea that the magazine is a machine for making fashion and one that, moreover, as Hilary Radner gnomically expresses it, is 'a cultural reservoir that functions as literacy within a certain arena'.[2] In turn, the general argument concerning word and image that is elaborated here is consolidated in Part 2 with a more specific analysis of Barthes' semiological text *The Fashion System*, a problematic work, but one that propounds probably the most incisive analytical model for deconstructing the verbal and visual elements of fashion publishing.

Notes

1. See J. Briscoe, 'Chic, worthy, sexy, successful', *The Observer Review Section* (22 August 1993), p. 1, and 'Femme Ordinaire', *The Observer Review Section* (21 January 1996), p. 3, for an assessment of *Marie Claire* and its editor Glenda Bailey.
2. See R. Barthes, *The Fashion System*, trans. M. Ward and R. Howard (California, 1990), p. 51 and H. Radner, *Shopping Around – Feminine Culture and the Pursuit of Pleasure* (London and New York, 1995), p. 130.

Vogue

You don't look to *Vogue* to pop the bubble. It is not just there to create desires but to sell, sell, sell them.

Anna Wintour, *The Guardian*, 1991.

Introduction: Style and Sensibility

Vogue had originally been launched in 1892 in America as a society magazine aimed at all those whose names were recorded on the Social Register.[1] It did not come into its own as a fashion periodical, however, until 1909, when a young tycoon called Thomas Condé Nast took over the running of the title in partnership with its first editor Edna Woolman.[2] A British edition subsequently followed in 1916, and French and Italian versions in 1920 and 1950 respectively. During the period January to June 1996 the inclusive circulation figures for British *Vogue* were at an all-time high of 193,539 copies, whereas when Nast purchased the American edition, the circulation of the magazine was more modest – approximately 14,000 copies per month.[3] For Nast, however, the issue was not one of aiming to increase *Vogue*'s readership, and during the 1920s and 1930s he deliberately continued to emphasise the magazine's social exclusivity. What was of more importance to him was its aesthetic appearance, and he was fully aware of the ways in which the layout of the contemporary magazine in Europe was being greatly transformed by new developments in typography and photomechanical printing.[4] The impetus of both the Arts and Crafts Movement and Art Nouveau at the end of the nineteenth century had implied that utilitarian objects like magazines could nonetheless be the subject of aesthetic production values, involving the quality of the paper used as much as a commitment to harmony in graphic design. This ideology was manifest in many periodicals published across Europe and America, including *The Studio*, *Jugend*, *Ver Sacrum* and *Inland Printer*.[5] In turn, the half-tone process, which had been patented by Meisenbach in Germany in 1882 and involved breaking down the image into a matrix of dots by photographing the subject through a screen of diagonal lines, began to be consistently incorporated into the illustrated press by the

1890s. Indeed, in 1892 the French magazine *La Mode Pratique* was one of the first periodicals to rely on half-tones in representing the latest fashions.[6] Significantly, it had also been realised in the nineteenth century that the potential for printing words and images simultaneously in illustrated texts would transform public attitudes towards literacy. An editorial in the first issue of the illustrated French weekly *L'Univers Illustré* (22 May 1858), for example claimed that:

> Our bustling century does not always allow enough time for reading, but it always allows time for looking; where an article demands half an hour, a drawing takes a mere minute. It requires no more than a rapid glance to uncover the message it conveys, and even the most schematic sketch is always easier to understand than an entire page of writing.[7]

The implied shift towards the image was to continue well into the twentieth century, and is discussed more fully in the next chapter. But it is perhaps also worth taking note at this stage in my discussion of a similar line of argument that was expressed by Kurt Korff concerning the popularity during the 1920s of photojournals like *Berliner Illustrirte Zeitung*:

> It is no accident that the development of the cinema and the development of [*BIZ*] run roughly parallel. To the extent that life became more hectic, and the individual was less prepared to leaf through a magazine in a quiet moment . . . it became necessary to find a sharper, more efficient form of visual representation, one which did not not lose its impact on the reader even if he only glanced fleetingly at the magazine page by page.[8]

Korff's sentiments also help to explain why Nast felt it important to revitalise the form and content of *Vogue* in keeping with the prevailing aesthetic values of modernism, and why, to this end, he employed a succession of inventive layout artists, editors and photographers. Between 1909 and 1939 the chief artistic contributors to *Vogue* in America and Europe were the photographers Edward Steichen, George Hoyningen-Huene and Horst P. Horst, and the graphic designer Mehemed Fehmy Agha, all of whom emulated the avant-garde art movements of New Objectivity and Surrealism in their stylistic tendencies.[9] Indeed, Nast took his role as arbiter of style and taste so seriously that he analysed sales returns from each issue of *Vogue* to help him determine whether photographic covers were more popular with the public than illustrated ones.[10] What was of significance in this respect was the way that fashion photographers during the early twentieth century began to transcend any straightforward or utilitarian interest in clothing itself. Rather, through a manipulative use of lighting, tone and scale, they used the garments in their images as the basis of fetishised fantasies of desirability and beauty. Horst's photograph of a Mainbocher corset for French and American *Vogue* (13 September 1939) has become one of the most seminal and iconic forms of this type of representation.[11] In this image, a minimum of detail has been used to dramatic effect. In it, we see a woman who has been photographed *contrapposto* and half-length from behind; her arms are raised and folded at chest height, and she tilts her head to one side in the manner of an expiring ballerina. The shelf in front of her, which forms a strong horizontal demarcation between the top and bottom halves of the photograph, seems to double up as a plinth on which her fetishised body rests like a sculpture bust, while the use of strong directional lighting creates subtle chiaroscuro effects that give emphasis to the sinuous curves of her figure and a textural sensuosity to her skin. Consequently, as Elizabeth Wilson has appositely argued: 'It was above all the camera that created a new way of seeing and a new style of beauty for women in the twentieth century. The love affair of black and white photography with fashion *is* the modernist sensibility.'[12]

Sex and Sensuousness

By 1943, the art direction of American *Vogue* was taken up by Alexander Liberman, who continued to occupy the post until 1961, and the work of a new school of indigenous photographers, including chiefly Irving Penn, Jerry Schatzberg and William Klein, began to appear in its pages.[13] In Britain also, the post-war period witnessed the revitalisation of fashion photography in *Vogue* by a younger generation of photographers including Tony Armstrong-Jones, Terence Donovan, Brian Duffy and David Bailey.[14] Summing up the work of these post-war photographers, Martin Harrison concluded that, while sex has always been intertwined with fashion photography, after 1945 it had become its very *raison d'être*.[15] This shift of emphasis was manifest in a new, sensuous form of iconography that represented men and women together in various acts of sexual flirtation, and that coincided with the impact of more relaxed attitudes towards sex among young people. We can see this attitude amplified in 'Amoureuse', photographed for *Elle* (16 June 1958) by Santoro, whose alpha-pictorial content is assessed in more detail in Part II, as well as in much of David Bailey's fashion and portrait photography during the 1960s.

In the early 1960s, Bailey had been specifically invited by British *Vogue* to shoot a regular fashion feature called 'Young Idea', for which he used his favourite model Jean Shrimpton. In Bailey's dynamic iconography, Shrimpton was shot on location as well as in the studio, and her gawky, gamine appearance offered an appropriately unconventional prototype in keeping with the new, playful fashions of the period designed by Mary Quant, Marion Foale, Sally Tuffin and others.[16] Bailey's fashion photographs often appear to be as theatrically contrived as do those of many of his forerunners in their use of artificial lighting and exaggerated poses (during his early period of production he admitted a stylistic indebtedness to the futuristic vision of *nouvelle vague* film directors like Godard).[17] Nonetheless, we can detect in them a freedom of expression and intimate sensuality that transcended the lofty grandeur of work by Irving Penn, for example, whose wife, the model Lisa Fonssagrives, was most commonly embodied as an aloof and unattainable goddess in his photographs for American *Vogue* during the 1950s.[18] At the same time, the informal intimacy that is implicit in Bailey's work is also indicative of the more ingenuous sexual relationships that had begun to spring up between the photographer and his model(s) by the early 1960s. He and Shrimpton, for instance, eventually became lovers until 1965.[19]

The foregrounding of sexual content in fashion photography persisted into the 1970s and 1980s in the work of Helmut Newton, Guy Bourdin, Patrick Demarchelier, Herb Ritts, Norman Watson and Bruce Weber (see Appendix I, which includes more specific details of work by Ritts, Watson and Weber, and Appendix II, which lists the chief photographic contributors to British *Vogue* between 1980 and 1995). On several occasions during the 1970s such imagery became the centre of debates on the objectification of women, to the extent that Ernestine Carter commented: 'Pornography having taken over films, the theatre and literature, took over fashion photography too.'[20] At the time of writing, Carter was referring particularly to the work of photographers like Helmut Newton, Guy Bourdin, Chris Von Wangenheim, Jeanloup Sieff and Deborah Turbeville, which had begun to appear in the American, French and Italian editions of *Vogue*, and in Britain in *Queen* and *Nova*.[21] It is important to stress here, however, that such work was rarely censored officially; rather, it contributed to an arena of ongoing debate concerning sexual politics after it had been published.

One of the chief criticisms made against fashion photography during the 1970s centred on the exploitation by the photographer (who was usually male) of his subjects (who were usually female). As Helmut Newton himself put it, 'we did a lot of naughty things and had a lot of fun'.[22] Newton, in particular, gained notoriety for the fashion work he produced for magazines like *Nova* and the continental editions of *Vogue*, with his images representing models ostensibly engaged in scenes of lesbian flirtation for French *Vogue* in March 1979 becoming something of a *succès de scandale*. In one scene, for example, we can perceive an interesting play on phallic symbolism as two women performing an intimate masquerade in a hotel lobby share a cigarette. One of them has long hair and wears a figure-revealing boob tube and split-knee skirt, while the other, with slicked back hair and dressed in a double-breasted suit, leans over her as their lighted cigarette ends provocatively touch. Feminists were quick to accuse Newton of producing work that was undeniably based on male fantasies of the psychosexuality of women (whether straight or gay), and that violated and degraded them.[23] But such criticism failed to take into account the meaning for the clothes intended by the designer – in this case Yves Saint Laurent, whose fashion at the time played deliberately on a *style androgyne*. It also overlooked the fact that even female photographers can objectify women in ambiguous terms. In American *Vogue* in May 1975, for instance, a photograph by Deborah Turbeville of five models in a communal shower wearing either swimsuits or dressing gowns was attacked by readers. Not only because they felt it portrayed a scene of lesbianism (even though the models had been posed separately and in no way appear remotely interested in each other) but also because they alleged it set up a symbolic association with the gas chambers at Auschwitz.[24] More cogently, as these examples serve to demonstrate, it would be myopic, if not erroneous, to say that sex was the only concern of either the photographers or editors of *Vogue*. Whenever we do encounter scenes of overt sexuality they also subscribe to various photographic genres, or take place in the context of other issues and ideas. As Hilary Radner attests: 'The use of fashion as a global signified is ... symptomatic of the *Vogue* discourse, in which the rhetoric of fashion is ubiquitous, applied indiscriminately to health, culture, and education .... "Fashionableness" becomes a story waiting to be told, a fiction of coherence ready to be assembled.'[25]

Between Art and Commerce

Between 1980 and 1995, a roll call of some 93 international photographers had contributed to British *Vogue* (see Appendix II), and several chief discursive or rhetorical themes recur in their work. These include principally: romantic nostalgia (for example, 'A la recherche du temps Bardot, photographed by Herb Ritts, October 1989, and 'Tinker Tailoring', by Paolo Roversi, October 1993); art ('A fashion splash', by Bruce Weber and borrowing stylistically from Abstract Expressionism, November 1984); literature ('New Morning Nebraska', by Bruce Weber and referencing *My Ántonia* by Willa Cather); class and tradition ('Great Classics – Margaret Howell's Moving Picture', by Bruce Weber, September 1981, and 'English Lessons' by Mario Testino, September 1993); and exotic travel (see Alex Chatelain's

'Sri-Lanka – fashion in the sun and serendip', May 1980, and 'Japan: New-fashioned departures', January 1984). These themes are not always elaborated independently, and, as we shall see below in my analysis of Bruce Weber's work for British *Vogue*, several of them may be found simultaneously in any given fashion shoot. In many respects, however, the iconography of the magazine has been somewhat limited in scope and relatively tame in comparison to its competitors in the style and youth culture market. Most fashion spreads in *Vogue* tend to be straightforward studio shots that represent the fashions in an uncompromising and clear-cut manner.

This much is due to the demands of many designers and manufacturers themselves, who regard *Vogue* as a showcase for their latest collections and expect the magazine to show their clothes off to their best advantage, whether directly in the form of advertising or indirectly in its fashion pages. In 1965, for example, *Time* ran the following editorial satirising what it saw as the gratuitous use of style over content in fashion photography:

> Who is that girl prancing on the hood of a Rolls, strutting along a beach on ice skates, fording a stream on a water buffalo, serving tea in a space suit, climbing a tree in a cocktail dress? Who else but that rag-bone-and-hank-of-hair known as a High-fashion Model. She is supposed to be showing off the new clothes for the readers of *Vogue*, *Harper's Bazaar*, and fashion pages of general magazines. Is she succeeding? No, scream a growing gaggle of fashion designers who claim their clothes are being downgraded to mere props for far-out photography.[26]

And more than 25 years later, when asked in an interview what she thought the function of the fashion photograph should be, the newly-appointed editor of American *Vogue* at that time, Anna Wintour, succinctly replied, 'Obviously . . . to show the clothes.'[27]

Indeed, as we have seen in the case of Helmut Newton and Deborah Turbeville, on the rare occasion that *Vogue* did publish more adventurous work, its editors incurred the wrath of readers and the fashion industry alike. Corinne Day's representation of Kate Moss wearing underwear in June 1993 is another good example of this, and is discussed in more detail in Part III. But the clout of advertisers and their power to influence the editorial bias and content of *Vogue* was also clearly demonstrated in June 1996 when Omega watches threatened to boycott the British edition of the magazine in protest against its photographs of the model Trish Goff, which they deemed made her look anorexic.[28]

Bruce Weber: A Nostalgic Interlude

In marked contrast, Bruce Weber, who has achieved a certain notoriety for producing egregiously erotic work that celebrates the male anatomy, is probably one of the few contributors to *Vogue* to have redefined the boundaries of what constitutes a fashion photograph without alienating potential consumers or producers. As Alexander Liberman, artistic director for Condé Nast publishing, affirmed in 1986: 'The fashion photograph is evolving. Weber may have been one of the first to have sensed it. As clothes grow simpler and less important, the human factor becomes dominant, and there Bruce is unique in daring to portray a reality that is seldom seen in fashion magazines.'[29]

Weber's professional debut came in 1973 when he was commissioned to make a portrait of the American fashion designer Ralph Lauren and his family for *Harper's Bazaar*. He is probably best known, however, for the series of underwear and perfume advertisements he photographed for Calvin Klein that hypostasise a monumental or classical ideal of the male body. As discussed in Part III, much of this work quite openly appears to trade on homoerotic desires and fantasies in its representation of phallic bodies. At the same time, it conforms to an avowedly eclectic, postmodern style that leans heavily towards both the mythopoetics of Leni Riefenstahl's images of the 1936 Berlin Olympiad and the male nudes that George Platt Lynes photographed in the 1950s (Figure 42).[30] But we have to take care to make a distinction between the iconography of Weber's advertising and fashion photographs. For, while Barbara Lippert could claim that his 1980s representations of the body for Klein and Ralph Lauren had given 'each one a distinct mythic image that's either beautiful or scary', Weber himself maintained he had more trouble in convincing magazine editors that a similar treatment of the male form would make for appropriate fashion editorial.[31] Speaking of his first photographs of Jeff Aquilon for *GQ* in America in 1978, for instance, he affirmed: 'They were really frightened of seeing men's skin, pushing up the sleeves was an amazing adventure.'[32] Thus it would be erroneous to pigeonhole his entire *oeuvre* as either erotic or homoerotic, and Weber's photography is certainly more semiologically complex than at first meets the eye. Indeed, it is debatable whether Weber on his own terms sets out to be the author of any one particular type of image:

> I really don't think "this is going to be a fashion photograph". I mean, you know, even if I'm doing a photograph of a girl in a dress or a guy in a suit, I don't think of it as being a fashion picture . . . I love fashion photographs, but I never think of them as fashion pictures . . . I look at a book by August Sander and I see lots of

fashion in those photographs. I think *National Geographic* has some of the best fashion I've ever seen. It's always people, if they're expressing a lifestyle or wearing something that is very personal. For me photographs like that bring something to life.[33]

To illustrate this point in more detail, it is worth briefly examining the stylistic content and narrative structure of a representative sample of the fifteen fashion spreads that he has photographed for British *Vogue* since January 1980 (see Appendix I). While to one degree or another all of them could be said to connote certain ideas concerning gender and the body, a closer reading reveals that this is not necessarily Weber's chief preoccupation. Rather, several other important themes emerge when we examine such work, most obviously a nostalgia for the past and a certain way of American living associated with nature and the land, that are themselves often imbricated with gender issues. This attitude is particularly in evidence in two fashion shoots that also reference the artistic and literary patrimony of American culture: 'New Morning Nebraska – Pioneers of 82 Wear Plain Clothes' (*Vogue*, January 1982), and 'Under Weston Eyes – Bruce Weber in a romantic encounter with Edward Weston and the pure and simple style' (*Vogue*, December 1982).

The first of these ostensibly pays homage to the lesbian American writer Willa Cather (1873–1947), and consists of thirty-one photographs of different dimensions taken by Weber in Red Cloud, Nebraska. Cather was raised there in the late nineteenth century, and the area formed the basis of many of her stories about farming communities.[34] In the fashion spread, Weber's lyrical photographs have in turn been interwoven into a prolonged narrative of fourteen pages with *Vogue* editorial and snippets of text from three of Cather's novels: *My Ántonia* (1918), *Death Comes for the Archbishop* (1927), and *Lucy Gayheart* (1931). The introductory paragraphs of editorial are highly evocative, and play on what Barthes would call the caritative nature of clothing by poetically relaying details of texture and sensation. Thus we succumb to the seductive look and feel of 'weathered woven and felty wools' and 'scrubbed cambric and linen, soft curling collars, laced, and button boots'.[35] Immediately, the conjugation of two historical moments in time is also established and we are told that, 'The look is strongly of the present and deeply reminiscent.'[36] But we need to ask, reminiscent of what exactly? For what we appear to be confronted with in this piece is nothing more than a mythical image of the 'ideal' American way of life that is bolstered by its relationship to the timeless ideals of rural dress, here worn for style's sake and not for labour. For example a group photograph of models wearing contemporary clothing by Paul Smith, Manolo Blahnik, Marc O'Polo and

Margaret Howell gathered around a combine harvester, which also includes on the right a young boy shrouded in the stars and stripes (Figure 4), is given the caption: 'Working together, the harvest and the strength of black, white, grey and brown'. The inclusion of the combine harvester, in turn, underscores the mythological conflation of past and present that is elaborated throughout the spread. For Cather sets the narrative of each of the three novels to which 'New Morning Nebraska' refers in either the nineteenth century (*Death Comes for the Archbishop*) or early-twentieth century (*My Ántonia* and *Lucy Gayheart*); in other words, before the mechanisation of farming became widespread in America.

Furthermore, segments of Cather's writing, wrested from their original contexts, are used figuratively and are not illustrated exactly as we might expect, appearing to serve no other purpose than to reinforce an idyllic moment that is also given in pictorial form. Thus a full-length portrait of a young girl in a cornfield with her head tilted back and her face welcoming the morning breeze appears alongside the following excerpt from *Death Comes For The Archbishop*: 'Something soft and wild and free . . . released the prisoned spirit of man into the wind, into the blue and gold, into the morning.' In the original novel the text describes the yearning for freedom and purity that Father Latour encounters during the last months of his life in New Mexico,[37] while in the fashion spread it seems to commemorate the matutinal beauty of Lena Lingard as it is related in *My Ántonia*: 'Lena was never so pretty as in the morning; she wakened fresh with the world every day, and her eyes had a deeper colour then, like the blue flowers that are never so blue as when they first open.'[38] Similarly, the following piece of text from *My Ántonia*, 'It was no wonder that her sons stood tall and straight. She was a rich mine of life like the founders of early races' takes on a nostalgic aspect in the fashion spread. The passage appears in the closing chapter of the novel, where its narrator, Jim Burden, renews his friendship with the Bohemian immigrant Ántonia Shimerda after a period of some twenty years. Burden also tells us that she 'was a battered woman now, not a lovely girl' and the mother of five children,[39] whereas in Weber's photograph we discern a young woman seated centrally, with a boy kneeling at her feet, and flanked on either side by young men of a similar age who stand tall and erect. The photograph seems to evoke, therefore, a vision of the young and beautiful Ántonia with whom Burden was infatuated as an adolescent, and symbolises the idea that the youths who flank her could be alter-egos for Burden, who was four years Ántonia's junior, and her brothers Ambrosch and Marek.

Indeed, in several cases, Weber's photographs and Cather's prose seem to be related as a series of ekphrases, and the tonalism of his pictures with their trajectory from pearly dawn light to the warm, scorched hues of sundown seem to trade on the temporal symbolic effects of her writing. As we have just seen, the extract cited above from *Death Comes For the Archbishop* has been used to illustrate a picture bathed in the glow of early morning, while the phrase, 'The blond cornfields were red gold, the haystacks turned rosy and threw long shadows' from *My Ántonia*, is accompanied by two pictures taken in the full glare of the sun.[40]

In certain ways, several of the photographs included in 'New Morning Nebraska' also appear to reference, if even unwittingly, the authorial ambiguities latent in Cather's *My Ántonia*, where, in the prologue, an anonymous and non-gender-specific storyteller introduces his/her relationship with one of the novel's central male characters, Jim Burden: 'He and I are old friends, we grew up together in the same Nebraska town, and we had a great deal to say to one another.'[41] Weber, likewise, suggests the possibility of homosocial bonding and confraternity with four images of young boys huddled together in a barn, and a smaller picture of two youths embracing each other (Figure 4).

But, not surprisingly, seen in the context of *Vogue* there is another important correspondence set into operation between text and image. That is, one through which the words and pictures have been mobilised to connote the harmonious parallel between fashion and nature, a correspondence which is also manifest in the second of Weber's photo-essays for British *Vogue* in 1982, 'Under Weston Eyes'. The title of the piece is a pun on Joseph Conrad's novel *Under Western Eyes* (1989 [1911]). The tropes contained in it, however, bear no similarity to the style or content of his narrative, which centres on the apocalyptic journey towards self-knowledge of a Russian called Razumov as it is recounted by a professor of English living in Geneva. Running across eight pages, the *Vogue* fashion shoot could not be further removed from this diachronic narrative about revolutionaries in Europe before the First World War, a novel that Conrad was later to describe as, 'an attempt to render not so much the political state as the psychology of Russia itself'.[42] Rather, as its subtitle states – 'Bruce Weber in a romantic encounter with Edward Weston and the pure and simple style' – the shoot ostensibly sets out to pay homage to the photographer Edward Weston (1886–1958), best known for his compositions that explore the idea of biomorphic form, and his images of the landscape of the American West.[43] This is not so say, however, that 'Under Weston Eyes' is itself a straightforward fashion narrative. For it also weaves back and forth in time, and in so doing it seems to elaborate a vision of both fashion and photography that is quintessentially tenseless. Thus at the very outset, we encounter a convoluted masquerade that comprises seventeen photographs of different dimensions, interlarded with editorial and quotations concerning Weston's technique and practice by himself and others, and that appears to work on three interconnected levels.

First, the piece seems to be about Weston himself, a point that is connoted not just by the biographical details and the style of the monochrome photographs, which have been lit and printed in such a way as to look like original Weston compositions, but also in the symbiotic relationship that is set up between text and image. Hence the photographs appear to function as illustrations to the opinions included about his work. In the first double-page opening, for example, a reference to Weston's method of production by his son Cole is accompanied by several images of a photographer at work, while comments about the seductive power of his photographic vision by Charis Wilson Weston, and the way that he can make ordinary people appear extra-ordinary, are juxtaposed with a cluster of portraits of models (Figure 5). This dialectic is pursued in subsequent openings. Thus a chiaroscuro portrait of a female model and two others highlighting the form and contours of the female body are accompanied by quotations by the photographic historians Nancy Newhall and Ben Maddow concerning, respectively, Weston's preoccupation with woman as muse, and his fetishistic interest in the look and form of the human face (Figure 6).

Second, the piece appears to be not about Weston at all but about Weber himself. On this level, the work of the two photographers exists in parallel. Thereby, Weston's creative vision has been invoked in order to legitimate Weber's status as an art photographer, even though he also happens to be working in a commercial sphere: 'These photographs are about a way of seeing and a way of life. They are Bruce Weber's tribute to photographer Edward Weston . . . a tribute to the intensity of Weston's relationship with the camera and particular beautiful women.'[44] In this way, it is not Weston and his Californian milieu that we see in the images, but Weber and a group of friends at his Long Island home. Indeed, the ambiguous masquerade of this *mise-en-scène* is given a metonymic twist in so far as the Bruce who is identified in the list of characters is not actually Weber himself, but 'a friend of the same name playing the photographer'.[45]

Finally, the honorific connection that has been established between Weston and Weber takes another turn in a set of symbolic associations that strike up a relationship between fashion and Weston's photographic vision. Consequently, not only has the atmospheric tonalism of Weston's photographs been used as an appropriate stylistic code to represent the black-and-white fashions included, but by extension, Weston himself is framed as a fashion photographer: 'Weston was the inspiration. This is a diversion in the style . . . They (the models) are dressed in the fierce and soft monotones of a Weston print – not only in homage, *this is a part of fashion now*' (my emphases).[46]

Clearly, in their treatment of the past as a set of styles that can be replayed at will, the two Weber fashion spreads we have just analysed have implications for the meaning of authorship and originality that are bound up in post-modern debates concerning hyperreality and simulation. As Frederic Jameson has argued, for example, in mobilising or referencing other sign systems the postmodernist deploys nostalgia in such a way that the past and the future appear to dissolve into what he calls the 'perpetual present'.[47] Now, it is no longer a case of simply quoting other texts, 'as a Joyce or a Mahler might have done', but of literally incorporating them into the very substance of one's own work.[48] More cogently for Baudrillard, in a world that is over-saturated with images, we no longer have the propensity to tell representation and reality apart: 'It is no longer a question of imitation, nor duplication, nor even parody. It is a question of substituting the signs of the real for the real.'[49] This idea of the hyperreal in Weber's work was not lost on picture editors, one of whom expatiated anonymously that: 'he makes magnificent scenes, moods and places, and conveys a sense of lost time, but reality is not quite transcended. You can taste the dust, but it never happened.'[50] But, as Baudrillard was also quick to point out, hyperreality is the condition of a society in crisis – one that takes refuge in images because it does not know how to mourn the loss of what it once regarded as truthful or real.[51] It is this idea of fake history that informs Dick Hebdige's critique of *The Face* and that is evaluated in closer detail, therefore, in the next chapter.

Notes

1. K. Fraser, introduction, *On The Edge: Photographs from 100 Years of Vogue* (New York, 1992), pp. 2–3: 'The magazine was launched by and for people whose names were in the Social Register, the city's élitist "Four Hundred" families. (Four hundred would fit in Mrs. Astor's ballroom at one go.).' See also, British *Vogue* (June 1991), special issue celebrating 75 years of publication.
2. K. Fraser, 'The tender trap', *Independent on Sunday Review* (11 October 1992), p. 45.
3. A. Billen, 'No one looks at Vogue and thinks "I want to look like that". No one is that stupid', *The Observer Review* (4 August 1996), p. 7.
4. In 1928, for example, Condé Nast toured Europe to find a replacement for the longstanding art director of American *Vogue*, Heyworth Campbell, whom he regarded as 'steeped in the old school of decoration, classical type and dense layout'. He appointed Mehemed Fehmy Agha, who had been chief layout artist for German *Vogue*. See S. Bodine and M. Dunas, 'Dr. M. F. Agha, Art Director', *AIGA Journal*, 3:3 (1985).
5. See H. Brill, 'Fin de Siècle' in *The Art Press* (London, 1976), pp. 23–31.
6. See P. Jobling and D. Crowley, *Graphic Design – Reproduction and Representation Since 1800* (Manchester, 1996), pp. 27–9.

7. 'Notre siècle affairé, n'a pas toujours le temps de lire, mais il a toujours le temps de voir; ou l'article demande une demi-heure, le dessin ne demande qu'une minute. Il suffit d'un coup d'oeil rapide pour s'approprier l'enseignement qu'il contient, et le croquis le plus sommaire est toujours plus comprehensible et plus explicite qu'une page de description.' Translation by the author.

8. *Berliner Illustrirte Zeitung* had been founded in 1891. See Kurt Korff in 'Die illustrierte Zeitschrift', *Fünfzig Jahre Ullstein 1877–1927* (Berlin, 1927), pp. 279–303, cited in A. Kaes, M. Jay, E. Dimendberg, *The Weimar Republic Sourcebook* (Berkeley, 1994), pp. 646–7.

9. See N. Hall-Duncan, *The History of Fashion Photography* (New York, 1979); Jobling and Crowley, *Graphic Design*, pp. 137–51 and 179–83; and W. Owen, *Magazine Design* (London, 1991), pp. 20–55.

10. C. Seebohm, *The Man Who Was Vogue: The Life of Condé Nast* (New York, 1982), p. 175.

11. The pose of the model in the photograph was mimicked by Madonna in her video 'Vogue' (1990), directed by Herb Ritts. It is also interesting to note two further examples of such mimicry – a fashion feature entitled 'Flesh' in *The Face* (April 1993), photographed by Mario Sorrenti and styled by Cathy Dixon, represented Nick Moss from behind wearing a lace-up-back white leather dress by The Glorious Clothing Company (p. 101); while in *Cosmopolitan* (January 1997) an advertisement for La Perla fragrance depicted a female model from behind wearing a laced corset similar to the Mainbocher in Horst's photograph. The last two examples are particularly intriguing since they imply a kind of double-coding. That is, we can no longer argue that they are based on Horst's original photograph alone, but need to take account of the idea that they could just as well be derived from Madonna's pastiche of it.

12. E. Wilson, *Adorned in Dreams: Fashion and Modernity* (London, 1985), p. 157.

13. See M. Harrison, *Appearances – Fashion Photography Since 1945* (London, 1991), Chapters 2 and 3; W. Klein, *In and Out of Fashion* (New York, 1994); M. Shanahan (ed.), *Richard Avedon – Evidence 1944–1994* (London, 1994); and J. Szarkowski, *Irving Penn* (New York, 1984). During the 1940s and 1950s Penn retreated to the studio as the ideal milieu for the theatre of fashion, whereas Avedon, Klein and Schatzberg also tended to photograph fashion on the street.

14. See Harrison, *Appearances*, Chapter 5 and M. Harrison, *Bailey: Black and White Memories* (London, 1983).

15. Harrison, *Appearances*, p. 14.

16. Ibid., Chapter 5.

17. D. Mellor and M. Harrison, *David Bailey Black and White Memories* (London, 1983), p. 8.

18. See Szarkowski, *Irving Penn*.

19. An article entitled 'The model makers – Bailey, Duffy and Donovan in the *Sunday Times Colour Magazine* (1964) contains the following observation: 'We try and make the model look like a bird we'd go out with.' Cited by T. Imrie, 'Double page dream', *BJP Annual* (1984), pp. 27–33. See also M. Gross, *Model – The Ugly*

Business of Beautiful Women (London and New York, 1995), p. 127, which cites the model Celia Hammond saying: 'Bailey and Terry were very sexually oriented. That's how they worked. They would just tell you to, you know, fuck the camera or something. That's what their message was, sex and raunchiness. You've only got to look at their pictures to see what was going on.'

20. E. Carter, *The Changing World of Fashion* (London, 1977), p. 146.

21. See Harrison, *Appearances*, Chapter 6 and D. Gibbs (ed.), *Nova 1965–1975 – THE Style Bible of the 60s and 70s* (London, 1993).

22. Helmut Newton, *Portraits* (London, 1987), p. 18.

23. See C. Evans and M. Thornton, *Women and Fashion: A New Look* (London, 1989), p. 87.

24. Amy Gross, 'Turbeville. An interview', American *Vogue*, (December 1981), p. 248.

25. H. Radner, *Shopping Around*, p. 136.

26. 'The furor over Fashions', *Time*, 86 (3 December 1965), p. 66.

27. M. Roberts, 'High Anxiety', *Independent on Sunday Review* (6 October 1991), p. 37.

28. A. Billen, *The Observer Review*, (4 August 1986), p. 7. Although production costs for each issue are more than a quarter of a million pounds, these are greatly offset by advertising revenue. In 1992, for example, production costs stood at £350,000 while advertising revenue was £1.5m (source: *The Look*, programme 3, BBC2, 1992).

29. M. Gross, 'Camera Chameleon', *Vanity Fair* (June 1986), p. 102.

30. See J. Crump, *George Platt Lynes – Photographs from the Kinsey Institute* (Boston and London, 1993), introduction, where Weber states: 'George Platt Lynes's photographs gave me [that] courage to ask for anything in a photograph.'

31. Gross, 'Camera Chameleon, p. 106.

32. Ibid., p. 116.

33. R. Carroll, 'An interview with Bruce Weber', *Bomb* (Spring/Summer 1985), pp. 40–3.

34. Cather wrote twelve novels between 1912 and her death in 1947. See H. Lee, *Willa Cather: Double Lives* (New York, 1989).

35. 'New Morning Nebraska – Pioneers of 82 Wear Plain Clothes', British *Vogue* (January 1982), p. 74.

36. Ibid., p. 74.

37. W. Cather, *Death Comes for the Archbishop* (London, 1981), p. 276.

38. W. Cather, *My Ántonia* (London, 1980), pp. 281–2.

39. Ibid., p. 353.

40. *Vogue* (January 1982), pp. 82–5.

41. See J. Butler, *Bodies That Matter – On the Discursive Limits of "Sex"* (London and New York, 1993), Chapter 5 for an incisive assessment of the gender and sex ambiguities in Cather's prose.

42. Boris Ford, 'Introduction', p. 27 in J. Conrad, *Under Western Eyes* (Harmondsworth, 1989).

43. See B. Maddow, *Edward Weston, His Life and Photographs* (New York, 1979).

44. 'Under Weston Eyes', British *Vogue* (December 1982), p. 195.

45. Ibid., p. 195.

46. Ibid., p. 195.

47. F. Jameson, *Postmodernism; or, the Cultural Logic of Late Capitalism* (London and New York, 1991), p. 311: 'Now everything is new; but by the same token, the very category of the new then loses its meaning and becomes itself something of a modernist survival.'

48. Ibid., pp. 2–3.

49. J. Baudrillard, 'The Precession of Simulacra', in *Simulacra and Simulation*, trans. Sheila Faria Glaser (Ann Arbor, 1994), p. 2.

50. Gross, 'Camera Chameleon', p. 117.

51. Baudrillard, 'The Precession of Simulacra', p. 26.

2

The Face

Why should *Vogue* have a monopoly on the best paper?

Nick Logan, *Media Week*, 1988.

Introduction: The Search for an Identity

Whereas for *Vogue* the issue has always been how to harness the photographer's creative autonomy to the demands of advertisers and designers alike, alternative magazines like *The Face* have enjoyed relative freedom in both their choice of subject-matter and the way that they represent fashion. *The Face* first appeared in May 1980, the brainchild of Nick Logan, who had formerly edited *New Musical Express* and *Smash Hits*, and published by Wagadon on an allegedly shoestring budget of £4,500. Along with *i-D*, founded by Terry Jones and published by Levelprint Ltd, and *Blitz*, founded by Carey Labovitch and published by Jigsaw, it was one of three youth-culture magazines launched during the recession of 1980–81 to tap both the imagination and the wherewithal of young adults who had grown up in the shadow of punk. This was achieved by emphasising music, club culture and, more notably, the idea of street style as a way of mixing, for example, army surplus store items with the accoutrements of high fashion.[1] Indeed, the avowed aim of Logan was to emulate the look and production values of the glossy fashion magazines while breaking away from their more hidebound and exclusive convention of lionising *haute couture*.[2] From a creditable first-issue sale of 56,000 copies, the circulation of *The Face* grew exponentially thereafter, selling on average 75,306 copies per annum between 1981 and 1995.[3] During the 1980s it also went on to garner various design awards and to be the focus of several exhibitions. In 1983 it was elected Magazine of the Year in the Magazine Publishing Awards; in 1985 it was the subject of an exhibition at the Photographer's Gallery in London; and in spring 1988 the work of its chief designer, Neville Brody who was responsible for the magazine's distinctive style between 1981 and 1986, was showcased in the Boilerhouse at the Victoria and Albert Museum. As a result of this activity, the professional journal *Design and Art Direction* went on to claim that:

'from a design point of view [*The Face*] is probably the most influential magazine of the 1980s'.[4]

While *The Face* billed itself as 'the world's best dressed magazine', it was essentially something of a schizophrenic ragbag of ideas during its early run, seemingly still in search of a cohesive identity. Thus in the October 1982 issue the leading editorial portrayed the magazine as a kind of chrysalis, and underscored its transitional status by tentatively inquiring whether *The Face* was, 'a downmarket arts journal, or an upmarket music magazine'. Furthermore, if fashion was to be a large part of *The Face*'s editorial remit, in the early years of its run both the fashion and fashion photography that appeared in its pages were restricted quantitatively as well as qualitatively speaking. Music had a much larger part to play in its content and editorial direction, and until October 1981 the magazine's express aim was to act as 'rock's final frontier'. From the very outset, however, Logan determined to patronise the work of mostly young or aspiring photographers rather than relying exclusively on the same well-established producers who were employed by *Vogue*. Between 1980 and 1996, seventy-seven photographers had their work published in *The Face*, but only eighteen of them had also published in *Vogue*, the majority after they had already made a name for themselves in the youth press (see Appendices I and II). The latter include Martin Brading, Corinne Day, Michel Haddi, Nick Knight, Greg Luchford, Andrew Macpherson, Schoerner, David Sims and Juergen Teller. The reliance on so many tyros, as well as the rapid turnover in the number of photographers employed, is for *The Face* a matter of fiscal expediency as much it is to do with pioneering artistic vision. In stark contrast to the astronomic fees paid to photographic *causes célèbres* like Herb Ritts, whose basic rate of remuneration was $30,000 in 1992, or Newton, whose rates were £20,000 per day plus expenses in 1994,[5] the majority of contributors to *The Face* appear to work for fame rather than fortune, and are paid in accordance with the basic rates stipulated by the National Union of Journalists. In 1989, for example, commission fees for one day's work (i.e. over four hours) stood at £110, while daily earnings for studio and location work stood at £480.[6] Thus, according to Sheryl Garratt, the magazine's editor in 1993, in most cases photographers were lucky if they managed to cover their costs for the production of large fashion spreads.[7]

In the early days, the magazine's chief photographers were Sheila Rock, Graham Smith and Peter Ashworth, and in their fashion work we can discern how music was *The Face*'s principal lodestar. Not only were most of the fashions portrayed intended to be worn as club gear, but the individuals who modelled them were also often rock stars, such as Suggs of Madness (*The Face*, January 1981) and Spandau Ballet (*The Face*, February 1981). Rather than pioneering a distinctively new form of publishing for youth culture, *The Face* appeared instead to have revived the format and editorial policy of the best-selling 1960s pop pin-up magazine *Fabulous* (from June 1966 known as *Fabulous 208*). Thus Dave Hill could refer to the early 1980s as 'The Fake Swinging Sixties', declaring that 'fashion faces, far out places, conspicuous consumption, so much more fun than the real thing had ever been' were the order of the day.[8] Just as *The Face* had been generated during a period of renewed interest in the British music industry with the incipient New Romantic movement, exemplified by the likes of Adam Ant, Steve Strange and Spandau Ballet in their 'sub-elementary electronic thud-funk'[9] and camp, narcissistic appearance, so *Fabulous* profited from the phenomenon of what it called 'Merseymania', spearheaded by The Beatles. From its inception in 1964, *Fabulous* aimed to typologise pop singers as leading lifestyles that were close to, if not exactly the same as those of their fans. Hence, stars were semiotically democratised by the magazine, appearing alongside its readers in fashion spreads, and wearing the same expendable mod outfits – witness 'Sugar Sweets', which represented Marianne Faithfull with one of her male admirers in Regent's Park.[10] In 'Style: A West Side Story' (*The Face*, October 1981), conceived and photographed by Sheila Rock (Figure 7), we can see a similar democratic ideology at play as performers from various groups congregate by night in the vicinity of Chelsea Bridge, London to model affordable, 1950s-style clothes from street-cred outlets like Robot and Za-Zuza.

The Stylist and the Photographer

By the Spring of 1983 a more defined and distinctive approach to fashion photography began to surface in *The Face*. At the same time, however, tensions appeared to arise concerning the need to produce original-looking work and the formal emulation of contemporary and past masters of the art. Its first designated fashion feature, 'All Black – All White – But No Nostalgia', photographed by Peter Ashworth and published in April 1983, for example, appeared to fly in the face of the style-raiding of the likes of Bruce Weber, while the following month the first themed fashion spread, 'The Last Daze of the Raj', photographed by Sheila Rock and styled by the American designer Stephen Linard, seemed in contrast to harp on a retro style and feel similar to that in Weber's work (Figure 8). Yet, in either case, we can also detect the aesthetic dynamics of what was to become the quintessential *Face* fashion layout for much of the 1980s. Here we find Neville Brody deconstructing the rigid logistics of the magazine grid by deploying colourful, asymmetric typography in different fonts and weights (many of them were, in fact, hand-drawn by him) and laying it down in different directions.[11] As a result, the typographic elements were taken as seriously as the photographs, and fully integrated with them to produce a holistic piece of design. In addition, the idea of creatively styling each fashion feature according to a particular theme so as to optimise the types of fashion represented was also increasing in importance, and with the advent of Ray Petri in the summer of 1983 seemed to become an art form in its own right. As Nick Logan and Dylan Jones attested in their obituary for Petri after his untimely death at the age of forty-one in 1989:

> At its most prosaic, a stylist is the person on a fashion shoot who selects the clothes for the models. Ray Petri was never prosaic, and 'styling' was always an inadequate term to describe what it was he excelled at. Ray used clothes to create a mood, to construct an 'attitude', and in so doing he defined the look of men's fashion in the Eighties.[12]

Before joining *The Face* Petri had had a somewhat chequered career in London's rag trade, becoming a stylist 'almost accidentally'.[13] Between 1983 and 1989 he worked freelance for *The Face*, *i-D* and *Arena*, evolving the Buffalo Boy series of fashion spreads in collaboration with the photographers Jamie Morgan, Martin Brading, Roger Charity, Marc Lebon and Norman Watson (Figure 9), which was to become known as his signature style (see Appendix I). Buffalo Boy was an interesting concept that both made a direct appeal to the large young male readership of *The Face* – by 1987, 62 per cent of its readers were men, almost exclusively in the 15–34-years-old age profile[14] – and configured a renewed interest in male appearances and fashions, spearheaded in the early 1980s by the hybrid character of new man and retail outlets such as Next and Hyper Hyper. The impact of these phenomena and the queer politics of new man are discussed in more detail in Part III of this study; but what is important to note here is the way that Petri's style had engendered the sharpening up of attitudes to the form and content of the fashion shoot. Henceforth and without exception, photographers worked in conjunction with a chief stylist and his/her assistants in the conceptualisation and production of any given fashion shoot.

In addition to Petri's collaboration with Morgan and others, therefore, a number of prolific partnerships have emerged since 1984. These include principally: Simon Foxton and Nick Knight, working for *The Face* in 1986 and for *Arena* in 1989; David Bradshaw and a cluster of photographers, including Alan Beukers, Paolo Roversi, Christopher Griffiths, and in particular Randall Mesdon and Norman Watson, whose work appeared in *Arena* between 1987 and 1994; Melanie Ward and Corinne Day for *The Face* between 1990 and 1993; Venetia Scott, who has worked with both Michel Haddi (*The Face*, 1989) and Juergen Teller (*The Face* between 1991 and 1996); Karl and Derick (UTO) and Norman Watson for *The Face* between 1991 and 1993; and finally, Inez van Lamsweerde and Vinoodh Matadin for *The Face* since 1994 (see Appendix 1). At the same time, the iconography of *The Face* also became much more diverse, and the photographer–stylist collaboration generated an eclectic range of *mises-en-scènes* in which both male and female bodies were very much in the foreground as objects of spectatorial pleasure. By 1985 a more consistently discursive treatment of fashion and the body in terms of style and narrative structure, much like *Vogue*'s, was established. The types of themes and ideas represented by *The Face* were, however, larger in number and, generally, more avant-garde in treatment. In summary, therefore, the following identifiable major themes emerged between 1985 and 1996: gender, sexuality and androgyny; race and nationality; alien bodies; the waif look; anti-fashion; fetishism; the cinema; surrealism; history and nostalgia; and the millennium (see Appendix 1 and Figures 9–22). The form and content of many of these fashion features are analysed in more detail in subsequent chapters. However, at this point of my discussion, it is worthwhile investigating how such texts were being received, and to take note of the fact that the burgeoning style press and the consumer culture it espoused did not go entirely unopposed. Judith Williamson, for instance, speaking on the Radio 4 programme *The Stylographers* in 1988, lamented the vapid economy of capitalist chic that the style press had engendered, stating: 'It's the supercilious way that people look in places like the Soho Brasserie. They look like that in the magazine photos and they look like that in the street. They don't look as though they could be open to any experience. It's as though the whole world is a market.'[15] And two years earlier, the cultural historian Dick Hebdige, writing in the left-wing photographic journal *Ten.8*, had proffered one of the more incisive, if antagonistic, critiques of the style politics of *The Face*.[16]

Style Versus Substance

Hebdige's analysis of *The Face* had been conducted in the wider context of postmodern debates concerning the shift in popular consciousness from the primacy of the word to that of the image. Consequently, he maintained that *The Face* was: 'a magazine which goes out of its way every month to blur the line between politics and parody and pastiche; the street, the stage, the screen; between purity and danger; the mainstream and the 'margins': to flatten out the world'.[17]

To get this point across, he weaves an imaginative allegory that invites us to contemplate and to compare how life is lived in two different galactic worlds, each with its own distinct epistemology. In the first world, priority is given to written and spoken language. Here, language and knowledge are almost sacred entities, protected by a priesthood of male and female scribes. Images have some part to play in this world in the form of illustrations, but their status is always subordinate to the written text. As Hebdige explains it, these scribes each appear to function in somewhat Hegelian terms to assist history to unfold and to enable us to link a past that is known and understood to a future that is 'eternally uncertain'. By comparison, in the second world the hierarchy of word and image has been abolished and now it is the latter that holds sway: 'Truth – in so far as it exists at all – is first and foremost pictured: embodied in images which have their own power and effects.'[18] Language, if it is used at all, serves to supplement the image and the priesthood of scribes has been supplanted by an army of advertising copywriters and image consultants who create a 'reality as thin as the paper it is printed on'.[19] The turnover of images in this world also becomes more rapid and kaleidoscopic, so that the present or the New are perpetually celebrated, and history, seemingly, evaporates. Hebdige, therefore, goes on to mark the contrast between the two worlds by relating them to different types of periodical journalism, 'For the sake of argument, let's call the First World, *Ten.8* and the Second *THE FACE*', and he exhorts us to 'imagine a war between these two worlds'.[20]

From its postmodern perspective on the battlements *The Face*, somewhat predictably, is argued to have renounced the social realism that is at the heart of *Ten.8*'s project and, not only this, but to gloat over the depoliticisation of material culture that worship of the *eidos* implies. To justify this criticism, Hebdige quotes a comment by Paul Virilio that had appeared in *The Face*, May 1985, 'Classless society, social injustice – no-one believes in them anymore. We're in the age of micro-narratives, the art of the fragment', and he quips, 'Who, after all, is Paul Virilio anyway?'[21] Thus to Hebdige's way of thinking, *The Face* can be seen to prioritise style over substance and representation over reality in so far as it appears to resist the idea that anything exists prior to representation. Everything appears as if on the surface and, consequently as Hebdige argues: 'We are left in a world of radically "empty" signifiers. No meaning. No classes. No History. Just a ceaseless procession of simulacra . . . The only history that exists here is the history of the signifier and that is no history at all.'[22] In framing his discussion in this way, Hebdige appears to execute an interesting deconstructive tactic in at one and the same time referencing the ideas of Baudrillard, while also undermining them. As has already been mentioned, it was Baudrillard who had first spoken about the idea of hyperreality, or a world that exists only as an economy of images and reproductions, in several texts, most notably, 'The Precession of Simulacra' and 'The Beaubourg Effect: Implosion and Deterrence'. In the latter, he comments on a world which has literally been turned inside out, calling the Beaubourg Centre in Paris, 'a monument to the games of mass simulation', that 'functions as an incinerator absorbing all cultural energy and devouring it . . . a machine for making emptiness'.[23] It is in this world of floating signifiers and depthlessness that Hebdige locates *The Face*, contending that it is 'not read so much as wandered through'.[24] Likewise he opposes its ludic treatment of history as nothing more than 'a series of masks' through which: 'the past is played and replayed as an amusing range of styles, genres, signifying practices to be combined and recombined at will'.[25]

And yet, one is still left to ask, is such gratuitous style-raiding and the seamless recycling of images *all* that is left for us in postmodern photographic discourse? Indeed, is *The Face* itself just a superficial production that looks aesthetically pleasing, but has nothing serious to say about anything? The evidence would suggest otherwise, and even Hebdige has to concede that, while *The Face* is hardly the *Picture Post* of the 1980s, it is 'about looking at popular social history in the making'.[26] For Hebdige, of course, such history resides in the way that *The Face* does not exactly create a tendency from scratch. Rather it is relative to the way in which it represents the very espousal of the image by society at large, and the general drift into a putative atomisation and *culte du soi* that postmodern consumer culture implies. In arguing his case against this tendency, therefore, Hebdige invokes the role of advertising and its influence on the form and content of *The Face*, concluding:

> Advertising – the eidos of the marketplace – is pressed into the very pores of THE FACE . . . THE FACE habitually employs the rhetoric of advertising: the witty one-liner, the keyword, the aphorism, the extractable (i.e. quotable) image are favoured over more sustained, sequential modes of sense-making.[27]

Yet this is to overdetermine *The Face*'s investment in consumer culture and to overlook the other, 'more serious' side of the magazine, such as its annual critical round-up of the past year's cultural and political events, as well as its forays into documentary practice. This aspect of the magazine is manifest in articles such as, 'Hoax! Scoop: How We Fooled The Red Army' (*The Face*, April 1984), dealing with the role of Russian propaganda in the war with Afghanistan, and its comparative analysis of youth culture across Europe (*The Face*, September 1983), which included an interview with the offspring of the Baader-Meinhof terrorists. Subsequent issues also investigated the pernicious rise of racism and homophobia, and the effect of social ills like bad housing and unemployment on young people, the latter painting an uncompromising picture of the growth of teenage prostitution and drug-taking.[28]

One of the main problems for *The Face* in this respect has been its heavy reliance on deconstructive, typographic layouts and graphic invention that have tended to level out its content with regard to form and meaning. This tension between word and image was, however, fully realised by the magazine's chief stylist Neville Brody, who claimed that: 'Style culture was an expression of individualism and an anti-establishment position. *The Face* dealt primarily with a visual culture. This was greatly misread, so that it appeared we were dealing with a superficial culture.'[29] This ambivalence certainly applies to the magazine's fashion content, and it is interesting to observe that Hebdige pays scant attention to it in specific terms. By 1985, the year in which his article was first published, there were already many spreads that would have fitted into his general critique concerning hyperreality, and the theology of appearances that he saw subtending the general ethos of the magazine. But to state things as baldly as this would simply be to reiterate the fatal error of regarding fashion photography as too superficial and devoid of any meaningful content for serious analysis, the very antithesis of documentary reportage. Two examples, both of them photographed by Andrew Macpherson and styled by Amanda Grieve, will suffice here to illustrate this tension between style and content. Moreover, in their referencing of the past, they serve as an instructive comparison with the simulacral effects of the two pieces by Bruce Weber discussed earlier.

Retro-chic Goes Political

The first, 'Apparitions', appeared in *The Face*, December 1984, while the second, 'Veiled Threats', was published in January 1985 (Figures 20 and 21). On the surface, each of these shoots appears to be nothing more than a hollow masquerade that trades on a mock gothic sensibility, and whose purpose is to revive a romantic interest in the style of past fashions. 'Apparitions', for example, comprises four large photographs of a female model wearing clothes by Scott Crolla that have been customised with pieces of old, diaphanous fabrics made of lace and silk. The sensation of evanescence that the images conjure up is, in turn, compounded by the editorial, which speaks of 'echoes of country house gatherings of a distant time and the gothic imagination of Edgar Allen Poe', and of a feeling that is, at one and the same time, 'haunted and ethereal'. The texture of fabric also looms large in

'Veiled Threats', only this time the photographs place an emphasis on the substance and opulence of the velvet and damask clothing by Crolla, Gaultier, Galliano and Richmond/Cornejo that the female model wears. As is the case with 'Apparitions', the accompanying text complements the style and content of the pictures. But in contrast, it also portrays improvisation not as a way of getting back to the past but of making a decisive break with it, and accordingly, it is worth quoting at length:

> The hunt is for dusty relics in a museum culture cluttered with the dusty artefacts of European decline and Anglo Saxon lyricism. An ill wind carries the secret of reinventing the tired style of spent wealth and opulence. Sidestep the clinical chic of modern nations: the keys to pin on your hat open the door to customisation not nostalgia. Do it your own way – progress on your own terms, fin de nothing . . . keep it moving ahead.[30]

We could, of course, argue that history has been used in each of these features as an alibi for dressing up that conflates two distinct periods in time, in much the way that Hebdige suggests: 'The then (and the there) are subsumed in the Now.'[31] At the same time, however, we need to question the more specific signification of this type of masquerade in Britain during the mid-1980s, and to analyse it in the context of his idea that: 'Amongst its other services, *THE FACE* provides a set of physical cultural resources that young people can use in order to make some sense and get some pleasure out of growing up in an increasingly daunting and complex environment.'[32] Put this way, we could argue that these features are not just simply about being *à la mode*; rather they connote the social and political spheres of experience that help to determine what is in fashion and when. For the retro-chic and interest in the nineteenth century that are manifest in them also found a contemporaneous ideological parallel in prime minister Margaret Thatcher's patriotic appeal to Victorian values. Through this she hoped to inspire a renewed sense of the greatness of British identity on both a national and an international basis by championing industrial entrepreneurship, family values and imperial triumphalism. Such historicist flag-waving is typically and gnomically encapsulated in her reply to those who doubted the hasty dispatch of British forces to the Falkland Islands in the Spring of 1982 after their invasion by Argentina: 'Do you remember what Queen Victoria said? "Failure – the possibility does not exist."'[33]

The way that nineteenth-century history is referenced in the visual and verbal rhetoric of both 'Apparitions' and 'Veiled Threats' appears to harp very much on a sense of society in crisis. Indeed, it portrays the past as an impediment to forging a cohesive or stable identity, an attitude that is also compounded during the 1990s in fashion features such as 'Head Hunters', photographed by Jean Baptiste Mondino and styled by Judy Blame (*The Face*, August 1993; Figure 15), and 'Stone Rangers', photographed by Marcus Tomlinson and styled by Kim Andreolli (*The Face*, November 1993). In 'Apparitions', for example, the general pull is not just backwards in time to something that is known and quantifiable, but to a more dream-like milieu made up of the traces of memory and provisional states of being. Here, fabrics float and people are ghosts or ciphers who seem to be destined to drift aimlessly through life; while in contrast, the rhetoric of 'Veiled Threats' paradoxically appears to be concerned with customising past styles in terms of self-empowerment, as a way of defying destiny and of resisting the idea of turn-of-the-century degeneration: 'Do it your own way – progress on your own terms, fin de nothing . . . keep it moving ahead.'[34] Indeed, the entire text of this piece appears to be a thinly disguised metaphor that encrypts youth culture's opposition to the prevailing Thatcherite political dogma. Hence the references to 'dusty artefacts of European decline and Anglo Saxon lyricism', and the contention that: 'an ill wind carries the secret of reinventing the tired style of spent wealth and opulence'.

Finally, it should be noted that several of the photographs in both pieces also underscore the ambivalent androgyny of the glamorous New Romantic fashions by the designers featured. As such, they seem to connote another type of youth-cultural improvisation that destabilised the idea of distinct masculine and feminine sexualities for much of the 1980s. Henceforth, as Dave Hill appositely argued: 'You dressed *up*, not down, to express your dissent. Glamour could be subversive after all.'[35] The subversion of gender that this form of masquerade implied, however, meant not just that boys could look like girls but vice versa, something that was amplified in the cross-dressing of pop singers like Annie Lennox and Prince, and that is also established, for example, in the pose and mock-Byronic dress code of very first picture we encounter in 'Apparitions'. Here, the same female model whom we perceive in the remaining photographs is represented sitting in a window seat with her eyes closed and her arms raised as if in a trance, and wearing the narcissistic habiliments of the dandy – breeches, frilly shirt and waistcoat (Figure 20). Likewise, the indirect gaze and dandyism are instrumental tropes in one of the central photographs in 'Veiled Threats'. Here, the strategic use of lighting and the large brim of a fedora obscure the face of the model wearing a white shirt, red waistcoat and black frock-coat, so that we do not know for certain whether his/her gender identity is male or female (Figure 21).

The historicism that is depicted in the two features from *The Face*, therefore, differs from that in the work of Bruce Weber in a number of significant respects. Weber's is altogether a much more self-conscious deployment of the simulacral, for example, and one that is based on a more specific referencing of the alternative styles of a past author and photographer. That is to say, in the case of the Cather piece, text and image seem as if they connote a timeless and mythopoetic idea of American history, while in the case of the Weston piece, the photographs seem as if they are one and the same thing as his own work. In comparison, *The Face* is far less reverential of the past, and certainly far less determinate in its response to history. If anything, *The Face* is a much more complex and ironical affair than Hebdige's critique at first makes out, and as its subsequent development testifies, it is also certainly more difficult to pigeonhole than just a style magazine. More importantly, it should be realised that the critique that Hebdige mounts against *The Face* is not exclusively to do with postmodern culture. Instead he compounds an ongoing debate that had begun in the nineteenth century with the development of the popular illustrated weekly,[36] and persisted into the twentieth with the consolidation of the same and the evolution of other forms of mass media like the cinema. Siegfried Kracauer, for example, identified such forms of spectatorship as the remit of *die Angestellten* (the white-collar workers) in his essay of the same name and in various essays written for the *Frankfurter Allgemeine Zeitung* during the 1920s and 1930s.[37] As Kracauer viewed it, these were people who were ideologically 'hollow' and intellectually 'homeless', and the popular culture industry enabled them to compensate for their lack of worth by pandering not just to their needs but to their dreams and desires as well.

But time, of course, moves on, and, as both Baudrillard and Hebdige argue, so too has the image explosion intensified and proliferated in terms of production and consumption. For now, in addition to cinema, we have images generated by electronic media such as television and computers, a development that is reflected in the production of many fashion shoots listed with code M in Appendix 1.[38] Furthermore, while Kracauer had, in somewhat paternalistic terms, insisted that the consumers of mass media were quintessentially women, as the readership figures for *The Face* attest, in postmodern culture they are just as likely to be men.

Notes

1. By the late 1980s only *Blitz* remained independent. *The Face* was by then backed by Condé Nast and *i-D* by Time Out. See M. Honigsbaum, 'Blitz – no time to grow up', *The Guardian Media* (2 September 1991), p. 23.

2. 'The Face that launched a hundred', *Media Week* (22 July 1988), p. 29.

3. See the following ABC circulation figures for *The Face* in *Benn's Newspaper Directory* (London): 60,000 (1981), p. 271; 60,000 (1982), p. 289; 60,000 (1983), p. 267; 57,050 (1984), p. 266; 60,819 (1985), p. 279; 80,032 (1986), p. 286; 91,660 (1989), p. 397; 65,163 (1991), p. 320; 68,655 (1992), p. 334; 73,202 (1993), p. 403; 89,615 (1994), p. 370; 105,592 (1995), p. 354; 107,192 (1996), p. 345.

4. D. Hebdige, 'The bottom line on Planet One – Squaring up to THE FACE', *Ten.8*, No.19 (1985), p. 41.

5. See British *Vogue* (July 1988), p. 6 concerning Herb Ritts, who had been working for the magazine since 1980, and 'Hot shots', *Observer Magazine* (15 November 1992), p. 37; for Newton see Z. Heller, 'At Home with Helmie', *Independent on Sunday Review* (3 July 1994), p. 12.

6. See National Union of Journalists, Freelance Fees Guide (London, 1989), pp. 24–5. This also states that reproduction fees would accrue to the photographer for black and white photographs on the following A4 page basis for use in Britain only: up to 1/4 page, £35; 1/4 to 1/2 page, £51; and 1/2 to full page, £67. Reproduction of colour work was paid double the rate and there was also a mark-up for foreign language rights of plus 50 per cent and World rights of plus 150 per cent. Similar figures are listed in the *Freelance Fees Guide* for 1987. These are the only two NUJ guidebooks available for analysis in the Trades Union Congress Library Collections at the University of North London.

7. S. Garratt, 'The making of Kate', *The Face* (March 1993), p. 42.

8. D. Hill, *Designer Boys and Material Girls – Manufacturing the 80s Pop Dream* (Poole, 1986), p. 53.

9. Ibid., p. 47.

10. See P. Jobling and D. Crowley, *Graphic Design* (Manchester, 1996), pp. 219–26.

11. J. Wozencroft, *The Graphic Language of Neville Brody* (London, 1988) and *The Graphic Language of Neville Brody 2* (London, 1994).

12. N. Logan and D. Jones, 'Ray Petri', *The Face* (October 1989), p. 10.

13. Ibid., p. 10.

14. D. O'Donaghue, *Lifestyles and Psychographics* (London, 1989), p. 64.

15. *The Stylographers*, BBC Radio 4 (Thursday, 29 September 1988, 7.30 p.m.), produced by Peter Everett and presented by Nigel Fountain.

16. Hebdige, 'The bottom line on Planet One'.

17. Ibid., p. 42.

18. Ibid., p. 41.

19. Ibid., p. 41.

20. Ibid., pp. 41–2.

21. Ibid., p. 42. When Hebdige's article was published much of Virilio's writing had still not been translated into English. Since 1975 he has, in fact, authored fifteen books, including *Vitesse and Politique* (1977) and *L'Espace Critique* (1984). In 1997, *Open Sky*, translated by J. Rose, was published by Verso.

22. Ibid., pp. 44 and 47.

23. J. Baudrillard, 'The Precession of Simulacra', in *Simulacra and Simulation*, trans. Sheila Faria Glaser (Ann Arbor, 1994), p. 43.

24. Hebdige, 'The bottom line on Planet One', p. 43.

25. Ibid., p. 47.

26. Ibid., pp. 47–8. *Picture Post* (1938–57) was one of the most successful weekly photojournals in Britain during the first half of the twentieth century. See S. Hall, 'The social eye of *Picture Post*', *Working Papers in Cultural Studies*, 2 (Spring 1972), CCCS, University of Birmingham, pp. 71–121; Jobling and Crowley, *Graphic Design*, pp. 183–209; and T. Hopkinson, *Picture Post 1938–50* (London, 1986).

27. Hebdige, 'The bottom line on Planet One', p. 47.

28. 'Love sees no colour', special issue, *The Face* (May 1992) and 'Strategies for the unemployed', *The Face* (January 1986).

29. N. Fountain, 'Just a light facelift', *The Guardian Media* (1 August 1988), p. 21.

30. 'Veiled Threats', *The Face* (January 1985), p. 52.

31. Hebdige, 'The bottom line on Planet One', p. 47.

32. Ibid., p. 47.

33. Cited in R. Kee, 'The Falklands Garrison', *Observer Magazine* (23 April 1989), p. 23.

34. 'Veiled Threats', p. 52. Janice Winship, 'Back to the future – a style for the eighties', *New Socialist* (July/August 1987), pp. 48–9, has argued a similar point about the fascination with 1950s style that was evident in advertising campaigns for Levi 501s during 1986 and 1987 and films such as *Absolute Beginners* (1986), contesting that in the Thatcher era of Youth Training Schemes and high unemployment amongst young people, 'fifties myths strike a vulnerable chord. They speak both of possibilities contemporarily denied the young and of problems still experienced today ... "Back to the fifties" is then a sign of young people's need both for conformism and rebellion' (p. 49).

35. D. Hill, *Designer Boys and Material Girls*, p. 36.

36. See, for example William Wordsworth's sonnet against the illustrated press of the nineteenth century, 'Illustrated books and newspapers': 'Avaunt this vile abuse of pictured page!/Must eyes be all in all, the tongue and ear/Nothing'. In W. Wordsworth, *Complete Poems* (Oxford, 1965), p. 383.

37. S. Kracauer, 'Shelter for the homeless' (first published as 'Asyl fÿr Obdachlose' in *Die Angestellten*, Frankfurt, Societäts-Verlag, 1930), in A. Kaes, M. Jay and E. Dimendberg (eds), *The Weimar Republic Sourcebook*, pp. 189–91, and 'Girls and crisis' (first published as 'Girls und Krise', *Frankfurter Zeitung*, 26 May 1931), ibid., pp. 565–6.

38. See A. Barbieri, 'Doing the Cybercatwalk', *Independent on Sunday Review* (4 June 1995), p. 48 and for Lee Swillingham, 'Exposed', *Creative Review* (September 1997), p. 55.

3

Arena

I think there's a problem with men's magazines . . . the one area there might be a gap is for a style magazine – but in that area Englishmen are uneasy, they don't admit to taking fashion seriously.

Mark Boxer, *The Observer*, 1987.

Introduction: Defining the Market

Although the new youth culture magazines launched in the 1980s had successfully managed to latch on to the male consumer, there was nonetheless still much leeway in the market for the circulation of at least one title that would be devoted exclusively to male fashions and lifestyles. There had been earlier attempts in Britain to produce a general-interest periodical for men that would depart from the one-sided view of masculinity promoted in pin-up magazines like *Men Only*. In 1953, for example, *Man About Town* was launched as a vehicle for males who were interested in fashion and the arts as well as politics. Michael Heseltine and Clive Labovitch bought the title in 1960, rechristening it *About Town* and later *Town*, and it ran until 1968. By the mid-1980s men's fashion retailing had expanded considerably in Britain, with the popularity of mainstream outlets such as Next for Men, founded in 1984 by George Davies, and the more exclusive or radical chic of designer labels like Paul Smith, Jean Paul Gaultier (who produced his first menswear lines in 1983), Katherine Hamnett and Giorgio Armani. Encouraged by these developments, as well as the subsequent rise of the much-vaunted new man in the iconography of advertising, spearheaded in campaigns for Levi 501s, Calvin Klein and Brylcreem, publishers began to draw up plans for the ideal prototype for a men's magazine that would concentrate on dress and style. It was as a result of these initiatives that a crop of the first successful magazines like *Arena*, *FHM* and a British edition of *GQ* came into existence. Of course, such prototypes had already long been part of American and European print culture – the American edition of *GQ*, for instance, was first published in the 1930s, while *Vogue Pour Hommes* originated in France in 1979 and the Italian title *Per Lui* in 1983.[1] As Paul Keers, who had been involved with launching the *Cosmopolitan* supplement *Cosmo Man* in November 1984, argued, the survival of a male-oriented press in America during the 1980s had less to do with accruing a mass readership or with enlightened social and sexual attitudes than – much more decisively – with the narrow-casting of one's potential readership in terms of spending power. The ideal target audience was the Yuppies, and it was, 'By isolating the interests of this specific, large, wealthy, and image-conscious demographic bulge in the male market, a UK men's magazine could succeed.'[2]

While there is something in this thesis, it could not guarantee the longevity of any periodical publication on its own, and other instrumental factors such as advertising revenue and striking the right balance in content were also to prove paramount. This much is demonstrated by the failure of the British bi-monthly *Unique*, which had been launched in the summer of 1985 by Jonathan Obadia. The magazine was an elegant production, consisting on average of three-quarters editorial and one-quarter advertising, both of which tended to concentrate almost exclusively on men's fashion (Figure 36). As such, however, it appeared to be too limited in scope to compete with more broad-based rivals such as *The Face*'s stablemate *Arena*, and ceased publication in the winter of 1987. The first issue of *Arena* appeared in November 1986. It was published on a bi-monthly basis until February 1996 and thereafter on a monthly basis. From the outset, the magazine's publisher Nick Logan had set himself realistic targets – pitching the magazine at an adult readership aged between 25 and 35 years old, and aiming to accrue a circulation of between 45,000 and 50,000 readers.[3] As things turned out, it went on to far exceed these expectations, the first two issues selling over 60,000 copies each, and for the period January–June 1996 achieved average sales of 93,513.[4] *Arena* can, therefore, be regarded as the first title to have dispelled the taboo that a general-interest magazine for men was doomed to failure in Britain. It eclipsed the tentative plans of Condé Nast to launch a men's edition of British *Vogue*,[5] and generated subsequent scions including the British edition of *GQ* and *FHM*, and ironically, a cluster of backlash men's magazines devoted to 'new laddism' such as *Loaded* (founded May 1994) and *Maxim* (founded April 1995).[6]

The success of *Arena* was due in part to its high design and aesthetic values. Neville Brody had crossed over from *The Face* to become its first art director, evolving a series of distinctive typographic devices and layouts, including a masthead closely modelled on John Heartfield's cover for the January 1927 issue of the sports magazine *Die Arena*. Equally as important was a more realistic attitude to readerships and advertisers. Whereas the promotions in *Unique*, for instance, had centred largely on fashion, *Arena* ran campaigns concerning music, film, alcohol and tobacco, as well as clothing and grooming.[7] Moreover Rod Sopp, who was advertising manager on the magazine at that time, was astute enough to realise that by eschewing the National Readership Survey, which defined magazine readerships solely in terms of socio-economic class, he could tag 'the less clued-up agencies' along and, thus, maximize *Arena*'s advertising potential in media circles.[8] As a result, *Media Week* gave the magazine a special commendation in its 1987 Consumer Magazine Awards, and concluded that: '*Arena* has increased the advertisers' ability to target an extremely elusive consumer. Before its launch, young male fashion magazines were taboo. Its success is a credit to the judgement and nerve of a small publishing team which really knows its readers.'[9]

Hitting on New Man

The ideal *Arena* reader referred to in this instance by *Media Week* was someone who by the mid-1980s had been typologised as 'new man', and whose impact on fashion iconography is discussed more fully in Part III. Suffice to say for the moment, however, that new man was adland's dream male subject. In 1984, for example, the advertising agency McCann Erickson published their *Manstudy Report* and concluded that new man constituted 13.5 per cent of all British males. The constituency was made up of three distinct types: avant-guardians or nurturers, who were strongly contemporary and politically iconoclastic with regard to patriarchal notions of masculinity; self-exploiters, who were at the forefront of social and cultural trends; and innovators, who were style leaders in fashion and clothing. In addition, many advertisers at this time were intent on exploiting the hedonistic lifestyle of the gay scene and what came to be defined as the 'pink pound'.[10] However, in bringing the term 'new man' into popular currency, the media could also strategically transcend any overt connotations of homosexuality, and acknowledge that taking an interest in one's appearance could be an acceptable and feasible project for all men, regardless of their sexual orientation.

As we have already recognised, during the 1980s new man could be found in campaigns for Levi 501s and others for clothing and grooming products, but he also began to appear in advertisements for financial services (Nat West and Halifax), alcohol (Stella Artois), and health (most notably, HEA-sponsored campaigns for HIV/AIDS and related promotions for condoms). As Rowena Chapman went on to define him, therefore, new man was culturally diverse, the ubiquitous 'child of our time':

rising like Venus from the waves or Adonis from the shaving foam, strutting his stuff across posters, calendars, magazines and birthday cards, peering nonchalantly down from advertising hoardings, dropping his trousers in the launderette. He is everywhere. In the street, holding babies, pushing prams, collecting children, shopping with the progeny, panting in the ante-natal classes, shuffling sweaty-palmed in maternity rooms, grinning in the Mothercare catalogue, fighting with absentee mums and the vagaries of washing machines in the Persil ad.[11]

Since its launch in 1986, *Arena* has peddled a similarly eclectic ideology concerning new man, witness Nick Logan's contention at the outset that: 'I don't have any big philosophy of the new man . . . Take people like myself who became interested in fashion as mods in the sixties, or the soul boys and Bowie fans of the 70s and 80s. If you become involved in fashion with that intensity I think it stays with you.'[12] Thus its editorial policy has tended to stick to a tried and tested formula in terms of content that, until the early 1990s, made a deliberate appeal to the self-styled politics of new man and usually included many, if not all, of the following items: interviews with well-known personalities; articles concerning politics, culture, travel, cars, fitness, health, and sex; reviews of music, books, film and food; a section called 'Vanity' (later known as 'Eye') concerning matters of grooming, style and sartorial details; and, last but by no means least, themed fashion spreads. In 1990 this formulation was appositely satirised by one of the magazine's female readers in a letter called 'INSTANT ARENA MAN' that enumerated the seven basic ingredients she regarded as a 'recipe for success':

1. Take any man
2. Dress it up in a bit of designer foreign
3. Gel its hair back and put a hat on it
4. Watch it smirk (especially if it's got a big dick)
5. Dispense alcohol
6. Drive it about in a flash car
7. Add smartass title, e.g. der Wiederaufbahn Menschlich and allow to settle.[13]

Style and Nostalgia

With regard to its fashion content, several of the photographers who had already contributed to *The Face* graduated to *Arena*, including Enrique Badulescu, Martin Brading, Michel Haddi, Nick Knight, Andrew Macpherson and Juergen Teller. Yet at the same time, it became a spawning ground for other producers like Randall Mesdon, Norman Watson and Ellen Von Unwerth (see Appendix I). The majority of the fashion spreads in *Arena* since its inception have coalesced around different typologies of masculinity and are the focus of a more sustained analysis in Part III of this study. Nostalgia for the past has also occasionally cropped up in various spreads (Figures 23–4), as has surrealism (for example, 'Reflections in a Golden Eye', photographed by Stephane Sednaoui and styled by Paul Frecker, November/December 1988), and nature ('Faith', by Nick Knight and Simon Foxton, January/February 1989, and 'Nature Boy', by Martin Brading and David Bradshaw, November 1992). Similar themes can also be found in many of the fashion shoots in *Arena Homme Plus*, a lavish publication that was launched in the Spring of 1994 and that appears twice yearly to offer a seasonal review of the latest designer fashions. Like its stablemate, *Arena Homme Plus* has also become a showcase for innovative photographic talent and has featured work by several familiar contributors to *The Face* and *Arena*, including Jean Baptiste Mondino, Nick Knight (Figures 38–41), Juergen Teller and Norman Watson (see Appendix I). Since I have already set up a discursive trajectory in the preceding two chapters, however, analysing how both *Vogue* and *The Face* have represented a simulacral idea of history, for the purpose of comparison I would now like to consolidate my argument by assessing the extent to which *Arena*'s perspective on the past is either analogous or different to theirs. Thus I have chosen two representative examples for analysis. The first, 'fin de siècle', photographed by Michel Haddi and styled by Debra Berkin, was published in *Arena*, January/February 1988. The second, 'once upon a time', photographed by Randall Mesdon with assistance from David Shadee Perez and styled by David Bradshaw, appeared in *Arena* in November 1992.

'fin de siècle' runs across eight pages and comprises an introductory page of type followed by seven toned photographs of models wearing various dress suits. The historicist tropes here are economically effective, and we are on familiar simulacral territory from the outset. The mood is set, for instance, with the succinct opening text, which initiates a pair of oppositions – 'light and shade, decadence and formalism' – which are followed through in the images, both in the dress codes of the clothing represented and in their photographic style (Figure 23).[14] Rather than evoking the soft-toned pictorialist photography of the 1890s, however, the clear focus of the photographs, with their crisp attention to the weave and contour of fabric, the use of opulent backdrops and chiaroscuro lighting, is redolent of the form, if not the content, of modernist images by Steichen, Hoyningen-Huene and Horst that appeared in *Vogue* during the 1920s and 1930s. Such images reproduced on the one hand, the clear geometric lines of the *Neue*

Sachlichkeit (New Objectivity), and on the other, the more elaborate *trompe l'oeil* effects of Surrealism.[15] This formal and temporal oscillation is also anticipated in the opening text, which states in lower-case letters: 'sometime in the not-too-distant past, somewhere in the heart of europe. history repeats itself, with a modernist edge'.[16] Even the use of a lower-case, sans-serif type here appears to be a postmodern evocation of the modernist precepts for printing propounded in Central Europe after the First World War by the likes of Làszló Moholy-Nagy, Herbert Bayer and Jan Tschichold, which by the early 1930s had coalesced around the ideal of the New Typography.[17] Moreover, in reworking the idea of the turn of the century the piece appears to correspond to 'Veiled Threats' from *The Face*, but in many respects the links between them are superficial. As we have seen, although the latter has historicist connotations, it does not simply romanticise the past as a fashion statement or as an ideologically safe haven, but rather uses the past as a masquerade to suggest what is wrong with the present. Conversely, 'fin de siècle' envisages history somewhat lamely as repeating itself, and in its stylistic and formal analogies to the work of past producers is probably more akin to the simulacral effects of Bruce Weber's fashion photography for British *Vogue*.

A similar hyperreal tendency can be discerned in 'once upon a time – dressing the american dream'. In this case, the title and *mise-en-scène*, ostensibly shot on location in New York State, evoke Serge Leone's epic cinematic fable *Once Upon A Time In America* (1984), which deals with the fate of four Jewish boys from New York's Lower East Side as they grow up to become involved in gang warfare during the Prohibition era. Apart from the opening title, photo and retail credits, the feature consists exclusively of eight full-page toned photographs, representing one black and two Italianate models wearing woollen autumn fashions that have been loosely based on the 1920s and 1930s sequences in the film. Here, history operates at the level of metanarrative, in so far as what we perceive is a heavily sanitised, textual masquerade based on a cinematic representation of more criminal and bloodthirsty historical events. Indeed, Leone's film, adapted from Harry Grey's novel *The Hoods*, is a metanarrative in its own right. There are also oblique references to the macho, working-class culture portrayed in the film in the retro dress codes of the models, who wear lace-up boots, flat caps, and braces (Figure 24). Of course, here even class is a sham, for most of the garments they wear are actually by expensive designers like Ralph Lauren (braces for £60 and tweed overcoat for £600), Yohji Yamamoto (a double-breasted suit for £950), and Dolce e Gabbana (knitted sweater, approximately £400).

But in its eclectic cultural references the shoot also goes beyond the specifics of Leone's filmic narrative. One of the models, for instance, is black, and, although the film is clearly concerned with racial tensions between Jewish and Italian hoodlums, none of its protagonists are black, nor does it deal with the inherent racism against black people in American society. Indeed, there is only one black personage in the entire film, who appears fleetingly as a cleaner in a New York bus station. Of course, it would be naive to contend that the inclusion of a black model in this fashion shoot is necessarily a political statement, given that its grounding in the film is so simulacral, and that its pictorial emphasis is very much on dressing up. It is interesting to note, however, that 'once upon a time' pays lip service to the racial prejudice and segregation of the period. For the black model is represented exclusively in isolation, whereas in one of the pictures the white models have been posed fraternally at a birthday party in a way that evokes the comradeship between David ('Noodles') and Max, two of the gangleaders in the film.[18] Furthermore, while the retro-style fashions promoted in the shoot appear to be one of a piece with the 1920s and 1930s fashions that are worn by characters in the film, the historical parallels do not end there. In its opening sequence and overall monochromatic styling, for example, 'once upon a time' appears to pay homage not to Leone, who filmed in colour, but instead to Lewis Hine's heroic photographs of male construction workers and industrial labourers, produced in the 1920s and early 1930s.[19]

This brings us neatly to a comparison of 'once upon a time' with Weber's 'New Morning Nebraska' and 'Under Weston Eyes'. Clearly, all three pieces appear to converge in their interest in a mythical image of American history and confraternity, and this has been compounded in the creation of a meta-narrative that involves the linking of the past to the present through stylistic analogy. But there are also several important differences that emerge in comparing the three fashion spreads. Most obviously, we could comment on the use of colour in 'New Morning Nebraska'. In contrast, the other two pieces have been shot in monochrome, a stylistic format that seems to add to their nostalgic appeal. Also, while the 'working-class' dress codes are similar in all of them, the Weber pieces place these very much in an idyllic rural environment, and Mesdon's in the industrial, modern city. More notably, there is another play on colour concerning the gender and racial connotations of such work. 'once upon a time' represents an exclusively macho, homo-social world, as well as introducing the image of black America. By comparison, the two *Vogue* fashion shoots include both male and female subjects, who are conspicuously and exclusively Caucasian.

Finally, 'New Morning Nebraska' and 'Under Weston Eyes' are much more entropically wordy pieces than 'once upon a time', and depend equally on the symbolism of text and image in conveying their latent meanings. Thus, in borrowing stylistically from other producers and in referencing their texts, they elaborate a dialectic between the verbal quotations and the fashion images reproduced. As we have already seen, for example, one of Weber's shoots for *Vogue* incorporates various excerpts from Willa Cather's novels, which the photographs seem simultaneously to illustrate, while another pays homage in word and image to the life and work of the photographer Edward Weston in such a way that the end product could appear to have been authored either by him or by Weber. In contrast, 'once upon a time' is verbally laconic, and the simulated historical and textual references it sets up are, therefore, conveyed by the photographs. For all that, however, the tropes it deploys are neither more nor less artificial than those in the Weber texts and, indeed, in its double signification, referring at once to Leone's film and to Hine's photographs, it seems to compound a hyperreality in which, to quote Baudrillard, 'nostalgia assumes full meaning'.[20]

Notes

1. Indeed, rather than simply being a British version of an American title, *GQ* can be seen to continue a tradition of a general-interest men's magazine that had been established in London in the late seventeenth century. In 1692, for example, Peter Motteux launched *The Gentlemen's Journal*, which was not illustrated and lasted for 33 issues, folding in 1694. It reappeared three more times under different management – in 1735, 1869 and 1890 respectively. See J. Sale, 'Founding father of GQ', *The Guardian, Media* (20 April 1992), p. 3.

2. P. Keers, letter to the editor, *Campaign* (2 May 1985), p. 20.

3. 'Men's fashion is Logan's latest run', *Campaign* (15 August 1986), p. 18.

4. T. Douglas, 'Magazines that could explode the male myth', *The Observer* (26 April 1987), p. 37 and 'The information', *The Observer Review* (11 August 1996), p. 16.

5. R. Hill, deputy managing director of Condé Nast in 'Vogue Men gets set to stand on its own', *Campaign* (26 September 1986), p. 7: 'People are always saying that men are becoming peacocks and while that's certainly true in Europe, I'm not sure whether we've got the full plumage here yet. But we are almost there and what we want to find out is whether its enough to make a separate *Vogue* for men viable'.

6. D. Aaronovitch, 'Outrageous!', *Independent Section Two* (21 November 1995), pp. 2–3.

7. In the first issue of *Arena* (Nov./Dec. 1986), for example, the following ads could be found: Stella Artois (pp. 4–5); Brylcreem (p. 16); Benson and Hedges (pp. 56–7); Boots (pp. 68–9); David Byrne's *True Stories* (p. 83); and The Damned, 'Anything' (p. 122).

8. 'The ideal homme magazine', *Media Week* (12 February 1988), p. 43.

9. Ibid., p.43.

10. See H. David, 'In the Pink', *The Times Saturday Review* (13 June 1992), pp.

10–11. David cites gay tourism as the prime indicator of the 'health of the pink economy'; in 1991, for example, the International Gay Travel Association grossed £247 million. At the same time, however, in the wake of HIV/AIDS and the implementation of Clause 28 in 1988, which banned the promotion of homosexuality by any local government agency, gay consumerism can be regarded as an act of political solidarity, a way of expressing one's individuality and existence in protest against marginalisation and victimisation by heterosexual society.

11. R. Chapman, 'The Great Pretender: Variations on the New Man Theme', in R. Chapman and J. Rutherford (eds), *Male Order – Unwrapping Masculinity* (London, 1988), pp. 225–6.

12. *Campaign* (15 August 1986), p. 18.

13. *Arena* (March/April 1990), p. 29, letter from Jean Cave, Falmouth, Cornwall.

14. 'fin de siècle', *Arena*, No.7 (January–February 1988), p. 84.

15. See N. Hall-Duncan, *The History of Fashion Photography* (New York, 1979) and W. A. Ewing, *The Photographic Art of Hoyningen Huene* (London, 1988); W. Hartshorn and M. Foresta, *Man Ray in Fashion* (New York, 1990); M. Kazmaier, *Horst – 60 Years of Photography* (London, 1991).

16. *Arena*, No.7, p. 84.

17. See R. Kinross, *Modern Typography: An Essay in Critical History* (London, 1992), Chapter 8.

18. See H. Aptheker (ed.), *A Documentary History of the Negro People in the United States 1910–32* (Secausus, NJ, 1973).

19. See L. Hine, *Men At Work, Photographic Studies of Modern Men and Machines* (New York, 1977).

20. J. Baudrillard, 'The Precession of Simulacra', in *Simulacra and Simulation*, trans. Sheila Faria Glaser (Ann Arbor, 1994), p. 6.

Conclusion to Part 1

I have attempted in the preceding chapters to proffer an understanding of the production and circulation of three important magazines that deal with fashion and fashion photography by concentrating on their social, economic and historical contexts. At the same time, much has been made of their form and content with regard to postmodern debates concerning simulation and hyperreality, and in trying to construct a focused argument I have tended to analyse a series of fashion spreads that have historicist connotations. As we have seen, the texts discussed reference an idea or image of the past to differing effect and for diverging aesthetic and discursive purposes. But there is probably one significant respect in which they all overlap, and this lies in the way they deploy a mythological metanarrative to naturalize the past and to synchronize discrete historical periods. At this point in my analysis, therefore, I would like to draw some threads together by examining the representation of the past in contemporary fashion publishing in the context of Roland Barthes' ideas on mythology, and of the relationship that he propounds between history and nature.

In his essay 'Myth Today', first written for *Les Nouvelles Lettres* in 1956, Barthes takes great pains to demonstrate that signs in themselves are not hermetic entities but part of a wider signifying chain and, as such, prone to distortion and ambiguity. According to Barthes, therefore, every sign is not only polysemous or open to multiple readings, but may also form the basis of a second sign system, which he calls myth or *metalanguage*:

> Mythical speech is made of material which has *already* been worked on so as to make it suitable for communication ... it is a peculiar system, in that it is constructed from a semiological chain which existed before it: *it is a second-order semiological system* ... It can be seen that in myth there are two semiological systems, one of which is staggered in relation to the other: a linguistic system, the language (or the modes of representation which are assimilated to it), which I shall call the *language-object*, because it is the language which myth gets hold of in order to build its own system; and myth itself, which I shall call *metalanguage*, because it is a second language, *in which* one speaks about the first.[1]

Thus, *'myth is speech stolen and restored'*;[2] its purpose is not to make the original symbol disappear but to distort it, and in this way, the language-object or meaning and the metalanguage or myth can be seen to co-exist in one and the same text or image. This is achieved through an elision or slippage between the sign of the language system, which Barthes calls 'meaning', and the signifier of the mythical system, which he calls 'form': 'It is this constant game of hide and seek between the meaning and the form which defines myth.'[3] We have already seen, for example, how the kind of slippage that Barthes describes between the meaning of one sign system and the form of another is evident in all the fashion spreads included for analysis in the preceding chapters: Weber in the way that his images appear to quote the work of Cather and Weston; Macpherson in the way that he mobilises a romantic image of the nineteenth century; and Haddi and Mesdon in the way that they reference an image of the 1920s and 1930s that is based on the style of the photography from the period, and also, in the case of Mesdon, on Serge Leone's own filmic metanarrative, *Once Upon A Time In America*.

Furthermore, as Barthes expresses it, myth is invested with a potent motivational or persuasional force because its predilection is 'to work with poor, incomplete images.'[4] The motivational power of myth, however, is also one of degree; and, in achieving a double or secondary signification, Barthes suggests that myth functions on three different levels of complexity. These imply the spectator's share, and he categorises them as the empty signifier, the full signifier, and ambiguous signification, contending: ' I can produce three different types of reading by focusing on the one, or the other, or both at the same time.'[5] With the empty signifier, the meaning or original sign is taken over, usually by the producer, in a literal or unambiguous way as the basis of the form in order to legitimise the new signified, that is the mythical concept. This is achieved in such a way that we accept the link between meaning and form, appreciating how, if not why, the original sign has been chosen to correspond to the new text. With the full signifier, the intended symbolism is again unambiguous. But, in contrast, meaning and form are not so readily or easily confused by the reader or mythologist, who is able to detect the imposition and recognise the mythical concept as a distortion, an alibi or an excuse. Finally, with ambiguous signification, the meaning and form appear to be inextricably linked into a unitary sign that we find confusing, in so far as we can fully believe in and doubt its mythology at one and the same time. Accordingly, Barthes sees that: 'the first two types of focusing are static, analytical; they destroy the myth, either by making its intention obvious, or by masking it'. By comparison: 'the third type of focusing is dynamic . . . the reader lives the myth as a story at once true and unreal . . . everything happens as if the picture naturally conjured up the concept, as if the signifier gave a foundation to the signified'.[6] In his analysis of this tripartite system in 'Myth Today', Barthes invokes a photograph of a saluting black soldier that he had observed on the cover of *Paris-Match* as a paradigm of French Imperialism. But in other essays he turns his attention to the mythologies of various cult products and advertising campaigns. He writes, for instance, about the militaristic discourse of soap-powder advertisements that speak of 'killing' dirt and germs, and concludes: 'To say that Omo cleans in depth is to assume that linen is deep, which no one had previously thought.'[7] Thus the compulsion to believe in myth occurs because its ultimate objective, as Barthes contests, is to transform history into nature, and in so doing, to interpellate us as if we were individual or exclusive personalities: 'Myth has an imperative buttonholing character . . . It is I whom it has come to seek. It is turned towards me, I am subjected to its intentional force, it summons me to receive its expansive ambiguity.'[8]

Taken literally as nothing more than fashion shoots it could, of course, be argued that all six of the examples included in Part 1 will be automatically interpreted by the readers of magazines like *Vogue*, *The Face* and *Arena* at the level of either the empty or the full signifier. Hence either, on the one hand, their form and content will be regarded as nothing more than an appropriate stylistic fit for the clothes represented, or conversely, the overlap between form and content could be seen as a way of investing fashion (otherwise, an allegedly 'vacuous' sign system) with some discursive credibility by forging a symbolic association between it and art, literature, film, nature and history. But as I have also attempted to argue, in their very treatment of the past these are, by definition, ideological texts that, in one way or another, demonstrate a propensity towards ambiguous signification. Consequently, 'New Morning Nebraska' can be decoded as an idyllic representation of *both* fashion and nature; indeed, dress can be seen here to bolster an idea of clean-living and virtue. 'Under Weston Eyes' can be interpreted as an ambiguous statement concerning authorship, in which the identity of Bruce Weber, fashion photographer, is both bound up with, and legitimated by, that of Edward Weston, art photographer. 'fin de siècle' can be viewed as an essay that not only has class connotations, but that also deploys them to promote the timeless, high taste of modernism. And 'once upon a time' can be seen to portray retro-style fashions as a way of legitimising a mythic ideal of the work ethic and the heroism of industrial masculinity.

In contrast, and somewhat ironically, the two most obvious contenders for empty or full signification, 'Apparitions' and 'Veiled Threats', are also the most mythologically complex and contradictory pieces with regard to word and image. On the surface they each appear to harp on the past for no other reason than to find a convenient stylistic parallel for the New Romantic clothes portrayed. Nonetheless, the chromatic tonalism of their imagery is too contemporary to be a convincing match for the technical effects we would actually observe in nineteenth-century photographs. And, as we have also seen, the intratextual relationship between word and image in both pieces seems to transform politics into a form of depoliticised speech. Consequently, the stylish masquerade we witness in them acts as a smokescreen for their underlying opposition to the dangers of anchoring national and individual identity in the past, and of seeing history as an escape route from the present: 'A conjuring trick has taken place; it has turned reality inside out, it has emptied it of history and has filled it with nature.'[9] Furthermore, these two pieces can be seen to deconstruct the popular myth that masculine and feminine identities are naturally or perpetually distinct and stable phenomena. As such, they introduce a central aporia that is further assessed in Part 2 of this study, which is concerned with Barthes' *The Fashion System*, and more rigorously pursued in the analysis of the body in fashion photography in Part 3.

Notes

1. R. Barthes, 'Myth Today', in *Mythologies*, transl. A. Lavers, (London, 1973 [1957]), pp.119, 123 and 124.
2. Ibid., 136
3. Ibid., p. 128.
4. Ibid., p. 137.
5. Ibid., p. 138.
6. Ibid., p. 139–40 .
7. Barthes, 'Soap powders and detergents', in *Mythologies*, p. 41.
8. Barthes, 'Myth Today', p. 134.
9. Ibid., p. 155.

Part 2

Written Clothing and Image-Clothing: Roland Barthes' 'The Fashion System' in Perspective

Introduction to Part 2

To write the body. Neither skin, nor the muscles, nor the bones, nor the nerves, but the rest: an awkward, fibrous, shaggy, raveled thing, a clown's coat.

Roland Barthes, *Roland Barthes*, 1977.

In the spring of 1997 a double-page advertisement produced by Richard Smith for the design consultancy Area, representing a Japanese pop singer called Miju, appeared in several style and women's magazines, heavily disguised as a fashion feature.[1] The right-hand page of the work consisted of a mono-chrome head-and-shoulders portrait of the singer herself along with her name printed in sans-serif capitals. On the opposite page, two sets of text composed of the same type in different weights and contrasting shades of grey were printed on a black background, one superimposed over the other. The smaller in scale of the two texts conveyed information concerning the name of the photographer, dress designer and record company, but was eclipsed by the larger text in light grey on to which it was grafted, which stated provocatively, 'Images Travel Faster Than Words'. On one level we could regard such an act of textual mimicry as nothing more than a piece of harmless, postmodern simulation. While on another, I feel, the ad/fashion spread both raises and crystallises a number of interesting points concerning the relationship of words to images and vice versa in media texts such as the fashion magazine. In the image-saturated economy of Baudrillardean hyperreality, it is tempting to fall in line with the iconocentric sentiments that the piece enunciates, since the photograph of Miju is indeed quite straightforward to assimilate.[2] How-ever, this ad in itself also implies a paradox. For in the way that the work is laid out, the image is absorbed so quickly as to become virtually redundant, whereas the verbal elements seem more complex and interesting, and it is over them we tend to deliberate. Consequently, if images really do travel faster than words, then we need to examine why they do so, and at what aesthetic and intellectual cost. Indeed, *mutatis mutandis*, we could just as easily ask what is at stake by either prioritizing words over images or arguing for their interdependence?

We have already encountered some of the ways in which the intertexuality between word and image can operate in our analysis of a selection of fashion shoots in Part 1. At this stage of my argument, therefore, I should like to compound the issue of intertextuality and its implications for the discourse of the fashion magazine by concentrating on Roland Barthes' often neglected and much misunderstood and maligned text, *The Fashion System*, a work that has sometimes been called his 'bleakest book', and often 'dismissed as unreadably dull'.[3] Certainly Barthes' is a notoriously opaque analysis. Nonetheless, it is singular in the way that it explicates a particular methodology for the reading or decoding of the fashion magazine as a generator of what is fashionable and what is not, an idea he neatly sums up in the lapidary phrase 'the magazine is a machine that makes Fashion'.[4] In examining Barthes' text my aim here is twofold. Given the structural complexity of *The Fashion System*, and by way of clarification, I want first to proffer a synopsis of the work, and to identify the chief ideas that Barthes raises. Principally, I want to evince the dichotomy between what he calls written clothing (*le vêtement écrit*) on the one hand, and image-clothing (*le vêtement-image*) on the other. And second, I want to build on this overview, by attempting to unravel some of the textual knots and ambiguities in the work, and by critically evaluating how useful his methodology actually is in analysing the aims and objectives of word and image in the fashion spread in more specific terms.

In this regard, I do not wish simply to endorse Barthes' ideas, but more cogently to contest and re-contextualise them in terms of both the type of fashion publishing he encountered during the late 1950s and that produced since 1980. More particularly, my intention has been to locate his thesis into a broader methodological context concerning logocentrism, and to deconstruct the apparent inconsistencies of his predilection for written clothing. In so doing, I want to postulate a dialectic between words and images that seeks not to prioritise the one over the other, but to propound instead their complementarity. At the same time, Barthes speaks of the performative nature of the rhetoric of fashion and the poetics of clothing, not least in the way they construct a constant ideal for the woman of fashion. His analysis consequently frames the Fashion system in gender terms as a strictly feminine pursuit, a point that I also want to re-evaluate in this discussion. Again, in dealing with these issues and for the sake of clarity, I have tended to concentrate my analysis on a representative sample of fashion texts: an archetypal spread from the late 1950s entitled 'Amoureuse', published in *Elle*, 16 June 1958, with text by Denise Dubois-Jallais and photographs by Santoro,[5] and several more recent spreads that deal with the poetics of clothing with regard to gender and race – 'Sri Lanka – Fashion in the Sun and Serendip', photographed by Alex Chatelain for British *Vogue* (May 1980); 'borneo', photographed by Corinne Day and styled by Melanie Ward; 'Heavy

Metal', photographed by Jamie Morgan and Ray Petri; and 'Who's Shooting Who?', photographed by Oliver Maxwell and styled by Elaine Jones (Figures 9, 18 and 25).

Notes

1. See, for example, *Arena* (March 1997), pp. 106–7.

2. J. Baudrillard 'The Precession of Simulacra' in *Simulacra and Simulation*, trans. Sheila Faria Glaser (Ann Arbor, 1994).

3. Rick Rylance, Roland Barthes (London 1994), p. 42.

4. R. Barthes, *The Fashion System*, trans. Matthew Ward and Richard Howard (Berkeley, 1990), p. 51. The quotations from this translation cited throughout Part 2 are credited in parentheses (as *F/S* plus page number) in the main text. In keeping with Barthes' original text, fashion has also been capitalised throughout this Part.

5. Unfortunately, it has not been possible to trace either the photographer or the author of 'Amoureuse' for the purpose of clearing copyright for its reproduction in this book. The English translations from the text of 'Amoureuse' are my own.

Elle was edited at this time by Marguerite Duval with Roger Giret as art editor; contributing photographers included J. F. Clair as well as Santoro. *Jardin des Modes* was founded by Lucien Vogel (who had also been editor of the weekly photojournal *Vu*, founded 1928) and published by Condé Nast. It was edited by Marie-France de la Villehuchet with Jacques Montin as art editor, and contained a summary in English of the main text. During the late 1950s two of its contributing photographers were Helmut Newton and Frank Horvat.

4

'The Fashion System': A Synopsis

This dress, photographed on the right, becomes on the left: a leather belt, with a rose stuck in it, worn above the waist, on a soft shetland dress . . . in one the substances are forms, lines, surfaces, colours, and the relation is spatial; in the other, the substance is words, and the relation is, if not logical, at least syntactic; the first structure is plastic, the second verbal.

The Fashion System, p. 3.

Introduction: Defining the Corpus

Six years in the making between 1957 and 1963, and emanating from the research scholarship awarded by the *Centre National de Recherche Scientifique*, where Barthes had been appointed reader in sociology, *Système de la Mode* was eventually published in 1967, with the first English edition, *The Fashion System* (hereafter *F/S*), appearing in 1983. Although Barthes spent considerable time evolving his thesis, by the time it was published he felt compelled to write somewhat apologetically in the foreword that he felt the work was, 'already dated . . . *already* a certain history of semiology' (*F/S*, ix). In effect, Barthes' project was the first, and to date the only, large-scale study of the representation of fashion or, as he puts it himself, the 'translation' of clothing into language: 'without discourse there is no total Fashion, no essential Fashion' (*F/S*, xi). At the very outset of his discussion, Barthes postulates that the object of this discourse is to fetishise the object represented by drawing around it, 'a veil of images, of reasons, of meanings', with the ultimate aim of making Fashion speak to or about itself (*F/S*, xi–xiii). In undertaking his study, moreover, Barthes admits that he was under the sway of Saussurean structuralism,[1] and that he was originally inspired by 'une rêve euphorique de scientificité'.[2] *The Fashion System* mobilises a syncretic and somewhat indeterminate methodology, combining linguistics (or spoken language) with semiology (or written language). As such, it appears to transcend, or at least to confound, the analytical model adumbrated by Saussure in the *Course in General Linguistics*. This was intended to show the way to a more radical and comprehensive semiotic system, one that would be grounded initially in linguistics, but that would have the potential to embrace other forms of cultural representation.[3] Hence, as Barthes expresses it:

> this study actually addresses neither clothing nor language but the "translation", so to speak of one into the other, in so far as the former is already a system of signs: an ambiguous goal, for it does not correspond to the customary distinction which puts the real on one side and language on the other; thus it escapes both linguistics, the science of verbal signs, and semiology, the science of object-signs (*F/S*, x).

In *The Fashion System*, Barthes is highly selective of the material he chooses for linguistic and semiological analysis. The thrust of his argument is based chiefly on sampling two magazines between June 1958 and June 1959, namely *Elle*, published weekly, and *Le Jardin des Modes*, published monthly. In addition, he states that he also consulted sporadic copies of *Vogue* and *L'Echo de la Mode*, and the weekly fashion features of certain daily newspapers during the period prescribed. Barthes justifies his selection of titles on socio-economic grounds, and picking up on Crozier's research into the different readerships for women's magazines he claims that: '*Elle* and *L'Echo de la Mode* seem to have a more "popular" appeal than *Vogue* and *Le Jardin des Modes*' (*F/S*, 11).[4] But his decision to study the representation of Fashion in magazines, rather than the garments themselves, also affords him the methodological opportunity of framing Fashion as a kind of rhythmically reiterated language. What Barthes discerns in operation in Fashion publishing, therefore, is a general structural principle through which the Fashion system perennially appears to renew itself by prioritising different styles, fabrics and colours according to changes of season. Paradoxically, however, it is by conforming to the very same temporal pattern, year in and out, that he sees the Fashion System as tending towards renewal on the one hand, and regularity on the other: 'the synchrony of Fashion changes abruptly each year, but during the year it is absolutely stable' (*F/S*, 8). As he contends, both the magazines and period of his choosing, June 1958–June 1959, may delimit a particular corpus of representations for analysis, but in themselves they constitute at the very most an arbitrary paradigm: 'we are not attempting to describe some Fashion in particular but Fashion in general' (*F/S*, 10). Given that this is the case, then, we could just as easily subject any other annual corpus of representations to his structural imperative for understanding

Fashion as a distinct, though generalised, form of language: 'As soon as it is gathered, extracted from its year, the raw material (the utterance) must take its place in a purely formal system of functions . . . we have not sought to deal with any particular substance of Fashion, but only with the structure of written signs' (*F/S*, 10–11).

For Barthes, however, written signs form part of one of three chief ways of defining or conceptualising Fashion: 'the general system of Fashion clearly includes three levels theoretically available to analysis: the rhetorical, the terminological and the real' (*F/S*, 41). Hence, the vestimentary or real code is the garment itself (*le vêtement réel*, confusingly also referred to as *le vêtement technologique*). The terminological code (*système terminologique*) belongs to spoken language, while the rhetorical code (*système rhétorique*) concerns written clothing and images. In turn, Barthes anchors each of these three elements in distinct epistemologies. As he argues it, therefore, the real garment is the province of the sociologist, the terminological garment concerns linguistics, and the rhetorical garment must be decoded in terms of semiology: 'Semiology . . . describes a garment which from beginning to end remains imaginary, or if one prefers, purely intellective; it leads us to recognize not practices but images. The sociology of Fashion is entirely directed toward real clothing; the semiology of Fashion is directed toward a set of collective representations' (*F/S*, 9–10).

Shifters and Meanings

Barthes ultimately insists that each of the three structures of Fashion he outlines 'calls for an original analysis' of its own (*F/S*, 8), and that 'we must study either acts, or images, or words' (*F/S*, 7). At the same time, however, he regards the real code of clothing as a generative mother tongue, that deals with materials, measurements, types and styles of clothing, and through which actual garments become instances of 'speech'.[5] Thus the second and third structures/codes, that is the verbal and the iconic respectively, feed off the technological mother tongue, and derive their significatory value from it: 'In our society, the circulation of Fashion thus relies in large part on an activity of *transformation*: there is a transition (at least according to the order invoked by Fashion magazines) from the technological structure to the iconic and verbal structures' (*F/S*, 6). The meaning of Fashion is, accordingly, elaborated in the interpenetration that takes place between these three structures or codes, and that Barthes describes (expanding on terminology used by Jakobson)[6] as taking place through a series of *shifters*.

The first shift occurs in the translation of the real/technological garment to the iconic code, that is from the real to the rhetorical level. This is effected initially in the illustrative elements of sewing patterns, for example, and subsequently in photographs and other graphic illustrations. The second occurs in the shift from the real/technological garment to written clothing, as witnessed in the texts of sewing patterns and other descriptive formulae. Initially this seems to entail another unproblematic shift from the real to the rhetorical. But Barthes suggests that the real/language shifter implies a kind of indeterminate status for Fashion, midway between reality (the fabric or garment) and signification:

> It is generally a text quite apart from the literature of Fashion; its goal is to outline not what is but what is *going to be* done . . . As a shifter, it constitutes a transitional language, situated midway between the making of a garment and its being, between its origin and its form, its technology and its signification (*F/S*, 6).

Finally, and of more relevance for this study, there is a shift that takes place exclusively at the rhetorical level between the iconic and the verbal code, and that is the *sine qua non* of the fashion spread: 'Fashion magazines take advantage of the ability to deliver simultaneously messages derived from these two structures – here a dress photographed, there the same dress described' (*F/S*, 7). We shall be returning to a more detailed analysis of the implications of this rhetorical shift in due course with specific reference to the form and content of the fashion spread 'Amoureuse'. But at this point in my discussion, it is relevant to mention briefly two of the significant exchanges between word and image that are elaborated in it. First, the overall narrative structure of the piece has been arranged around four scenes in a drama, each of them consisting of its own short pieces of editorial and photographs that link love and fashion by representing respective typologies of the feminine: 'She who charms'('Celle qui charme'); 'She who surprises '('Celle qui étonne'); 'She who plays'('Celle qui joue') and 'She who bewitches' ('Celle qui ensorcelle'). And complementary to this, a strict directional relationship between the numbered captions and the corresponding photographs not only delineates a particular sequential movement from one textual element to another, but also helps to guide us from one act to the next.

The Case for Written Clothing

Thus far we have seen how Barthes sets up an elaborate chain of imbricated information systems, arguing that the real vestimentary code generates a language for Fashion that is operative on two separate but interconnected levels: the linguistic (or terminological) vestimentary system, and the semiological or rhetorical system. For Barthes, therefore, it is not so much the actual garments themselves that create the meaning of Fashion but the ways in which they are articulated in verbal and iconic forms of representation. Moreover, he explains the distinction between these two systems in terms of effect – the former being principally concerned with utility, and the latter with signification:

> The study of the garment "represented" (by image and text), i.e. the garment dealt with by the Fashion magazine, affords an immediate methodological advantage over the analysis of real clothing. . . . "Real" clothing is burdened with practical considerations (protection, modesty, adornment); these finalities disappear from "represented" clothing, which no longer serves to protect, to cover, or to adorn, but at most to signify protection, modesty or adornment (F/S, 8).

But he qualifies this statement by affording priority to written clothing, that is the verbal account of fashion, over image-clothing (photographs and illustrations), with the justification that words seem to proffer a purer reading of the fashion text than pictures:

> The choice remains between image-clothing and written (or, more precisely, described) clothing. Here again, from the methodological point of view, it is the structural "purity" of the object which influences the choice: image-clothing retains one set of values which risks complicating its analysis considerably, i.e. its plastic quality; only written clothing has no practical or aesthetic function . . . the being of the written garment resides completely in its meaning . . . written clothing is unencumbered by any parasitic function (F/S, 8).

And in the final analysis, he insists on a fundamental rule that will determine 'the constitution of the corpus', and through which, 'no other raw material for study other than the language provided by the Fashion magazines' will be subject to scrutiny (F/S, 12).

Written clothing, in the form of captions and/or editorial, goes beyond photographic representation for Barthes in several strategic ways, as demonstrated in the text of 'Amoureuse'. First, it can transmit information that is not evident in the photograph. Most obviously the colour of the garment if the print is monochrome ('Triangular dress in pale blue shantung with a round collar and white piqué strap'/ 'Robe trapèze en shantung ciel à col rond et patte de piqué blanc'), or those parts of the garment that are either not visible or in some way obscured in the photograph, usually the back of the garment and intricate decorative motifs. Second, it can endow the garment with a system of functional meanings ('For her every game, white poplin overblouse with turquoise pattern and turquoise trousers' / 'Pour elle, tous les jeux. Marinière de popeline blanche à dessins turquoise et pantalon turquoise'). And finally, it can isolate certain elements such as fabric, texture, buttons, and trim for specific attention, and thereby arrest the reading of Fashion at a certain level ('Sheath dress in chiffon, with braided flounces' / 'Fourreau en mousseline à volants gansés de satin'). Consequently, as Barthes extrapolates:

> it is the photograph of the real garment which is complex; its written version is immediately significant . . . Thus, every written word has a function of authority in so far as *it* chooses – by proxy, so to speak – instead of the eye. The image freezes an endless number of possibilities; words determine a single certainty . . . What language adds to the image is *knowledge* (*F/S*, 119, 13, 14).

The OVS Matrix

The language of Fashion is enunciated as a series of utterances, in which meaning is established through both the syntagmatic, or spatially linear, relationships between one word and another, and their paradigmatic, or oppositional, values. Hence, as Barthes argues: 'without its verbal limits, Fashion would be nothing other than an infatuation with certain forms or details, as has always been the case with costume; in no way would it be an ideological elaboration' (*F/S*, 49). By way of clarifying how the terminological, and by extension rhetorical, systems of signification work, Barthes insists that the verbal utterance needs to be deconstructed into smaller units within a signifying matrix. This involves an object (O), a variant (V) and a support (S), through which, 'the harvest promises to be immense and outwardly anarchic' (*F/S*, 59).

The matrix is constituted of the relationship between the object, variant and support, where 'O' and 'S' are material substances, and 'V' is a non-material entity. The variant is what Barthes also refers to as the *vesteme*, since it 'is the point of the matrix from which signification emerges and, as it were, emanates all along the utterance, i.e. the written garment' (*F/S*, 66). Accordingly, the OVS matrix should be conceptualised as a metaphor in which 'O' acts as a door, 'V' a key, and 'S' a lock: 'In order to produce meaning, we must "introduce" the variant into the support' (*F/S*, 68). Finally, Barthes also demonstrates that the order of the three elements may be expressed in different combinations or permutations, and in differing degrees of complexity, as exemplified in the two following models that he furnishes:[7]

(i) OVS
a blouse with a large collar
   O   V   S

(ii) OSV
a cardigan with its collar open
    O   S   V

It is the object, in the form of the entire garment itself, that is the constant element in the matrix, and upon which meaning is built. Only the object cannot be multiplied, since the matrix functions to make meaning converge on the object: 'the very aim of the fashion system is this difficult reduction from the many to the one' (*F/S*, 79). Barthes includes the following two more complex OVS structures to illustrate this idea. In diagram (iii), O (the garment in its entirety) is unuttered or paradigmatic, but still forms, as in diagram (iv), the base of a pyramidal superstructure:[8]

(iii) *white braid and white buttons*
  SV   O   SV   O
      S1   V   S2
        O (unuttered garment)

(iv) a cotton dress with red (checks) and white checks
   VS   O   VS (O)   VS   O
                  S1   V   S2
      O   V   S

The Rhetorical System and Connotation

While the OVS matrix is the logical starting-point for placing Fashion into a linguistic chain of signification, it is more particularly through the phraseology or tone of the magazine or fashion editor that it is incorporated into the rhetorical system. Thus the rhetorical system is instrumental, in so far as it qualifies or inflects the terminological or linguistic code by revealing hierarchies of class or economic and social status, a point that Barthes reinforces with reference to his own sample of magazines. He claims, for instance, that magazines that are intended for a socially and economically higher audience such as *Vogue* and *Jardin des Modes* tend towards denotation, since their readers are already 'in the know' concerning fashion, and do not need to be persuaded to buy what they can already afford. By the same token, if we look at the opposite end of the market, and magazines intended for readers with the lowest level of income (in his sample *Echo de la Mode*), we find once more a tendency toward denotation. Only this time the garments will be cheaper, and the way that they are described will emphasise utility. In contrast, it is the 'middle-ground' or aspirational magazines such as *Elle* that are stronger on rhetoric and connotation. Barthes concludes: 'The denotation of the popular magazine is poor, for it apprehends a cheap garment which it regards as obtainable: utopia occupies, as it should, an intermediary position between the praxis of the poor and that of the rich' (*F/S*, 245).[9]

It is the rhetorical system of written clothing, then, that appears to be the most significant code, since it puts fashion into a given context, affording it not only a voice but also a tone: 'With the rhetorical system, we broach the general level of connotation' (*F/S*, 225). But, as Barthes is at pains to demonstrate, the rhetoric of fashion is in effect a mythological syntax, always setting up arbitrary oppositions between what is to be approved and what is not, while appearing to make this sound natural:

> the meaning the magazine gives to the garment does not come from any particular intrinsic qualities of form, but only from particular oppositions of kind: if the *toque* is in Fashion, it is not because it is high and has no brim, it is simply because it is no longer a bonnet and not yet a hood; to go beyond the nomination of species would thus be to "naturalize" the garment and hence to miss the very essence of Fashion (*F/S*, 48–9).

It is on this basis that he exhorts us to consider the statement, 'white accents on daytime clothes are a sign of the city', and to commute *blue* for *white*. In effect, when we change the two words the imputed reality of the statement does not change, even if its signification does (*F/S*, 48).[10] His thinking at this stage of the argument evinces some of the chief ideas that he had already raised in his comparatively more cohesive and clearly structured essay on semiology, 'Myth Today', published in *Mythologies* (1957), where he sums up the motivational force of such forms of ambiguous signification in the following terms: 'Mythical speech is made of material which has already been worked on so as to make it suitable for communication . . . myth is neither a lie nor a confession: it is an inflexion . . . driven to having either to unveil or to liquidate the concept, it will naturalize it.'[11]

The Rhetorical System: Poetics, Reality, and Fashion

The verbal limits of the Fashion system, as much as any form of motivated speech, therefore, must be understood in semiological terms. Thus, as Barthes remarks, even without enunciating the words 'fashionable' or 'in fashion', it is fashionability, and by extension unfashionability, that its rhetorical system implies. As we have already seen, in achieving this association, the sign of Fashion is 'elaborated each year . . . by an exclusive authority' (*F/S*, 215), the avant-garde, for example, or the editors of magazines. But it is also connoted by making Fashion refer either to the real world or to itself. As such, Barthes contends that the rhetoric of Fashion is circumscribed by three smaller constituent systems: the poetics of clothing (*poétique du vêtement*); the worldly signified (*rhétorique du signifié mondain*); and the reason of Fashion (*la "raison" de Mode*).

With regard to the first, the real function of the garment represented is shrouded in metaphors that suggest an equivalence between sensation, mood, time and place. In this way, the garment is affective, dealing with 'the idea of seduction, more than protection', and 'the garment is sometimes loving, sometimes loved', to the extent that: 'we would call this the "caritative" quality of clothing' (*F/S*, 241). In 'Amoureuse', we can see how this correspondence is made explicit through a series of metaphoric verbal exchanges that draw a parallel between the condition of being in love and of being fashionable: 'Love is a merry-go-round . . . and women make it go round . . . Fashion is a merry-go-round . . . and dresses make it go round' ('L'amour est un manège . . . Et les femmes mènent la ronde . . . La mode est un manège . . . Et les robes mènent la ronde'). In this context, garments literally take on the status of 'romantic dresses' ('robes à romances'), and their very materiality is lyrically connoted thus: 'a dress with roses . . . decorated dresses' ('robe à roses . . . robes enrobées').

At the same time, within the poetic signifying chain, cultural or cognitive models are referenced, such as nature, geography, history, literature and art. In this way, the fashionable garment and the notion of being in fashion, and, by extension, of being superior to those who are not, will frequently be associated with tropes of good taste, refinement and egregiousness. As we have already noted, for example, the narrative of 'Amoureuse' has been organised as if it is a play with four acts. Each one mobilises a certain female stereotype or set of feminine attributes and attitudes that, in turn, have been complemented by an apposite photographic *mise-en-scène* and text. Thus, 'She who surprises' ('Celle qui étonne'), does so by dressing *à l'avant-garde*. While, 'She who bewitches' ('Celle qui ensorcelle'), is a red-headed vamp who is a 'public danger', a 'psychologist', 'dramatic' and 'a little perverse'. Moreover, in many instances of poetic signification, indigenous subjects and exotic locations are used as nothing more than props or background for the white models in fashion shoots. This is particularly evident in British *Vogue*, where fashion spreads taken overseas are often intertwined with a complementary travelogue about the country in question. A key example is 'Sri Lanka – Fashion in the Sun and Serendip', photographed by Alex Chatelain for the May 1980 issue and supplemented with an article by Polly Devlin. In several pictures from the spread, the female model is seen surrounded by natives, who, while they seem to realise they are taking part in a fashion masquerade, have nonetheless been represented as being coincidental both to her and to the clothes she wears. In one sense, she comes close to going native in these images, with her bare feet, her hairstyle and the cut and fabric of her garments. But the spread also raises another problem concerning racial identities, and how the nature of whiteness can be defined in relation to the non-white Other when, as black writer and critic Kobena Mercer has appositely argued: 'one of the signs of the time is we don't really know what "white" is'.[12] The model's dusky skin, dark hair and eyes suggest, for example, that she also is not necessarily a 'white' European. Nonetheless, throughout the spread her skin tone is represented as being lighter than that of the Sri Lankans who surround her, and thereby she is connoted as being superior to and more civilised than them. In the spread this is maintained both by the way she holds centre stage and the verbal rhetoric of the piece, which, in the name of Fashion, serves to contrast civilisation and exclusivity with collective primitivism. Thus even in 'the jungled countryside' she is seen modelling a 'very short puffed dress, elasticated waist, big sleeves', while the Sri Lankan family who pose with her are seen in sarongs and simple tops. Indeed, her Jap outfit, retailing at £65, would probably alone cost enough to feed this entire family for at least several months.

Yet *Vogue* is not alone in deploying this type of paternalistic tokenism, and somewhat surprisingly, we find a similar act of subordination in so-called alternative magazines like *The Face*. In 'borneo', photographed by Corinne Day for the August 1991 issue, for example, Kate Moss has been represented on several occasions with Bornean children. In the majority of the pages from the spread, however, natives and tribesmen have also been literally relegated to the margins as primitive Others (Figure 25). The nature of this exploitation was not lost on several of the magazine's readers, one of whom wrote to complain that: 'While I feel that it is acceptable to use other cultures to contrast with our western fashions, I find it disgusting to use people's poverty, which is demeaning to all those who suffer from it, in something as facile as a fashion shoot.'[13] Likewise, Barthes himself is disparaging of poetic signification, regarding it as too eclectic and immature, since it seems merely to be interested in: 'the divisions of a high-school girl's learning ... the models Fashion proposes pell-mell are borrowed from the intellectual baggage of a young girl who is *"on the go and in the know"* (as Fashion would say)' (*F/S*, 240).

Both 'Amoureuse' and 'borneo' also trade on the second internalised rhetorical Fashion system, the worldly signified. With the worldly signified, the referencing of the real world we witness is bogus or hollow, and, as in the case of poetic signification, this type of association serves to connote everything that Fashion relates to, or draws from the world, as being subordinate to it. Consequently, life is played as if it were no more than a game performed in honour of Fashion. Barthes maintains that this ideology is manifest in statements like, 'Prints win at the races' ('les imprimés triomphent aux Courses'); but we can also see it underscored in closer detail in the narrative of 'Amoureuse'. This implies that not even scientific discovery and revolutionary or political events can deter the sempiternal progress of love/fashion: 'La science et les évenements politiques peuvent bouleverser le monde, cela n'arrêtera rien', (*rien* here refers to the dual *manège* of *l'amour* and *la mode*). The equivalence between love and fashion is especially acute in the Fashion system's sequestration of work. For, as Barthes contends, 'the world of Fashion is work in reverse' (*F/S*, 248). Thus:

> jobs are defined not by their technical conduct but by the situation they confer . . . This explains how Fashion can speak of work and leisure in the same manner; in Fashion, all work is empty, all pleasure is dynamic, voluntary, and, we could almost say, *laborious*; by exercising her right to Fashion, even through fantasies of the most improbable luxury, woman always seems to be doing something (*F/S*, 253–4).

On the rare occasions we do observe women – or men for that matter – 'at work' in the fashion spreads from Barthes' prescribed period, the work they perform is always concerned with stereotypically feminine and masculine professions. Women, for instance, frequently assume the role of the secretary or the shop assistant, while men appear predominantly as white-collar workers, as in 'Monsieur J. M. A La Côte' ('Monsieur J.M. at the Stock Exchange'), featured in *Jardin des Modes* (February 1959), with photographs by Frank Horvat.[14] Additionally, women's 'work', when it is connoted, virtually always appears to be performed in the service of a male subject, or in the hope of captivating a male partner. In the context of the fashion spread, however, as Barthes suggests, it is probably more accurate to speak of work as having an indexical relationship to Fashion. That is, shopping or shareholding take place as an alibi for wearing a new outfit. Accordingly, the idea of work represented in the rhetoric of Fashion is euphoric and, as Barthes maintains, never tainted by real concerns with money or adultery: 'Fashion's *bon ton*, which forbids it to offer anything aesthetically or morally displeasing . . . is the language of a mother who "preserves" her daughter from all evil' (*F/S*, 261).

Finally, we have the reason of Fashion, where the rhetoric of Fashion is self-reflexive and self-supporting, dwelling on supports and variants such as the texture, size and detail of garments. Thus Fashion maintains its exclusive authority by speaking to and about itself, and deploying its own arbitrary terms of reference on a dialectic basis in statements like 'This year blue is in fashion.' In this regard, Barthes compounds an idea he had already expressed in *Essais critiques* in 1964, where he had drawn an analogy between literature and fashion in terms of their propensity to reiterate textually homeostatic or self-regulatory forms of expression and signification.[15] As a corollary, he maintains that the Fashion System exists to give a great deal of semantic power to "nothing": '"*nothing*" can signify "*everything*" . . . one detail is enough to transform what is outside meaning into meaning, what is unfashionable into Fashion' (*F/S*, 243). The language of Fashion is therefore a conceit. It proclaims small differences as if they were a matter of life or death by stating things like, 'This year fuzzy fabrics replace shaggy ones', or by asking questions like, 'Do you have this year's face (or body)?' Moreover, while Fashion appears to represent different times of the day or week, or the different seasons of the year, Barthes claims that 'the time of Fashion is unreal' and 'essentially festive' in the way that it grants precedence to weekends, vacations, springtime (*F/S*, 250). This is evidenced repeatedly in the fashion spreads of both *Jardin des Modes* and *Elle*.[16] Indeed, the entire *mise-en-scène* of 'Amoureuse' is given over to playful or recreational activities, such as walking the dog or dancing, which take place out of doors, by day and night, in town and countryside.

Ultimately, this leads Barthes to reaffirm the terminological rule that he postulated at the start of his investigation: the temporal signified of Fashion is always the same thing. That is to say, Fashion is always the equivalent of this year's Fashion: 'In fact, Fashion postulates an achrony, a time which does not exist; here the past is shameful and the present is constantly "eaten up" by the Fashion being heralded' (*F/S*, 289). The language of Fashion may appear to be new each season. But this is not because it always has something new to offer or worthwhile to say, but rather because it exploits the limits of our own memory in a perpetual recycling of retro styles. In Part I we saw how this was operative in several fashion spreads that formed a symbolic association with the past. It is also evident in 'Amoureuse', for example, in its reference to an organdy dress 'with a wide collar "draped" in the style of Marie-Antoinette', or in 'Le Prêt A Porter Et La Haute Couture' (*Jardin des Modes*, March 1959) in the way that gold buttons are invoked to describe the timeless or classic appeal of a woollen navy jacket.[17] In common with the texts assessed in Part I, therefore, the fashion details that are emphasised in these two examples seem to function on a simulacral level and, as such, they imply a temporal paradox. What is at stake here, of course, is not just a matter of style for style's sake, but the very existence of the Fashion system itself. Accordingly, in simultaneously inaugurating 'this year's Fashion' and ostensibly trading on an ideal of timelessness, Fashion aims to perpetuate both its own economic and cultural authority:

> Fashion is structured at the level of history: it is destructured at the only level at which it is perceived: actuality . . . the number of Fashion features is high, it is not infinite: we could very well conceive of a Fashion-making machine. One function of this rhetoric is to blur the memory of past Fashions, so as to censure the number and return of forms (F/S, 299–300).

Notes

1. Roland Barthes, *Roland Barthes* (London, 1995), p. 145.

2. Barthes, 'Réponses', *Tel Quel*, 47 (1971), p. 97.

3. Ferdinand de Saussure, *Course in General Linguistics*, trans. Roy Harris (Chicago and La Salle, Illinois, 1986), p. 17: 'By considering rites, customs, etc., as signs, it will be possible, we believe, to see them in a new perspective. The need will be felt to consider them as semiological phenomena and to explain them in terms of the laws of semiology.'

4. R. Barthes, *Système de la Mode* (Paris, 1967), p. 21, n. 3 references M. Crozier, *Petits fonctionnaires au travail* (CNRS, Paris, 1955), p. 126, Appendix, as a source of information concerning the popularity of the magazines he consulted. This detail is missing from Barthes, *The Fashion System*, p. 11, n. 19. The idea of selecting a corpus of finite materials for the purpose of analysing a particular issue is also discussed in Barthes' earlier work, *Éléments de Sémiologie* (Paris, 1964). See *Elements of Semiology*, trans. A. Lavers and C. Smith (New York, 1973), pp. 96–8.

5. Barthes, *Elements of Semiology*, p. 27 expresses a similar point: 'Finally in clothes as worn (or real clothes) . . . we again find the classic distinction between language and speech.'

6. Barthes, *The Fashion System*, p. 6, n. 6.

7. Ibid., p.73.

8. Ibid., pp. 81 and 83. Thus, we could break down the sentence, 'Robe trapèze en shantung ciel à col rond et patte piqué blanc' ('Amoureuse', Elle, 16 June 1958, p. 34) into the following pyramidal OVS matrix:

Robe trapèze en shantung ciel à col rond et patte de piqué blanc

O	VS		V	VS		S	V
O			V	S1		S2	V
	O		S	V			

9. In *Elements of Semiology*, p. 26, Barthes makes a similar point about the denotation of written clothing, contending that in the context of the fashion magazine it often appears to be a language in its pure state in so far as it 'does not emanate

from the "speaking mass" but from a group which makes the decisions and deliberately elaborates the code.'

10. Ibid., pp. 65–7, where he discusses the implications of the commutation test in linguistics and semiology.

11. R. Barthes, *Mythologies*, trans. A. Lavers, (London, 1973 [1957]), pp. 119, 140.

12. K. Mercer, 'Skinhead sex thing', *New Formations*, 16 (1992), p. 20. Other authors who have also recently begun to deal with the problems of regarding whiteness as if it were an already pre-defined or blank canvas include A. Bonnet, '"White Studies": the problems and projects of a new research agenda', in *Theory, Culture and Society*, 13:2 (1996), pp. 145–55; D. W. Stowe, 'Uncoloured people: the rise of Whiteness Studies', *Lingua Franca* (September/October 1996), pp. 68–77; and R. Dyer, *White* (London, 1997).

13. Lucy and Kate Gillett, letter to *The Face* (October 1991), p. 10. The editors replied: 'Far from "receiving a huge sum", the model, stylist and photographer all helped fund their trip to Borneo . . . from their own pockets.'

14. *Jardin des Modes*, pp. 76–7.

15. Barthes, *Essais critiques*, (Paris, 1964); *Critical Essays*, trans. R. Howard (Evanston, 1972) – see p. 156.

16. See also 'Boum-patrons toutes vacances', *Elle* (27 April 1959), pp. 76–89 with photographs by J. F. Clair.

17. Translation by the author from *Jardin des Modes*, p. 126: 'Sa veste est allongée, croisée, son allure classique accentuée par les boutons dorés.'

5

Going Beyond 'The Fashion System': A Critique

Words and language are not wrappings in which things are packed for the commerce of those who write and speak. It is in words and language that things first come into being and are.

Heidegger, *An Introduction to Metaphysics*, 1959.

Introduction: An Indeterminate Project?

At the outset, Barthes embarked on writing *The Fashion System* because he claimed to have been inspired by a 'euphoric dream of scientificity'. Yet in the final analysis he felt compelled to conclude that the same system is governed by its own arbitrary internal logic, that its chief goal is to be self-reflexive, and that its *raison d'être* is to perform nothing more than a masquerade of trivial transformations by, for example, suggesting that the length of a skirt or the width of a tie are a matter of life or death. What, then, are we to make of his project as a totality? And to what extent could we claim that Barthes has engineered a useful and apposite paradigm for analysing the discourse of fashion publishing in general terms?

Reviewing *The Fashion System* for *Paris-Normandie* on 19 May 1967, Pierre Lapape commented favourably on the work, even going so far as to make the claim that: 'semiology under Barthes was just as important as Marxism or psychoanalysis in changing man's view of the world'. And Baudrillard, not for the first time, also seemed to endorse one of Barthes' theoretical standpoints, putting a spin on his idea concerning the self-referentiality of the Fashion system thus: 'Fashion is one of the more inexplicable phenomena . . . its compulsion to innovate signs, its apparently arbitrary and perpetual production of meaning – a kind of meaning drive – and the logical mystery of its cycle are all in fact of the essence.'[1]

Other critics, however, have tended not to be so accommodating. Thody and Jonathan Culler, for instance, both concede that Barthes' exploration of the rhetorical system of Fashion, and the symbolic effects such as the poetics of clothing with which it deals, was successfully and cogently argued. Nevertheless, they take him to task for lack of clarity and specificity in his analysis of the vestimentary code. Thody, for example, remarks in *Roland Barthes, A Conservative Estimate* (1977) that the first two hundred pages are a 'head-splitting analysis' and concludes that the book is not 'any more translatable than a grammar book, complete with all its examples would be. It is equally impossible to summarise.'[2] Certainly, as we have already identified in Chapter 4, it is not always easy to follow the thread of Barthes' argument. The inspissated prose in some of the sections concerning the vestimentary code and the seemingly endless inventory of genera that one finds there are testimony to this.

In a similar vein, Culler (*Barthes*, 1983) remonstrates with Barthes for his lack of exactitude in dealing with the vestimentary code.[3] Culler has a valid point here in several important respects. As we have seen, for example, at one stage in his analysis Barthes postulates that the study of real clothing is the province of sociology rather than semiology. However, even though real clothing is, as he puts it, 'burdened by practical considerations', there is no reason why its materiality cannot or should not also be the substance of, or at very least form the basis of, a semiological inquiry. Thus a pin-striped navy blue suit may be worn by white-collar professionals, but at the same time it is this social convention itself that serves to imbue the actual garment with connotations of, say, class and status. We find a similar definitional ambivalence compounded by Barthes himself on two occasions. First, when he assesses the real or vestimentary code of clothing as the bedrock of a signifying chain, and hence as one that inaugurates its own set of signifiers and signifieds (*F/S*, Chapter 3). And second, when he refers to the real vestimentary code as a pseudo-real code, since, as he contends, the garment can only gain legitimacy in the context of an utterance that is either spoken (the terminological system) or written (the rhetorical system) (*F/S*, 49–50). The essential thing to realise about real clothing is that the practical considerations Barthes raises would of necessity lead to a different order of signification than the linguistic or rhetorical codes of the Fashion system. They would not, therefore, exclude real clothing from semiological analysis altogether.

Moreover, in another convoluted passage concerning the tension between written clothing and image-clothing (which he explicates in terms of Saussure's oppositional dialectic between language and speech), he seems to be arguing both for and against the structural purity of the former. Here he states somewhat baldly and ambiguously that written clothing now belongs to two systems.[4] And he claims, somewhat confusingly, that written clothing is both an institutional 'language', with regard to clothing, and a form of 'speech', in terms of writing. Thus he appears to revert back to the idea that the linguistic and semiological verbal codes both derive their meanings from a generative mother tongue, which is the garment itself. He insists that, 'This paradoxical status is important: it will govern the entire structural analysis of written clothing' (*F/S*, 18), although, as Culler rightly attests, he proves 'unwilling to follow a formal method through to the end'.[5]

Culler also found Barthes' methodology flawed because it fails to 'provide rules which distinguish the fashionable from the unfashionable', and he concluded that it is this that 'makes his results indeterminate'.[6] For Culler, it would have been much clearer and more logical had Barthes attempted to distinguish the fashionable from the unfashionable by setting up a diachronic method of analysis. This would entail comparing what was regarded as fashionable by magazines in different years, rather than postulating a general synchronic principle based on the study of one year's fashion alone. Clearly, Culler's methodology would be fruitful in analysing the periodic or cyclical transformations in Fashion on a comparative basis. In some ways, however, he also unnecessarily seems to capsize Barthes' central thesis that the meaning of fashionability and the exclusions it maintains conform to a perennial and repetitive logic that is outside the control of the readers of fashion magazines.

Plus Ça Change, Plus C'est la Même Chose

Rather more, Barthes is concerned with how, if not why, such preferences or oppositions are arbitrarily negotiated and immanent in the way that language itself is mobilised to describe Fashion. To put this slightly differently, what he observes is that the messages the linguistic (terminological) and rhetorical systems of Fashion encode appear to conform to a sempiternal structural logic, irrespective of the seasonal or annual differences they enunciate. It is the authoritative nature of the phrases themselves that is strategic here, and the way that they repeatedly tend to conform to a similar pattern or formula in which the words can be changed, but the underlying message ('this is what is fashionable') remains the same. Thus we could argue that, as far as Barthes is concerned, the phrase 'Prints win at the races', taken in isolation, is both self-sufficient and prototypical in the way that it signifies what is and is not fashionable. It would not matter if at another point in time a magazine either reiterated the same proposition, or stated instead that, 'Linens win at the races.' For, in either case, we are not dealing with facts but with mythological linguistic or semiological statements. These attain a sense of urgency and reality, both by representing a structural or ideational isology between apparently disconnected elements ('fabric' and 'races'), and connoting paradigmatically what should and should not be worn in the name of Fashion. Thus we understand that 'prints win at the races' because they exclude or stand in opposition to linens or silks, and vice versa. In the utterances and codes it proclaims, therefore, Fashion is encrypted perennially as a kind of unspoken law: 'the *fashionable* is almost never enunciated: it remains implicit, exactly like the signified of a word' (*F/S*, 22).

This inexorable logic is particularly underscored in his deployment of the 'commutation test' (discussed in Part One, Sections Two and Three of *The Fashion System*). Thereby Barthes demonstrates that any garment is literally invested with certain qualities and attributes in the translation from the real vestimentary code to the terminological and rhetorical systems of language. The point is that neither the word 'fashionable' nor 'unfashionable' is mentioned *per se*; rather, the opposition between them is always implied in the terminological and, more acutely, in the rhetorical systems we use. If, for instance, we state that a halter neck garment is buttoned in front instead of at the back, we not only commute the normative logic of the garment, but also enunciate a difference, or mistake, that connotes how much we do or don't know about Fashion. Consequently, as Barthes himself insists, any changes or variations that we introduce to the language of Fashion would also result in a parallel commutation in the meaning of the terms 'fashionable' and 'unfashionable' themselves.

From the Margins

As critics like Thody and Culler concur, therefore, Barthes' theory is both a difficult and an inconsistent one. Consequently, it has much to offer in the way that it analyses Fashion as discourse, and it also lays the foundations for understanding the differences as well as the correspondences between the technological, terminological and rhetorical codes of the Fashion system in general terms. By the same token, however, his method is clearly prone to some re-adjustment and qualification, and not only as a tool for analysing the fashion content of the magazines produced in the period he dealt with himself, but also for those produced at any point in time. Not least, therefore, we still need to ask, where are we to find the kind of linguistic and rhetorical utterances he includes for analysis? And why does Barthes concentrate on certain phrases to the exclusion of others? Indeed, what are the semiological implications of prioritising written clothing over image-clothing? As we shall see, these are not just discrete questions that necessitate individual responses of their own, but in many respects they are interconnected in terms of the issues and ideas they raise concerning the rhetoric of the Fashion system.

In the first place, it is important to note that phrases or utterances like 'a cardigan sporty or dressy, if the collar is open or closed' are, ironically, not credited by Barthes to their original sources. He contends that the rhetorical system of Fashion operates on a hierarchical or class basis, and thus that it is the aspirational fashion magazine that tends towards connotation ('utopia occupies, as it should, an intermediary position between the praxis of the poor and that of the rich' *F/S*, 245). On this basis, it would be only fair to assume that the examples of written clothing he cites could be traced back to either *Elle* or *Jardin des Modes*, both of which retailed for the same monthly outlay of 200 francs during the late 1950s.[7] In researching the rhetoric of the two magazines between June 1958 and June 1959, however, it has not been possible to identify the exact samples that Barthes used. Instead, what becomes evident is that they are paraphrases, approximating to the kind of statements that he would have originally encountered. Thus, 'A cardigan sporty or dressy, if the collar is open or closed' appears to be based on a fashion spread in *Elle*, 15 September 1958, entitled 'Deux Bons Magiques, Un Bon Automne' that commented: 'This cardigan will always be comfortable . . . the large collar has interwoven stitching and can also be worn open, lightly off the shoulders.'[8] And the sentence, 'daytime clothes in town are accented with white' appears to be derived from 'À Toi, À Moi, À Nous La Toile', which appeared in *Elle* on 20 April 1959 with the following commentary: 'One wearer, two dresses: on the left, in navy, complete with white piping for the town; on the right, in white, piped in blue for the beach.'[9]

It is not that such paraphrastic transformations are inadmissible in themselves (we find a similar tactic, for instance, in an earlier essay, where his referencing of the way that food is represented in *Elle* is equally non-specific).[10] And, even if they do reveal a lack of scientific exactitude in an otherwise exacting study, Barthes' paradigmatic utterances, ('women will shorten skirts to the knee' or 'This year blue is in fashion', *F/S*, 77), still seem to convey the performative tone and sense of the kind of original rhetoric he would have encountered. What is more interesting to note is the way that he gravitates towards the small print of the late 1950s fashion feature and eschews the more obvious headlines or taglines. In this way, he appears to perform a deconstructive tactic, recuperating for analysis the marginal details of a text, or the *parergon*, that is, what would usually be considered as being 'outside' or incidental to the main work. As Derrida has argued, these very marginalia are neither secondary nor extrinsic to the flow of texts, but essential for a fuller understanding of them:

A *parergon* is *against*, beside, and above and beyond the *ergon*, the work accomplished, the accomplishment, the work, but it is not incidental; it is connected to and cooperates in its inside operation from the outside . . . Aesthetic judgment must concern intrinsic beauty, and not the around and about. It is therefore necessary to know – and this is the fundamental proposition, the presupposition of the fundamental – how to define the intrinsic, the framed, and what to exclude as frame *and* as beyond the frame.[11]

Indeed, by virtue of his emphasis on the rhetoric of Fashion as opposed to its terminological or linguistic code, Barthes similarly appears to make a proto-deconstructive gesture. For the hypostasisation of writing that he elaborates in *The Fashion System* subverts the logocentric tradition of philosophy that, since Antiquity, has upheld the authority and purity of the speech act over the written word.[12] Hegel, for instance, had dealt with the difference between reason and irrationality in terms of the visibility and invisibility of thought in several of his writings, and he clearly betrays a logocentric attitude to both subjectivity and objectivity. For him, language as speech is the necessary, embodied medium of reason. In *Philosophy of the Mind*, for example, he writes: 'Given the name lion, we need neither the actual vision of the animal, nor even its image: the name alone, if we understand it, is the simple imageless representation.'[13] The nomination 'lion' is, therefore, sufficient means for rendering the quality of 'lion-ness', and its textual representation, whether verbal or pictorial, would only obfuscate the purity of the concept.

The Photographic Message

However, it would be erroneous to regard *The Fashion System* as a fully-fledged deconstructive text on account of Barthes' investment, so to speak, in written clothing, and his concomitant emphasis on its rhetorical marginalia. Certainly, Barthes appears to nod in the direction of Derridean deconstruction, but his methodology is too prone to enunciating its own system of exclusions to fit in with Derrida's ideal of deconstructive inter-texuality, which must: 'through a double gesture, a double science, a double writing, put into practice a *reversal* of the classical opposition *and* a general *displacement* of the system'.[14] Not least in this regard, we would seriously have to argue whether Barthes' predilection for written clothing is, objectively speaking, the most profitable way of analysing Fashion at the expense of photographic representation. In *The Phenomenology of the Spirit*, Hegel repudiates the baseness of the iconic in the strongest of terms, likening 'picture-thinking' to urination.[15] While Barthes does not express his own ambivalence concerning photographic representation in terms as strong as this, as we have already seen, nor does he reveal himself as an advocate for it. Thus Barthes is patently at odds with forms of photographic representation in *The Fashion System*.[16] As such, his sentiments are redolent of the ideas that he had expressed a few years earlier in his essay 'The Photographic Message', first published in 1961, in so far as they appear to hinge on the question of photographic reference.[17]

Ever since its invention in the nineteenth century, there has been a strong tendency for many people to regard the photographic image unquestioningly as a slice of reality. It is precisely this perspective, and the ontological status of photography as a form of realism, that Barthes compounds in 'The Photographic Message'. Hence he refers to the way that photographs work at the level of denotation as nothing more than traces or signifiers of reality: 'What is the content of the photographic message? What does the photograph transmit? By definition the scene itself, the literal reality.'[18] In the same essay, however, Barthes raises the idea of the photographic paradox, arguing that while photographs depict only what exists, as much as any other form of representation, their meanings become less obvious according to the context in which they appear. That is, photographs also function as signs in which a signifier (the material substance constituting the image, the photographic likeness itself) stands in a symbiotic relation to a signified (a form, idea or concept that we arbitrarily associate with the signifier, as in the case of red roses symbolising either passion or sorrow). As such, photographs work at the level of association or connotation, and are replete with cultural meanings or codes we have to interpret: 'All images are polysemous, they imply, underlying their signifiers, a "floating chain" of signifieds, the reader able to choose some and ignore others.'[19] In much the same way, therefore, we could argue that the fashion photograph can be read at both the level of denotation and connotation. But while Barthes is obviously aware of this point, he relegates it to one of the footnotes in *The Fashion System*.[20]

Photography, therefore, occupies an ambiguous space for Barthes in the chain of signification of the Fashion system, since, as he contests: 'Fashion (and this is increasingly the case) photographs not only its signifiers, but its signifieds as well, at least in so far as they are drawn from the "world"' (*F/S*, 301). And, at the very start of his investigation, he defines what it is about the Fashion photograph that makes it different to other forms of photography, asserting: 'the Fashion photograph is not just any photograph, it bears little relation to the news photograph or to the snapshot, for example; it has its own units and rules; within photographic communication, it forms a specific language which no doubt has its own lexicon and syntax, its own banned or approved "turns of phrase" (*F/S*, 4).

But the chief problem with the Fashion photograph, according to him –

and this is where he appears truly Hegelian – is that it is intrusive and pleonastic, confounding rather than compounding the clarity of the verbal code. Thus Barthes regards the photograph as a supplement that can be overlooked. It functions usually as nothing more than a decorative element, furnishing a scene or background so as to transform the garment in a theatrical sense. In achieving this, he comments that Fashion photography embraces three chief styles, which he calls the objective or literal, the romantic, and mockery. Their ultimate objective, however, is always mythological, serving to render the signifier (the garment) more real than the verbal signified ('prints win at the races'), either by appearing to invest the garment with a life of its own, or else by bringing the garment to life through the activity of the wearer.

Reconsidering Intertextuality

Barthes' resistance toward the Fashion photograph is underscored by the fact that there is not one single fashion spread reproduced in the entire book. But surely his argument would have gained more weight had he demonstrated to the reader the wider context for verbal statements such as 'prints win at the races', rather than simply representing them in isolation? If the fashion spread in which this kind of phrase appeared were reproduced in its entirety, we would be able to adjudicate more accurately whether words and images are either conflicting or competing elements or mutually reinforcing ones. At the same time, we would need to know what other verbal elements have been incorporated into the layout. Is the sentence 'prints win at the races', for instance, the title of a fashion feature or is it a caption for a particular idea or page opening? Is the text divorced from the pictures, or is it printed on top of them? And, finally, consideration of the size, weight and direction of the typography, as well as of any other graphic devices deployed, is necessary in arguing how and what the rhetoric of the Fashion system is intended to connote in its fullest sense. Barthes is not forthcoming on any of these points. If, for example, we were to analyse only the captions accompanying the photographs in the fashion feature 'Amoureuse', our impression of what the entire piece intends to signify would be both seriously limited and skewed.

First, we would fail to take into account the crucial way that the design elements contribute to the sequential or intertextual structure of the narrative as a series of four complementary acts in a unifying drama. By this I mean the asymmetric, dynamic layout of the text and images, the different dimensions of each of the photographs, and the way that two of them have been mortised into larger images. Such editorial decisions concerning scale and arrangement are not merely accidental, and the pictures have been laid out thus for practical as well as aesthetic reasons. Obviously, the larger pictures have been given precedence because they are technically and compositionally stronger images; but they also appear to convey the narrative thrust of the piece more cogently by crystallising a particular attitude or gesture associated with it. In comparison, the captions on their own seem to afford equal weighting to each of the photographs by following a similar pattern of wording. In 'Celle qui étonne', for example, each of the captions poses a different question, which is then followed by the details of the fashions depicted. What I am arguing here is not that the photographs should take priority over the captions, for that would merely be to establish another false opposition. Rather, I wish to restate the case that, in deconstructing the meaning of any fashion shoot, we need to decode both words and images *in tandem*. Indeed, in 'Amoureuse', the photographs and captions must be regarded as mutually reinforcing, since all the captions begin with a phrase that refers directly to the gesture or pose we observe being struck in the photographs, rather than simply being descriptions of the garments represented in them. In the first tableau, 'She who charms' ('Celle qui charme'), for instance, we are verbally directed to 'the power of a smile' ('le pouvoir d'un sourire') while we observe the model smiling, and to 'the power of a look' ('le pouvoir d'un regard') while we see a couple tenderly exchanging glances.

Second, and by no means unrelated or subordinate to the aesthetic flow of the piece, we also need to take into account many of the textual nuances implied by both the introductory paragraphs and the titles and descriptions of the acts themselves. As we have already identified, a general equivalence is being set up between love and fashion in the main body of text. But so too is a carnivalesque, Bakhtinian masquerade being elaborated that appears to empower women (if only intermittently) in both their sexual and social relationships with men. For Bakhtin, carnival culture represents the possibility of a world turned upside down – hierarchical positions are temporarily exchanged, so that the king plays the part of the peasant, the peasant that of the king, and so on.[21] The carnivalesque body exceeds itself in a grotesque and transgressive fashion, and thus it becomes a 'contradictory, perpetually becoming and unfinished being'.[22] But, as Bakhtin also assesses it, carnival culture is a collective and regenerative entity, portending the possibility of social and sexual liberation.[23] It is precisely this dialectic between individual and universal transformation that we observe at play in 'Amoureuse'. Here, the idea of fashion has been encoded as a merry-go-round that women not only may ride under different disguises (in this context, the charmer, the vamp, etc.), but that they are also positively enjoined to regard as a game or an act they should take part in: 'So! Why don't you play the game? Here's Barbara . . . In each instance, all she has to do is change her hair (by use of wigs), her behaviour, her clothing and words to embody in turns the woman who you are or who you would like to be' ('Alors! Pourquoi ne pas jouer le jeu? Voici Barbara . . . Il lui suffit de changer chaque fois ses cheveux (en un tour de perruque), son allure, sa robe et ses paroles pour incarner tour à tour la femme que vous êtes ou celle que vous aimeriez être').

Indeed, much of the terminology of 'Amoureuse' appears to trade on a deliberate semantic ambiguity, with the idea, 'to take a ride'/'mener la ronde' implying connotations of diversionary, anodyne *plaisir* and sexual *jouissance*. By this token, no matter which part a woman is seen to be playing in such a *ronde*, it is she who appears both to motivate the game of love and fashion ('And women make it go round' / 'Et les femmes mènent la ronde'), and to exploit it to take the man in her life for a ride: 'And the merry-go-round turns, and hesitant boys listen until the tune knocks them out . . . And the merry-go-round turns, and hesistant boys look until the colours make them turn their heads' ('Et le manège tourne, et les garçons indécis écoutent jusqu'à ce que le refrain leur martèle la tête . . . Et le manège tourne, et les garçons indécis regardent jusqu'à ce que les couleurs les fassent tourner la tête').

Yet the alpha-pictorial rhetoric of 'Amoureuse' does not only appear to compound a sense of the Bakhtinian carnival. For it also seems to trade on Luce Irigaray's idea that, through a process of ironic mimicry, women will be able to contest and undermine the dominant, patriarchal codes of femininity and representation: 'One must assume the feminine role deliberately. Which means already to convert a form of subordination into an affirmation, and thus begin to thwart it . . . It also means that, if women are such good mimics, it is because they are not simply resorbed in this function. *They remain elsewhere.*'[24]

None of this intertextual complexity of meaning could emanate from Barthes' method of analysis. For him fashion photography appears to function in the capacity of the *pharmakos* or 'scapegoat', which in Antiquity was intended to purify the city, but whose ambiguous status Derrida also exploits as a metaphor for the deconstructive strategy of breaking down binary oppositions such as pure/impure and within/without: 'The ceremony of the *pharmakos* is thus played out on the boundary line between inside and outside, which it has as its function to trace and retrace repeatedly. *Intra muros/extra muros*. Origin of difference and division, the *pharmakos* represents evil both introjected and projected.'[25] The *pharmakos* or 'evil one', therefore, originates within the city before being expelled from it, and as a corollary Derrida references it to parallel the way that philosophers have cast out writing as an inferior or debased form of language. Equally as much, we could argue that the photograph is intrinsic to the Fashion system before it is ostracised by Barthes for being more trivial than the written word. Indeed, the entire analytic of *The Fashion System* can be seen to elaborate a somewhat compromised model of supplementarity, of dealing with what is legitimately inside or outside the system. Consequently, on the one hand, it serves to reverse (if not to dismantle) the opposition between spoken and written language, while on the other, it introduces and insists upon its own set of arbitrary oppositions, not only between written clothing and image-clothing, but also between those types of written clothing that are to be included for analysis and those that are not. The types of phrases he mobilises, such as, 'This year blue is in fashion' or 'a blouse with a large collar', may all conform neatly to the OVS matrix he elaborates. As such, they serve to compound his general thesis that the Fashion system exists predominantly to signify the dichotomy between what is in fashion and what is not. At the same time, however, they tend to overdetermine the case. As we have already seen in the case of 'Amoureuse', the figurative devices and tropes of the fashion spread are much more polysemous than this. The metaphor of the merry-go-round does indeed appear to underscore the idea of fashionable circularity Barthes evinces. But by no means can the entire narrative structure of the piece be reduced to the OVS matrix, and both text and image lead us to consider other equally important issues concerning the masquerade of Fashion and its relationship to sexual politics.

Furthermore, when it comes to interrogating the rhetoric of the postmodern fashion spread since 1980, it becomes patently obvious in many respects how outmoded the methodology of *The Fashion System* is. After this point in time, we appear to be dealing with a phenomenon that does not necessarily grant precedence to the verbal code in the way that Barthes insists. Obviously, verbal details relating the names of the photographer, stylist and designer, or the price of the clothes represented, are still of relevance in fashion publishing today. Also, there are occasional instances of the kind of rhetoric that Barthes identified in the captions from the late 1950s, most notably in *Vogue* (see, for example, 'Under Exposure' (May 1983), and the American edition of *GQ*.[26] In the main, however, this type of phraseology is otherwise redundant in, or absent from, the contemporary fashion spread. Indeed, as we have already determined in Part 1, verbal and visual rhetoric now function on a number of significational levels. Frequently, for example, it is the photographs that have relative autonomy in the chain of signification.[27] Text may be included, but it is minimal, operating chiefly at the level of an opening title that both sets the tone for and establishes the chief theme of the narrative sequence of the pictures (witness 'fin de siècle' and 'once upon a time'). In addition, we have seen how in this kind of fashion feature not only is Barthes' ideal of written clothing reversed, but also, in the way that images reference other images, a hyperreal metanarrative is elaborated.[28] Finally, text and photographs are much more holistically integrated in many contemporary layouts. As such, they also operate within a more fluid definition of supplementarity. In common with 'Amoureuse', for example, words and images may be interwoven into a harmonious narrative structure (witness 'New Morning Nebraska' and 'Under Weston Eyes'). Or a conflictual tension can be set up between word and image (witness 'Veiled Threats'). In such instances, we are closer to the Barthes of *Image, Music, Text*, (1978) who writes of the interplay of word and image in terms of anchorage and relay.[29]

Gender and Identity in The Fashion System

Barthes, likewise, has some interesting points to make concerning the relation-ship of the Fashion system to gender and sexuality, although his discussion is also somewhat desultory and characteristically contentious. In the first instance, he briefly touches on these issues in his assessment of the 'woman of Fashion', who, as he puts it, dreams 'of being at once herself and another' (*F/S*, 256), and whom we have typically encountered in 'Amoureuse'. Here, Barthes appears to frame the Fashion system in psychoanalytical terms. Thus he states that the masquerade we observe in fashion texts resists the construc-tion of a solid, meaningful identity: 'we see Fashion "play" with the most serious theme of human consciousness (Who am I?)' (*F/S*, 257). In expressing things in this way, Barthes seems to anticipate Judith Butler's theory of gender as performativity, which has, since the early 1990s, become one of the most influential tools for exploring the meaning of identities. Butler's central thesis implies that gender and sexuality are provisional constructs. She argues, therefore, that an individual's identity both is dependent on and can only be consolidated through the constant reiteration of certain speech and body acts. Consequently, it is pointless attempting to define some kind of natural and pre-discursive masculine or feminine gender identities that exist outside acts and deeds: 'gender is not a fact, the various acts of gender create the idea of gender, and without those acts there would be no gender at all'.[30]

Barthes does not sustain the same perspective on identity for long. Indeed, he renounces it in favour of a more reactionary approach to gender, con-cluding, for example, that sex is 'a given' entity (*F/S*, 258). But even during the late 1950s sex and gender were more fluid and complex entities than he seems ready to admit. At that point in time, a burgeoning youth culture had begun to contest the rigid sexual mores of pre-war society. Culturally, this was manifest in more pluralistic and self-conscious attitudes towards style and consumption and, in terms of clothing, a shift away from haute-couture to expendable, ready-to-wear fashions.[31] Nor were these social values conveyed exclusively by fashion periodicals. Rather, they form part of a broader context for sexual objectification that was compounded in other media texts such as the cinema as well.[32] Accordingly, the fashionable or ideal bodies he mentions, all of them female stereotypes, can be seen to signify a particular change of attitudes toward sex and gender that emanated from society itself. In contrast, Barthes seems to imply both in *The Fashion System* and in subsequent pieces of writing on fashion that femininity, in the specific guise of the model, must take its place in a general cosmology of signs as nothing more than a hollow cipher:

> Fashion is not erotic; it seeks clarity, not voluptuousness; the cover-girl is not a good fantasy object: she is too concerned with becoming a sign: impossible to live (in the imagination) with her, she must only be deciphered, or more exactly (for there is no secret in her) she must be placed in the general system of signs that makes our world intelligible, which is to say: 'livable'.[33]

To a certain degree Barthes does acknowledge the impact of youth culture on fashion, mentioning the role of androgyny, for instance, when he discusses the concept of the 'junior', a popular prototype of the period.[34] However, he finally claims that what was being affirmed by this prototype was age or youth rather than more ambiguous sexual identities, and in turn overlooks the significant inroads that the new style culture had made on masculine identities. Hence, male bodies have no place in his epistemology, even though they had begun to appear in fashion spreads at the same time he was researching and writing *The Fashion System*. In February 1959, for instance, *Jardin des Modes* launched the first of its intermittent series featuring male fashion, 'Monsieur J. M.' Here, the French fashion press seemed to be dealing with men's interest in fashion in much more ingenuous and relaxed terms than in Britain or America during the same period, encouraging a positive attitude towards seasonal dress and accessories.[35] Moreover, in many of the 'Monsieur J. M.' fashion features, the male subject does not simply appear as an accessory or escort in a female world, as he does in 'Amoureuse'. Rather we observe him participating in an exclusively male, homo-social world, witness Frank Horvat's photograph representing a stylish young man at the stock exchange.[36] Clearly, the objectification of gender and sexuality since the time Barthes wrote *The Fashion System* has become more diverse and pluralistic, and we now have to take into consideration not only different typologies of the feminine but of the masculine body as well.

What is particularly interesting to observe in general terms is the way that normative bodies and sexualities have been subverted in the fashion pages of style magazines for youth culture since the mid-1980s. The masquerade we witness in many fashion photographs after 1980, therefore, is not simply something that concerns women, as Joan Riviere had suggested much earlier, but is equally relevant to men.[37] As already discussed in Part 1, in this regard British magazines such as *i-D*, *The Face* and *Blitz* became the stamping-ground for young, inventive photographers and stylists who, working in collaboration, pioneered a more overtly narcissistic, if sexually ambiguous, form of fashion iconography.[38] By 1987, it was also possible to identify a discernible shift of emphasis on the sexuality of the male body in a cluster of new titles intended for fashionable male readers – *Unique*, *Arena*, *FHM* and the British edition of *GQ*.[39] In the fashion pages of contemporary magazines, it is not so much the case that well-worn stereotypes such as the thin, vampish female or the muscular, predatory male have vanished, but a matter of their being objectified in more ambiguous terms. The furore surrounding Corinne Day's representation of Kate Moss in her underwear for British *Vogue* in 1993, and the ensuing debate concerning the alleged paedophilic connotations of the work, is testimony to this kind of recodification, and is assessed in closer detail in Part 3 of this study.[40] Similarly, the character of new man became one of the most frequent, if somewhat putative, masculine tropes to be found in both the iconography of fashion and advertising after 1984. This type included the Buffalo Boy, a hard, urban, streetwise individual originally conceptualised by the photographers Jamie Morgan and Norman Watson and the stylist Ray Petri.[41] Most commonly represented as inhabiting a muscular or phallic body, Buffalo Boy and his derivatives also revealed, however, the ambiguous status of masculinity as a site of narcissistic or scopophilic pleasure, and the tension between active and passive sexual identities that this seems to imply.

We can see how this ambiguity has been objectified in Figure 9, 'Heavy Metal', photographed and styled by Ray Petri and Jamie Morgan for *The Face*, April 1986. Here, the model's hard physique is uncompromisingly masculine, and in the top right photograph the Nikos posing pouch exaggerates his genital bulge or 'packet'. But his pouting gaze and body poses adopt the provocative attitude usually struck by female models on the catwalk as they intermittently stop to demonstrate particular details of the garments they wear. Moreover, in the bottom right photograph, the model tantalisingly raises his jacket to reveal his buttocks, while swivelling round to look seductively at the spectator as he does so. In the juxtaposition of the two pictures, this image also appears to act as the 'passive' pendant to the 'active' image placed directly above it, in which the same model stands facing us, body erect, proudly showing off his packet. The combination of the photographs, therefore, implies a gender paradox, and the antinomial fashion tropes of biker boots and posing pouch seem to undermine the binary opposition between hard/soft and active/passive. Indeed, the overall camp narcissism of the photographs subverts the very idea of 'Heavy Metal' that the title connotes, and casts doubt upon the imputed fixity of normative codes of gender and sexuality in such a way that, as Richard Dyer has argued: 'If that bearded, muscular beer-drinker turns out to be a pansy, how ever are you going to know the "real" men anymore?'[42] The hard bodies we see in contemporary fashion publishing, therefore, could be either straight or gay, since, by the mid-1980s, both many straight and gay men had begun to patronise gym culture and to espouse the ideal of pumping iron.[43] As such, the phallic prototype can be regarded as making a direct appeal to hetero-sexuals and homosexuals alike, a point underscored by fashion photographer Nick Knight when he professed: 'The men in my photographs aren't overtly heterosexual or homosexual. There's so much sexual pigeon-holing.'[44]

Notes

1. Baudrillard, *For A Critique of the Political Sign* (St Louis, MO, 1981), p. 47.
2. P. Thody, *Roland Barthes: A Conservative Estimate* (London, 1977), pp. 100 and 108.
3. Jonathan Culler, *Structuralist Poetics – Structuralism, Linguistics and the Study of Literature* (London, 1975), pp. 34–8; and *Barthes* (London, 1983), p. 75.
4. F. de Saussure, *Course in General Linguistics* (Chicago and La Salle, IL, 1986), pp. 13–14: 'By distinguishing between the language itself and speech, we distinguish at the same time: (1) what is social from what is individual, and (2) what is essential from what is ancillary and more or less accidental.'
5. Culler, *Structuralist Poetics*, p. 38.
6. Ibid., p. 35.
7. *Elle* retailed at 50F per issue until 2 March 1959, when it increased its quantity of pages (on average 172 pp. per issue) and its price to 70F. *Jardin des Modes* retailed at 200F per monthly issue.
8. Translation by the author from *Elle* (15 September 1958), p. 55: 'Cette veste cardigan sera toujours confortable . . . Le grand col est en maille unie deux fils, il se porte aussi roulé, légèrement décollé.'
9. *Elle* (20 April 1959), p. 75: 'Un seul patron, deux robes: à gauche, marine et toute surpiquée de blanc pour la ville; à droite blanche et surpiquée de bleu pour la plage.'
10. See 'Ornamental Cookery' in R. Barthes, *Mythologies*, trans. A. Lavers (London, 1973), pp. 85–7. Barthes' study of the magazine clearly led him beyond the exclusive consideration of its fashion pages, and he called *Elle* 'a real mythological treasure' (p. 85).
11. J. Derrida, 'The Parergon', *October*, 9 (1979), pp. 20 and 26.

12. Plato, for instance in *Phaedrus* records how Socrates condemned writing as a bastard or parasitic form of communication, privileging speech as the purest form of communication. See Plato, *Phaedrus and Letters VII and VIII*, trans. W. Hamilton (Harmondsworth, 1973) pp. 95–9.

13. G. W. F. Hegel, *Philosophy of the Mind*, trans. W. Wallace (Oxford and New York, 1971), p. 220.

14. J. Derrida, 'Signature Event Context', *Glyph*, I (Baltimore, 1977), p. 195.

15. G. W. F. Hegel, *The Phenomenology of the Spirit*, trans. A.V. Miller (Oxford, 1977), p. 210.

16. Martin Harrison, *Appearances – Fashion Photography Since 1945* (London, 1991), p. 14 appears to misrepresent this tension in his brief assessment of Barthes' text, where he implies that Barthes' analysis refers to specific photographs taken by Horvat and Newton for *Jardin des Modes*. A similar misapprehension appears in F. Mort, *Cultures of Consumption: Masculinities and Social Space in Twentieth Century Britain* (London and New York, 1996), p. 55, where he states: 'The language of the fashion plate – what Roland Barthes termed the 'fashion system' – is underpinned by an elaborate commercial infrastructure.'

17. R. Barthes, *Communications*, No. 1 (1961), pp. 127–38. See also R. Barthes, *Image, Music, Text*, trans. S. Heath (Glasgow, 1978), pp. 15–31.

18. Barthes, *Image, Music, Text*, pp. 16–17.

19. Barthes' 'Myth Today' was first published in *Les Lettres Nouvelles*, 1956 and subsequently in *Mythologies*, (Éditions du Seuil, Paris, 1957). The English translation by Annette Lavers was first published in *Mythologies*, (London, 1973) – see p. 39.

20. Barthes, *The Fashion System*, p. 4, n. 2.

21. M. Bakhtin, *Rabelais and His World* (Cambridge, MA, 1968).

22. Ibid., pp. 118 and 316.

23. Ibid., 'The unfinished and open body (dying, bringing forth and being born) is not separated from the world by clearly defined boundaries; it is blended with the world, with animals, with objects. It is cosmic, it represents the entire material bodily world in all its elements.'

24. L. Irigaray, 'The Power of Discourse and the Subordination of the Feminine' in *This Sex Which Is Not One*, trans. Catherine Porter (Ithaca, NY, 1985 [1977]), p. 124.

25. J. Derrida, *Dissemination*, trans. Barbara Johnson (London, 1981 [1972]), p. 133.

26. See, for example, 'Acapulco bold', American *GQ* (December 1991), pp. 236–45; 'Give in to the sensation', British *Vogue* (December 1981) and 'Skin on Skin', British *Vogue* (January 1989) pp. 108–11. Hilary Radner offers an interesting deconstruction of the word/image relationships of a specific fashion/beauty article entitled 'Looking Good: The Double Standard' from the American edition of *Vogue* (April 1987) in *Shopping Around – Feminine Culture and the Pursuit of Pleasure* (London and New York, 1995), pp. 135–40.

27. Examples of this kind of iconocentric fashion spread are legion, but see the following for a good indication of its effects: 'Fashion – Punk', *The Face* (Feb. 1986;

photographer, Nick Knight; stylist, Simon Foxton); 'The Lady from Shanghai', *The Face* (Oct. 1986; Eamon J McCabe/Simon Foxton); 'Grooms and Gamblers', *Arena* (Jan.–Feb. 1989; Marc Lebon/Ray Petri); 'Wide West', *The Face* (June 1989; Enrique Badulescu/Malcolm Beckford); 'Weekenders', *The Face* (Nov. 1995; Nicolas Hidiriglou/Charlotte [TDP]).

28. See, for instance: J. Baudrillard, 'The Ecstasy of Communication' in Hal Foster (ed.), *Postmodern Culture* (London, 1985), pp. 126–34, and J. Baudrillard 'The Precession of Simulacra' in *Simulacra and Simulation*, trans. Sheila Faria Glaser (Ann Arbor, 1994). Typical of the line of argument pursued in the latter is the following statement: 'Because heavenly fire no longer falls on corrupted cities, it is the camera lens, that, like a laser comes to pierce lived reality in order to put it to death' (p. 28). D. Hebdige offers an insightful critique of Baudrillard in the context of *The Face* in his essay, 'The bottom line on Planet One' in *Ten.8*, No. 19 (1985), pp. 40–9.

29. Barthes, *Image, Music, Text*, pp. 39–41.

30. J. Butler, *Gender Trouble* (London and New York, 1990), p. 8.

31. See A. Marwick, *British Society Since 1945* (Harmondsworth, 1982), pp. 117–18; T. R. Fyvel, *The Insecure Offenders: Rebellious Youth in the Welfare State* (Harmondsworth, 1963), p. 45; M. Abrams, *The Teenage Consumer* (London, 1960); and D. Hebdige, 'Towards a cartography of taste 1935–62', *Block*, 4 (1981), pp. 39–55.

32. R. Dyer, *Stars* (London, 1979), pp. 59–61 discusses alternative and subversive male and female film stars of the 1950s and 1960s.

33. Barthes, preface to *Erté*, trans. by W. Weaver (Parma, 1972).

34. *Junior Bazaar*, for example, was first published in 1946.

35. 'Monsieur J. M. et La Haute Couture', *Jardin des Modes* (March 1959), p.117: 'Monsieur J. M. is already familiar with the names of couturiers . . . So not only does high fashion announce a new style for springtime, but it also thinks about the boutiques that, housed in several couturier outlets, have a men's department . . . . It is natural, therefore, that Monsieur J. M. went to look for ideas there and that he has chosen some amusing accessories to dress up the never-changing male garb, and to satisfy the desire for colour and youthfulness that spring inspires in him' ('Monsieur J. M. est déjà familiarisé avec les noms des couturiers . . . Non seulement la Haute Couture présente alors sa nouvelle mode de printemps, mais elle pense aussi à ses collections de boutiques qui, chez quelques-uns des couturiers, ont un rayon masculin . . . Il est donc naturel que Monsieur J. M. soit allé chercher des idées chez eux et qu'il ait choisi des accessoires amusants pour rendre plus particulier l'éternel costume masculin, et pour satisfaire les envies de couleur et de jeunesse que lui donne le printemps'). Translation by the author.

36. See also Frank Horvat's photographs in the American edition of *Vogue* (15 October 1958).

37. J. Riviere, 'Womanliness as masquerade', *International Journal of Psycho-analysis*, 10 (1929), pp. 303–13.

38. All three magazines were launched in 1980. For *The Face*, see Hebdige, 'The bottom line on Planet One'; also *i-D* (October 1995 – 15th birthday issue) and *Blitz*,

Exposure! Young British Photographers from Blitz Magazine 1980–1987 (London, 1987).

39. See S. Nixon, *Hard Looks, Masculinities, Spectatorship and Contemporary Consumption* (London, 1996), Part IV.

40. 'Under Exposure', British *Vogue* (June 1993). See L. Alford, 'Don't get your knickers in a twist over fashion', *The Observer* (30 May, 1993), p. 52.

41. See N. Logan and D. Jones, 'Ray Petri', *The Face*, (October 1989), p. 10. Examples of Buffalo Boy fashion features created by Morgan and Petri can be found in *The Face* between January 1984 and September 1986, and by Watson and Petri in *Arena* between May 1987 and June 1988.

42. R. Dyer, 'Getting Over the Rainbow: Identity and Pleasure in Gay Cultural Politics', in G. Bridges and R. Brunt (eds), *Silver Linings: Some Strategies for the Eighties* (London, 1981), pp. 60–1.

43. See K. R. Dutton, *The Perfectible Body: The Western Ideal of Physical Development* (London, 1995), Part III; L. O'Kelly, 'Body talk', *Observer Life* (23 October 1994), p. 32; and, for a broader discussion of the relationship of bodybuilding and gym culture to gender and sexuality since 1980, A. M. Klein, *Little Big Men: Bodybuilding Subculture and Gender Construction* (Albany: 1993).

44. Cited by V. Steele, 'Erotic Allure', in *The Idealizing Vision, The Art of Fashion Photography* (New York, 1991), p. 96.

Conclusion to Part 2

As I have tried to demonstrate here Barthes' *The Fashion System* is both a complex and a flawed, or at any rate a wanting, analysis of the verbal and visual codes of representation we encounter in fashion periodicals. However, although we may express serious reservations concerning the methodology elaborated in the work, most notably his cathexis on written clothing and his one-sided attitude towards the objectification of gender, many of the tendencies he discusses are still very much in evidence in contemporary fashion publishing. I am referring here to his ideas on the poetics of clothing (*poétique du vêtement*), the worldly signified (*rhétorique du signifié mondain*), and the reason of fashion (*la 'raison' de Mode*). In this regard, Barthes' comments concerning the nature of time and the relationship of past to present in fashion texts are especially illuminating when it comes to analysing the simulacral effects in many recent magazine spreads.[1]

Figure 18, for example, 'Who's Shooting Who – In Beirut It Pays To Know Your Terrorist?', photographed by Oliver Maxwell and styled by Elaine Jones for *The Face* (July 1986), is an extreme and polemical case of the cannabilisation of history and work that he sees taking place in both the poetics of clothing and the worldly signified. Across five pages, we are presented with a range of typical uniforms worn by the different factions involved in the Civil War between Muslims and Christians in the Lebanon. Each of the five photographs is explicated with two short pieces of rhetoric: the first giving a potted history of the role of the particular faction involved in the conflict; the second, in smaller print and affecting the style of written clothing, representing the details of the garments they wear as if they were modish objects of fetishistic desire.[2] The strategy of textual grafting that we witness in this spread appears, therefore, to transcend the implicit semantic contradiction between the 'serious business' of war and the 'frivolous business' of Fashion, and serves instead to conflate them in a chiasmic form of rhetoric.[3]

At the same time it is interesting to note the tension that ensued between producers and consumers with regard to the pastiche represented in the spread. For, judging from the response to it expressed in the letters printed in the following issue of *The Face*, the feature obviously met with some antipathy from certain readers: 'Your "fashion" feature, *Who's Shooting*

Who? . . . ends up as being merely an alternative fashion parade which has no connection with reality. Posing should have its limits.'[4] But their displeasure is not only indicative of the fragile moral status of the Fashion system itself, it is also a revealing manifestation of the resistance that 1980s youth was able to mount against a prevailing style culture or, at least, of its threshold of toleration for it.[5] This point brings me, finally, to another important way in which Barthes' study is still of particular use and relevance today: that is, his assessment of the different kinds of pleasure and spectatorship involved in the reading of fashion texts. If, as he suggests, the logic of the Fashion system serves to connote nothing beyond the world of fashion itself, shutting out anything painful, challenging or political, then what he seems to be dealing with at the outset is a cultural phenomenon that makes a direct appeal to bodily sensations and that involves little intellectual stimulation: 'Fashion's bon ton . . . forbids it to offer anything aesthetically or morally displeasing' (*F/S*, 261).

But Barthes does not express things as crudely as this. Consequently, he also speaks of the activity of Fashion as a 'dreamed pleasure' (*F/S*, 252–3), that is as something that involves both mental and physical energy. This idea was to be more fully expressed in *Le Plaisir du Texte*,[6] but it manifestly subtends the closing passages of *The Fashion System*, where he describes the pro-active reader or analyst as the agent who will attempt to explore the meaning of fashion on his/her own terms: 'the analyst inaugurates (or adopts) an infinite science: for if it happens that someone (someone else or himself later on) undertakes the analysis of his writing and attempts to reveal its content, that someone will have to resort to a new metalanguage, which will signal him in its turn' (*F/S*, 294). Indeed, as Hilary Radner attests in her evaluation of the female body in fashion publishing, rather than being an alienated form of experience, pleasure is both fundamental to and immanent in the process of spectatorship: 'Ultimately, the issue of display remains a primary imperative, and the ability to function within a regime that privileges display is underlined as crucial to the constitution of the *Vogue* subject – the subject position that it offers its reader.'[7] Moreover, spectatorial pleasure or displeasure is not just an issue for the (female) readers of *Vogue*, as Barthes himself argues, but for the readers of less élitist texts as well – in his own analysis, *Elle*, and more recently in style or youth culture magazines like *The Face*. It is in this respect that we are all of us, regardless of our sexual, racial and class identities, both subject and object in relation to the discourse of the Fashion System.

Notes

1. For examples of the *poétique du vêtement* see: 'Blue Mood', *Arena* (Winter 1990–1) and 'Hard Edged', *Arena* (Spring 1993), both photographed by James Martin

and styled by David Bradshaw; 'Flesh', *The Face* (April 1993; Mario Sorrenti/ Cathy Nixon); 'Stone Rangers', *The Face* (November 1993; Marcus Tomlinson/Kim Andreoli); 'High Tension', *Arena* (March/April 1994; Christopher Griffiths/David Bradshaw); for the *rhétorique du signifié mondain* see: 'Fallout', *The Face* (November 1993; Nina Schultz/Dodi Greganti); and for *la 'raison' de Mode* see 'Headhunters – Back to the No Future', *The Face* (August 1993; Jean-Baptiste Mondino/Judy Blame) and 'Weekenders', *The Face* (November 1995; Nicolas Hidiroglou/Charlotte [TDP]).

2. *The Face*, p. 83, for instance represents on the left a member of the Christian Phalange and on the right an Italian Marine in the Battaglione San Marco (Figure 18). The two interconnecting captions accompanying the latter read as follows: 'Italian, French and American troops were part of the Multi-National Force brought in to supervise the PLO withdrawal from Beirut. Pleated camouflage trousers, padded at knee and gathered behind; Star of Savoy on collar points; national arms shield on sleeve (worn by marines); Lion of St. Mark unit chest patch; M1952 pistol and belt; Heckler Koch SMG; ID bracelet'.

3. Derrida both discusses and elaborates the deconstructive implications of grafting in several of his texts – see, for example, 'The Double Session' in *Dissemination*, trans. B. Johnson (London, 1981 [1972]) and 'Tympanum' in *Margins of Philosophy*, trans. Alan Bass (Chicago, 1982 [1972]). In *Glas*, trans. John P. Leavey and Richard Rand (Lincoln, NB, 1987 [1974]), Derrida arranges the text into two columns – the first representing Hegel's ideas on family life, and the second citations from and comments on the writing of Jean Genet. In 'Living On: Border Lines', in H. Bloom *et al.*, *Deconstruction and Criticism* (New York, 1979), p. 107, Derrida argues: 'Each text is a machine with multiple reading heads for other texts'.

4. Joanna Briscoe, reader's letter, *The Face* (August 1986), p. 92.

5. *The Face* (August 1986), p. 92. The editor rejoined that the storyline had been supplied by its news department and laid out by the fashion department and that it was as deadly as its subject: 'The rash of complaint that it caused seems to have come from the juxtaposition on our cover of the words Beirut Fashion, an irony that escaped some readers . . . It was useful information presented in a challenging way. Our Beirut fashions were real. If they caused offence, it should have been because they caught the undeniable lure of Boy's Own military machismo.'

6. *Le Plaisir du Texte* (Éditions du Seuil, Paris, 1973); *The Pleasure of The Text*, trans. Richard Miller (Oxford, 1990). In the work, Barthes makes a distinction between *plaisir*, as a more generalised and unthreatening form of pleasure, and *jouissance* ('bliss'), which is a more sexually-charged and disorienting form of spectatorship, thus: 'Text of bliss: the text that imposes a state of loss, the text that discomforts . . . unsettles the reader's historical, cultural, psychological assumptions, the consistency of his tastes, values, memories, brings to a crisis his relation with language . . . it granulates, it crackles, it caresses, it grates, it cuts, it comes: that is bliss', (pp. 14 and 67).

7. H. Radner, *Shopping Around*, p. 137.

Part 3

Bodylines: Identity and Otherness in Fashion Photography Since 1980

Introduction to Part 3

The body is the irreducible difference, and at the same time it is the principle of all structuration.

Roland Barthes, *Roland Barthes*, 1977.

Let us begin with something of a truism: the body is the central trope of the fashion system; there would not be any fashion without bodies. Yet, however obvious this may seem, it does not necessarily follow that the relationship between fashion and the body is always a straightforward or unproblematic affair. For bodies not only wear clothing, but, as the history of fashion and dress demonstrates, in any given period fashion has also generated, or at least bolstered, particular somatic ideals of size and weight based on sex and gender, class and race.[1] Within such a regime of ideals, the fashion periodical has undoubtedly had a major part to play in the dissemination and promotion of body image – all 455 fashion spreads listed in Appendix I, for example, represent bodies of one type or another. Yet as we have already identified in earlier chapters, the fashion spread, as much as the catwalk show itself, does not simply exist to replicate the intentions of the designer, but to form a symbolic link with the desires and expectations of the spectator as well. Indeed, more often than not fashion itself seems to become subordinate to the context in which it appears in magazines, and frequently it is the gender, sexuality and/or ethnicity of the models depicted that appear to be the prime focus of interest. As Elizabeth Wilson appositely attests: 'fashion magazines come on rather like pornography; they indulge the desire of the 'reader' who looks at pictures, to be each perfect being reflected in the pages, while simultaneously engaging erotically with a femininity (and increasingly a masculinity) that is constantly being redefined.'[2]

The redefinition of gender referred to by Wilson subtends, for instance, the entire content of the September 1984 issue of *The Face*, the cover of which featured a portrait of Prince, 'The Cool Ruler'. At the time, Prince had gained a certain notoriety for deconstructing the binaries of black/white and straight/gay, melding the thrusting machismo of his music and an overtly camp fashion sense into an incongruous whole.[3] A similar deconstructive gesture is pursued in the three main fashion features contained in the issue: 'Another Country' (photographed by Robert Erdman and styled by Hamish Bowles), representing Colin Firth and Tristan Oliver, two of the actors in the eponymous film that dealt with conflicting sexual and political ideologies in a boy's public school; 'Suit Yourself' (by Martin Brading and Debbi Mason), portraying a female model wearing male attire and adopting mannish poses; and 'Role Over and Enjoy It!' (by Robert Erdman and Caroline Baker). This last consisted of several strategically cropped photographs of white and black male models, 'The Cocky Generation', who display fetishistic, figure-hugging leggings that put 'lumps and bumps on show', and an article by Marek Kohn, intended to steer male readers through the murky waters of post-feminist sexuality with the following advice: 'The best thing to do is seize the opportunity of the changing times ... You have to be more of a man than ever before nowadays – and that opens up the possibility of all sorts of pleasures.'[4]

Thus, we can regard both fashion and the fashion magazine as central institutions for the discursive production and circulation of sexualities, as ways of 'putting sex in the picture', to paraphrase Foucault. Moreover, to take the Foucauldian analogy further, fashion photography mobilises the body in a dialectical form of spectatorship based on the 'double impetus of pleasure and power',[5] and involving those who see yet who are not visible (photographers, readers), and those who are seen and subjected to 'a principle of compulsory visibility' (models).[6] It is in this respect that we could argue that the rhetoric of fashion implies not just an act of surveillance (*scientia sexualis*) but also one of spectatorship or voyeurism (*ars erotica*).[7] But this nexus between power and pleasure in the production and consumption of fashion photography needs further explication. We still need to ask, for example, who are the producers and spectators of such images – male or female, straight or gay, black or white?: 'Rather than seeing narcissism and exhibitionism as inevitably feminine, and fetishism and voyeurism as inevitably masculine, as many theorists have tended to do, it has to be recognised that these tendencies are interdependent, albeit differently, for men and women.'[8] Furthermore, not only is the body a discursive entity whose gendered and sexual identity is subject to shifts in the exercise of power through which it may both survey others as the Other, and be surveyed by others as the Other, but one that Foucault argues will also eventually turn the gaze inward on itself so that: 'each individual under its weight ... is his own overseer'.[9]

The interiorising of the gaze that Foucault refers to here, in turn seems to point us in the direction of the psychoanalytical ego as it is discussed by Lacan in his essay, 'The Mirror Stage'. Lacan had suggested that one's specular image produces simultaneously a sense of jubilation and alienation: the former because what one sees in the mirror and in images appears to be a cohesive, fully-formed body; and the latter because the same imaginary body implies a material lack in the actual body, which in comparison to its mirror-image is a body in pieces (*le corps morcelé*). Thus one's ego appears to be shattered or haunted by the presence/absence of what it desires to be or have: the other.[10] What is more, this search for a cohesive ego is something that, as Judith Butler cogently argues, implicates us all into negotiating our identities, whether they are sexual, racial, social or political, through a series of oppositions and exclusions: 'This marking off will have some normative force and, indeed, some violence, for it can construct only through erasing; it can bound a thing only through enforcing a certain criterion, a principle of selectivity.'[11]

These, then, are the issues concerning the general condition of identity and otherness, and the complexities of what may be called the body double, that I wish to pursue in this part of my study. In elaborating my argument I shall be ranging over a wide spectrum of ideas; but at the same time, given the overwhelming quantity of bodies on display in the fashion periodicals consulted in the course of this study, I have been deliberately selective of the fashion spreads included for discussion. The material that is included in the following chapters has also been arranged thematically, and images of different body types have been mobilised in order to analyse other specific ideas and issues. Thus Chapter 6 deals with the portrayal of the woman-child and related debates on pornography, censorship, mimicry and the female photographer, and eating disorders and abjection; while Chapter 7 examines the persistence of the phallic male body as both a straight and gay, and white and non-white ideal, and its relationship to theories of performativity of sex and gender. Finally, in addressing the various ways that fashion photography deals with identity formation, the representation of the body as an object of desire, and the diverse pleasures of spectatorship this involves, each of the two chapters also aims to consolidate our analysis of the intratexuality between words and images in the fashion spread, and the intertextuality between the fashion spread and other media.

Notes

1. Two recent histories of fashion that offer a succinct but relevant assessment of clothing in relation to changing body ideals are C. Breward, *The Culture of Fashion* (Manchester and New York, 1994), and J. Craik, *The Face of Fashion, Cultural Studies in Fashion* (London and New York, 1994).
2. E. Wilson, *Adorned in Dreams, Fashion and Modernity* (London, 1985), p. 158.

3. See D. Hill, *Designer Boys and Material Girls – Manufacturing the 80s Pop Dream* (Poole, 1986), Chapter 10.

4. 'Role Over and Enjoy It!', *The Face* (September 1984), pp. 22–3.

5. M. Foucault, *The History of Sexuality: Vol. 1, An Introduction*, trans. R. Hurley (Harmondsworth, Middlesex, 1990), p. 47.

6. M. Foucault, *Discipline and Punish, The Birth of the Prison*, transl. by A. Sheridan (New York, 1977) p. 187.

7. M. Foucault, *The History of Sexuality*, Volume 1, pp. 70–1.

8. A. Partington, 'Popular Fashion and Working Class Affluence', in J. Ash and E. Wilson (eds), *Chic Thrills* (London, 1992), p. 156.

9. C. Gordon (ed.), *Power/Knowledge: Selected Interviews and Other Writings 1972–77 by Michel Foucault* (Brighton, 1980), p. 156.

10. For Lacan the development of the ego is dependent on the infant's identification with itself as an image, first glimpsed in reflection at around the age of six months, which leads to the alienated mirror-image, that is, an internalised and fantasised imaginary construction of oneself that provides the 'threshold of a visible world'. See J. Lacan, 'The Mirror Stage' (1949) in A. Easthope and K. McGowan, *A Critical and Cultural Theory Reader* (Buckingham, 1992), pp. 71–6 and 243–4.

11. J. Butler, *Bodies that Matter – On the Discursive Limits of "Sex"* (London and New York, 1993), p. 11.

6

Who's That Girl? Alex and Kate: A Tale of Two Bodies in Contemporary Fashion Photography

The ways in which female sexuality will be expressed are dependent not only on the context in which the image appears, but also on the intended target market for that image.

Kathy Myers, *Fashion 'n' passion*, 1982.

Introduction: 'The Girl'

By far the most common ideal of female sexuality represented since 1980 in the pages of *The Face*, *Vogue*, and to a lesser extent *Arena*, is that of the 'girl'. The 'girl' crops up in any number of contexts, but usually in one of two main guises: sometimes as the passive object of adoration or the gaze, as in 'Hotel Motel, Holiday In' (*The Face*, April 1991), photographed by Enrique Badulescu and styled by Mitzi Lorentz (Figure 26); sometimes as a castrating bitch, as in 'Crimes of Passion' (The Face, January 1990), photographed by Manfred Gestritch and styled by Jitt Gill. But in many instances the body of the 'girl' in fashion photography also implies a contradiction. For at one and the same time she is represented as a woman who is also a child, as someone who is sexually both knowing and innocent. Furthermore, she is not infrequently portrayed in somewhat gynandrous terms as a girl who could also be a boy, a transsexuality we have already identified at work in the case of 'Apparitions' and 'Veiled Threats' (Figures 20 and 21), but that is more explicitly evidenced in spreads like 'Oh You Pretty Thing', photographed by David Sims and styled by Venetia Scott for *The Face* (February 1993). In this, the waiflike supermodel Emma Balfour performs an interesting masquerade in which she appears simultaneously to mimic

111

Thus in 'The Daisy Age – The 3rd Summer of Love' (*The Face*, July 1990), Moss is seen smoking, and in one of the pictures happily shows off her breasts; while in 'borneo' (*The Face*, August 1991), she models figure-revealing swimwear and vests in poses similar to those in the subsequent *Vogue* piece (Figure 25). Moss likewise had become exponentially high-profile in America by the autumn of 1992. Patrick Demarchelier had photographed her for a spread called 'Wild: Fashion that breaks the rules', which appeared in *Harper's Bazaar* in September 1992, and he had also photographed her topless as she straddled the muscle-bound rap singer Marky Mark in ads for Calvin Klein's youth-oriented CK range of clothing.

As Dick Hebdige discusses it, in the usual flow of incorporation the subversive or shocking style and content of this kind of alternative imagery would normally be significantly sanitised or defused by the time it is absorbed into the hegemonic mainstream, through a process of commodification or ideological recuperation (as occurred during the late 1960s and early 1970s when the oppositional politics of underground graphics and music began to be treated as expendable commodities).[9] Not only do the images of 'Under Exposure', for example, subscribe to a style usually associated with the youth culture magazines, but so too does the use of language. Thus phrases like 'Hold me tights, don't let me go' and 'Madonna, eat your heart out' fit into the poetic signifying chain of written clothing that Barthes describes in their ironical referencing of popular music: the first alluding to songs by The Beatles ('Hold me tight', 1963) and David Essex ('Hold me close', 1975), the second to Madonna's penchant for wearing basques and corset dresses, designed by Jean-Paul Gaultier, during her 'Blonde Ambition Tour' in 1990. While they obviously complement the photographs with which they are juxtaposed, however, these phrases also seem to debunk the artifice of the fashion system. What we seem to witness in the case of the opposition voiced against 'Under Exposure', therefore, is the very reversal of the normative logic of incorporation. The criticisms of Hume *et al.*, rightly or wrongly, signal not just that *Vogue* readers might simply have been unprepared for what they saw, but rather that they would be too grown up or socially aware to find it acceptable.

Child Pornography: Reality and Representation

The critique mounted by Hume and others against 'Under Exposure' also tends to confuse and/or conflate Day's grunge-style representation of Kate Moss modelling underwear with the reality of drug abuse and under-age sex themselves. Consequently, they rehearse one of the commonest misconceptions

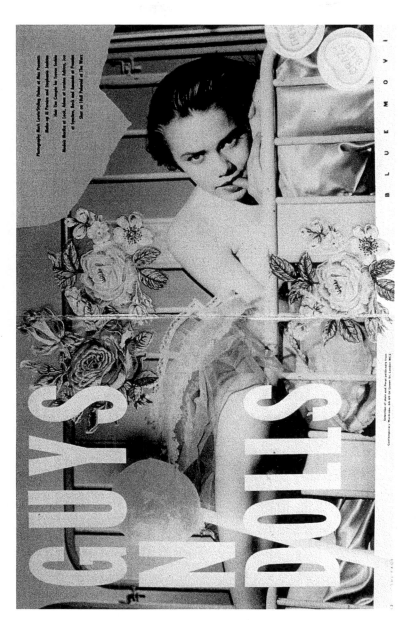

Figure 1. 'Guys N Dolls', photographer Mark Lewis, stylist Finbar at Max Presents, *The Face* July/August 1988, courtesy of *The Face*/Wagadon Ltd.

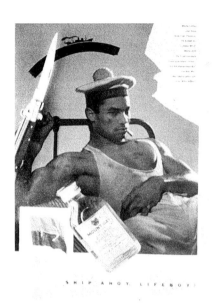
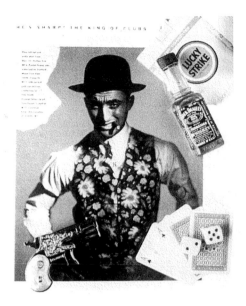
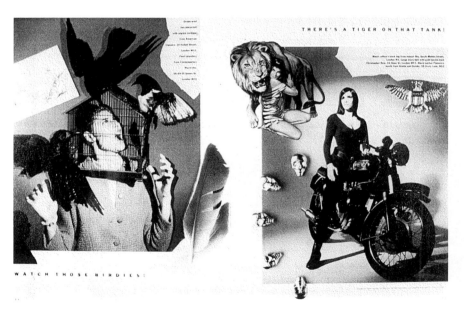

Figures 2 and 3. 'Guys N Dolls', photographer Mark Lewis, stylist Finbar at Max Presents, *The Face* July/August 1988, courtesy of *The Face*/Wagadon Ltd.

Working together, the harvest and the strength of black, white, grey and brown. Woman, *opposite and inset below*: pique bibbed cotton dress shirt, pinstriped waistcoat, at Margaret Howell; felt hat, at Herbert Johnson; man's hanky, at Liberty; circular skirt, by Chloé; frilled cotton apron, at Lunn Antiques.
Men, *below and below right*: Woollen waistcoats and trousers, at Aquascutum; collarless cotton shirts, striped, at Margaret Howell; plain, at Moss Bros; linen shepherd's smocks, at Lunn Antiques. Boy: flannel waistcoat and trousers, at John Lewis; tweed cap, by Burberry.
Right: Woman, *centre*, in woollen jacket, silk shirt, flannel circular skirt, by Chloé; rolled up apron, at Laura Ashley. *Far right, see page 82*: Men, *from left*: Fleck tweed jacket, wool shirt, flannel trousers, by Burberry. Tweed jacket, at Flip; collarless shirt, at Moss Bros; trilby at Herbert Johnson. Flannel jacket and trousers, by Burberry; collarless cotton shirt, at Moss Bros. Boys, in frilled and pintucked cotton shirts (see pages 80-81); cardigans, by Pringle; trousers at John Lewis. See Fashion Information for stockists. Hair by Howard Fugler of New York.

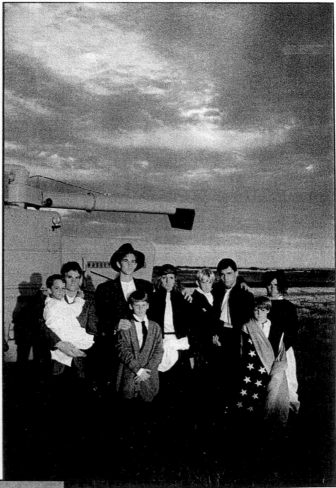

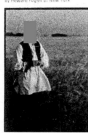

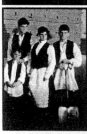

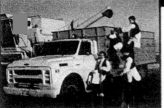

Virago Press have republished Willa Cather's work: *My Antonia, Lost Lady, Death comes for the Archbishop, The Professor's House* are now in print. *My Mortal Enemy, Song of the Lark, O Pioneers!* will be published in Autumn 1982. For further information on Willa Cather write to the Willa Cather Pioneer Memorial, Red Cloud, Nebraska 68970, USA. Vogue is very grateful for the Memorial's help in every way.

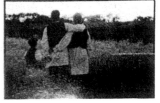

Figure 4. Bruce Weber, 'New Morning Nebraska – Pioneers of 82 Wear Plains Clothes', British *Vogue* January 1982, courtesy of Bruce Weber.

under WESTON eyes

Bruce Weber in romantic encounter with Edward Weston and the pure and simple style

The cast of characters. Tulsa in the field studio, opposite, pale grey wool laced hand-knit sweater, by Marion Foale, £58, at Paul Smith, 44 Floral St, W.C.2 and braces. Black and white hound's-tooth check woollen side-buttoned long skirt, £120 at Calvin Klein, 24 South Molton St, W.1.
In the studio, left, Bruce (not the photographer but a friend of the same name) playing the photographer, in sweatshirt, shirt and flannels from Browns and, below left, in white cotton Charvet shirt. The girls, from far left: Farrel in black cotton man's shirt from Paul Smith, black lined men's trousers from Crolla, black felt cloche, by Patricia Underwood for Calvin Klein. Natalie in white cotton man's shirt from Paul Smith, black gaberdine side-buttoned skirt from Calvin Klein. Tulsa dressed as opposite. Shelley in collared black cotton sweatshirt at Harrods, black woollen trousers by Comme des Garçons at Browns, black felt cloche as before.

these photographs are about a way of seeing and a way of life. They are photographer Bruce Weber's tribute to photographer Edward Weston (born 1886, died 1958), lived and worked in California, Mexico, and the American West. A tribute to the intensity of Weston's relationship with the camera and particular beautiful women — Margrethe Mather, Tina Modotti — to the qualities of his black and white prints, to his striving for a stripped but heightened reality and that glad Spartan existence that is a very American dream. Weston was the inspiration. This is a diversion in the style. The group are friends, spending time early fall 1982 in and around Bruce Weber's Long Island home. They are dressed in the fierce and soft monotones of a Weston print — not only in homage, this is part of fashion now.

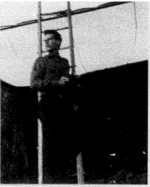

"You see, the image of Edward Weston that I will always have is of him with an 8×10 and tripod over his shoulder, ranging across Death Valley munching on a handful of dates and nuts – ready to pack his cameras to hell and back. . . "

Cole Weston,
Weston's youngest son

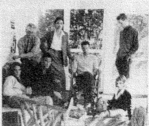

"The dramatic stone monuments at Point Lobos often turned out to be such insignificant bits of rock that even Edward had difficulty finding them again. People I had thought arrestingly handsome or fascinating in a Weston portrait seemed quite ordinary-looking when I met them. It seemed to me that I was being hoodwinked by a master illusionist. Then, as I continued to follow the process from the sighting of the photographic quarry to its being served up in a print, my beholding eye became conditioned, and I began to see things Edward's way; the dunes became dramatic, so did the small rocks he sought, and the people as handsome as their portraits.

Charis Wilson Weston

Indoors, left, from left: the girls—Tulsa in Margaret Howell grey skirt and jacket, Shelley in black cashmere by N. Peal, both with plain white cotton shirts, the men—Attila, Lance, Tommy, Bruce, Drew and Jeff, variously clad in Pringle sweaters, Calvin Klein flannels, pinstriped trousers from Browns.
Outside the darkroom, below left, Lance in water's cotton jacket from Denays, pinstriped wool trousers from Browns. Tulsa in grey knitted cashmere suit, white linen wide lapelled shirt from Calvin Klein; Bruce as above and top, plus foreman's white coat from Denays.
In the field studio, Shelley, below centre, in enormous black Kansai sweatshirt coat and, below right, Kimberley. The field studio was built by John Ryman.

Figure 5. Bruce Weber, 'Under Weston Eyes – Bruce Weber in a Romantic Encounter With Edward Weston', British *Vogue* December 1982, courtesy of Bruce Weber.

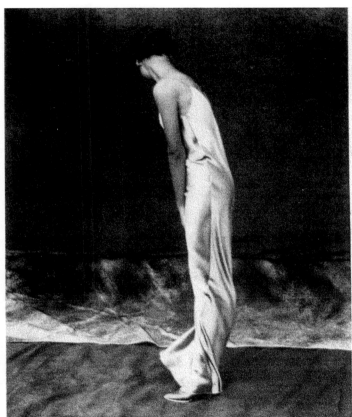

The label Bruce above
placing the photographer in
white cotton shirt from
Charvet at Paris and grey
trousers from a suit £198 at
Margaret Howell 29-29 St
Christopher's Pl W1
Posing in the field studio
Twiggy left in silver grey satin
kimono slip dress with silver
grey satin high heels both by
Anna Klein to order at Harvey
Nichols
Nude after Weston below
Natalie right in black gabar-
dine shirt with double wrap
overlap and long to mix scarf
by Zoran to order at Browns
27 South Molton St W1
Hair by Didier Malige for Jean
Louis David make up by
Marcela Smith-Masters both
of New York

"He now felt
strongly the impac
of the face itself,
the head as a
sculptured object,
within which
the springs of hate
and love
continually wound
and unwound. . ."

Ben Maddow
from Edward Weston,
his life and photographs
(Aperture, 1973)

*"h*e did not see her at first;
to the first casual glance
she looked mousy. Then he happened
to look at her direct, and was stricken -
she was exquisite. It was his first experience
of the power of understatement; he fell
in love with art and with Margrethe Mather
at the same time, and for some eight years
could not separate them. . ."

Nancy Newhall, introduction, Edward Weston's Daybooks

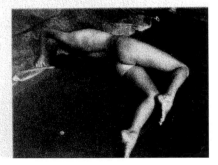

Figure 6. Bruce Weber, 'Under Weston Eyes – Bruce Weber in a Romantic
Encounter With Edward Weston', British *Vogue* December 1982, courtesy of Bruce
Weber.

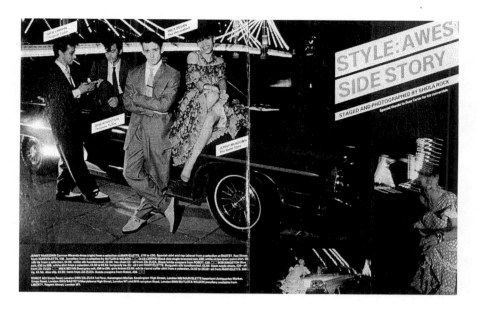

Figure 7. Sheila Rock, 'Style: A West Side Story', *The Face* October 1981, courtesy of *The Face*/Wagadon Ltd.

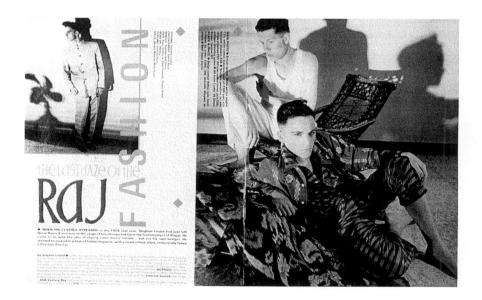

Figure 8. 'The Last Daze of the Raj', photographer Sheila Rock, stylist Stephen Linard, *The Face* May 1983, courtesy of *The Face*/Wagadon Ltd.

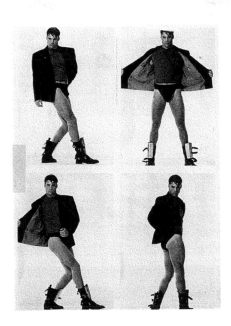

Figure 9. 'Heavy Metal', photographers Buffalo (Jamie Morgan and Ray Petri), *The Face* April 1986, courtesy of *The Face*/Wagadon Ltd.

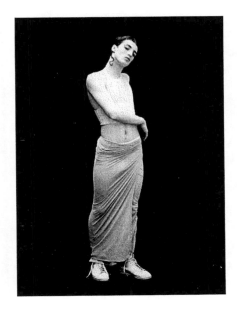

Figure 10. 'Flesh', model Nick Moss, photographer Mario Sorrenti, stylist Cathy Dixon, *The Face* April 1993, courtesy of *The Face*/Wagadon Ltd.

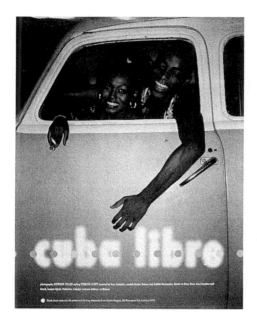

Figure 11. 'Cuba Libre', photographer Juergen Teller, stylist Venetia Scott, *The Face* February 1992, courtesy of *The Face*/Wagadon Ltd.

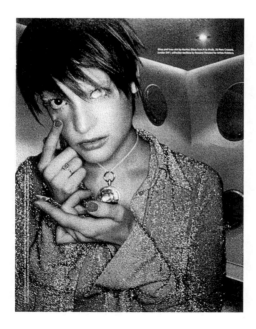

Figure 12. 'Leisure Lounge', photographer Andrea Giacobbe, stylist Maida, *The Face* October 1994, courtesy of *The Face*/Wagadon Ltd.

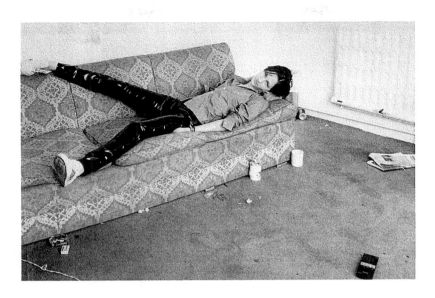

Figure 13. 'England's Dreaming', photographer Corinne Day, stylist Melanie Ward, *The Face* August 1993, courtesy of *The Face*/Wagadon Ltd.

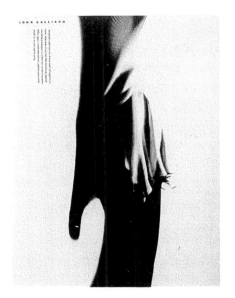

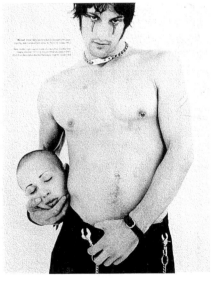

Figure 14. 'London March 88', photographer Andrew Bettles, stylist Paul Frecker, *The Face* May 1988, courtesy of *The Face*/Wagadon Ltd.

Figure 15. 'Head Hunters – Back To The No Future', photographer Jean Baptiste Mondino, stylist Judy Blame, *The Face* August 1993, courtesy of *The Face*/Wagadon Ltd.

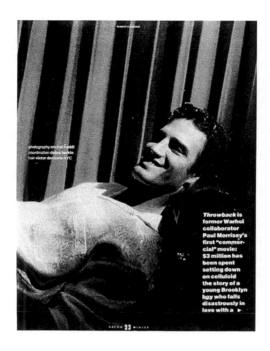

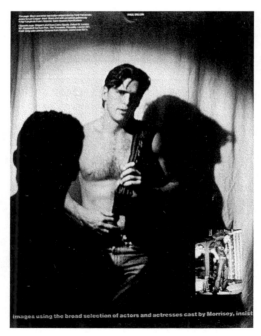

Figures 16 and 17. 'Throwback', photographer Michel Haddi, Arena January/February 1988, courtesy of Arena/Wagadon Ltd.

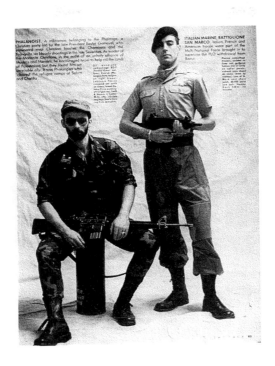

Figure 18. 'Who's Shooting Who?', photographer Oliver Maxwell, stylist Elaine Jones, *The Face* July 1986, courtesy of *The Face*/Wagadon Ltd.

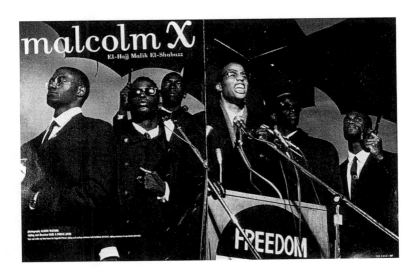

Figure 19. 'Malcolm X', photographer Norman Watson, stylists Karl and Derick (UTO), *The Face* November 1992, courtesy of *The Face*/Wagadon Ltd.

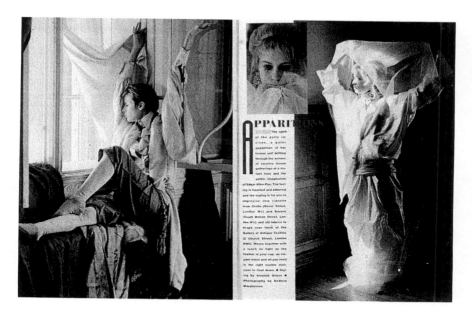

Figure 20. 'Apparitions', photographer Andrew Macpherson, stylist Amanda Grieve, *The Face* December 1984, courtesy of *The Face*/Wagadon Ltd.

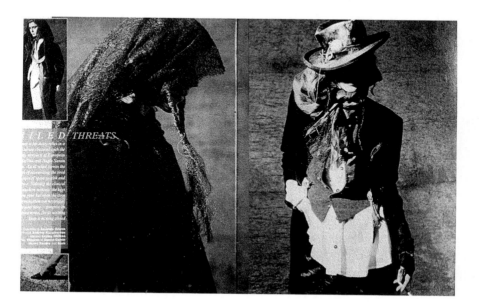

Figure 21. 'Veiled Threats', photographer Andrew Macpherson, stylist Amanda Grieve, The Face January 1985, courtesy of *The Face*/Wagadon Ltd.

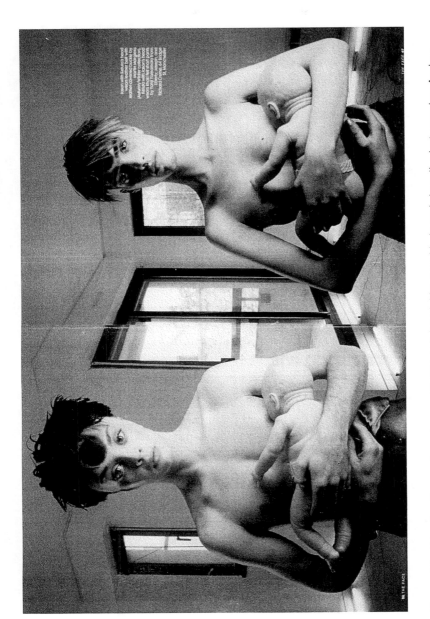

Figure 22. 'Simplex Concordia – Jason with Ketuta's head, Ketuta with Jason's head', photographer Andrea Giacobbe, stylist Maida, *The Face* July 1996, courtesy of *The Face*/Wagadon Ltd.

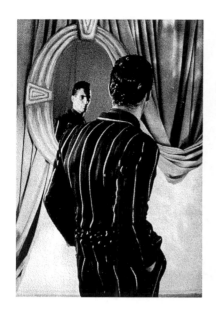
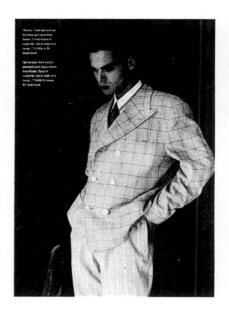

Figure 23. 'fin de siècle', photographer Michel Haddi, stylist Debra Berkin, *Arena* January/February 1988, courtesy of *Arena*/Wagadon Ltd.

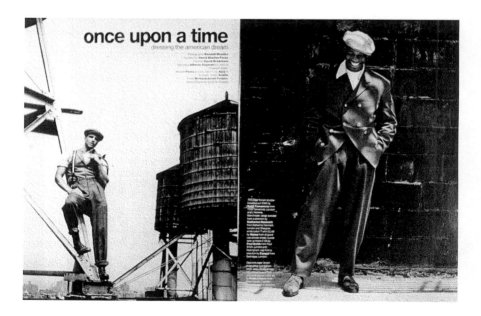

Figure 24. 'once upon a time', photographer Randall Mesdon, stylist, David Bradshaw, Arena November 1992, courtesy of *Arena*/Wagadon Ltd.

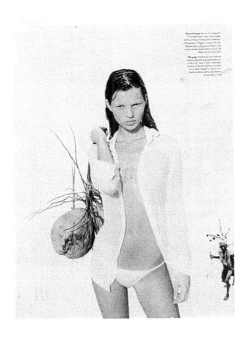

Figure 25. 'borneo', photographer Corinne Day, stylist Melanie Ward, *The Face* August 1991, courtesy of *The Face*/Wagadon Ltd.

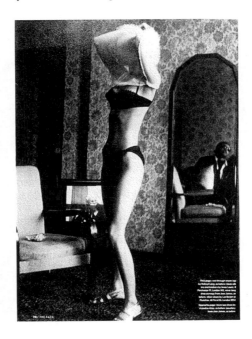

Figure 26. 'Hotel Motel, Holiday In', photographer Enrique Badulescu, stylist Mitzi Lorenz, *The Face* April 1991, courtesy of *The Face*/Wagadon Ltd.

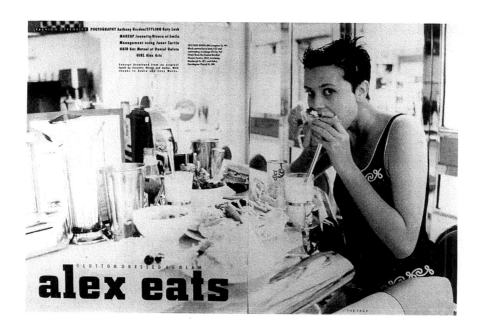

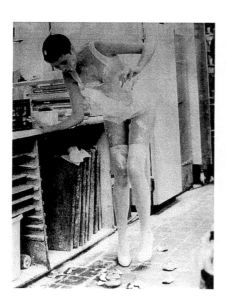
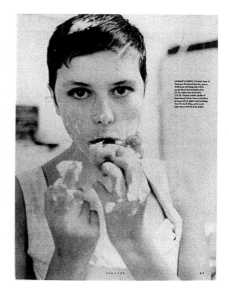

Figures 27 and 28. 'Alex Eats', photographer Anthony Gordon, stylist Katy Lush, *The Face* April 1988, courtesy of *The Face*/Wagadon Ltd.

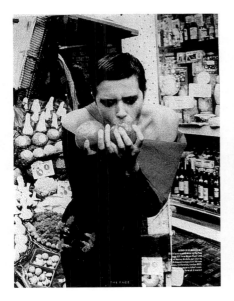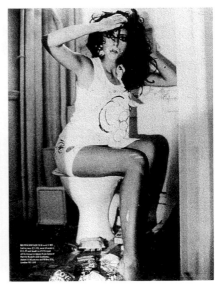

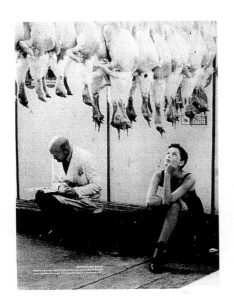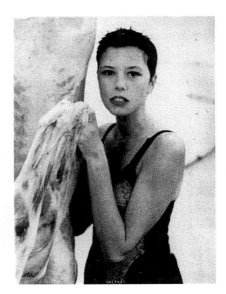

Figures 29 and 30. 'Alex Eats', photographer Anthony Gordon, stylist Katy Lush, *The Face* April 1988, courtesy of *The Face*/Wagadon Ltd.

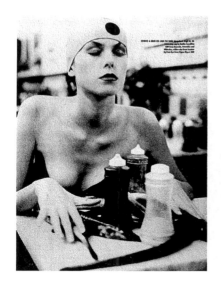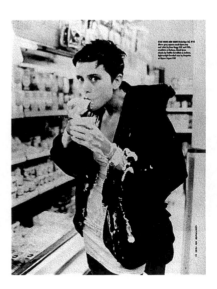

Figure 31. 'Alex Eats', photographer Anthony Gordon, stylist Katy Lush, *The Face* April 1988, courtesy of *The Face*/Wagadon Ltd.

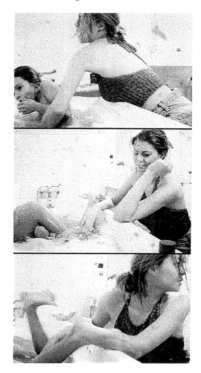

Figure 32. 'The Baby Sitter', photographer Bertrand Marignac, *The Face* March 1994, courtesy of *The Face*/Wagadon Ltd.

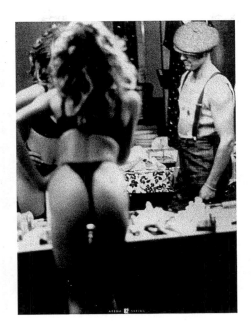

Figure 33. 'Idle Kitsch', photographer Ellen Von Unwerth, *Arena* March/April 1993, courtesy of *Arena*/Wagadon Ltd.

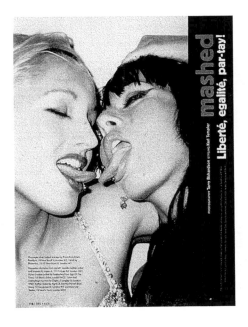

Figure 34. 'Mashed', photographer Terry Richardson, stylist Karl Templer, *The Face* June 1995, courtesy of *The Face*/Wagadon Ltd.

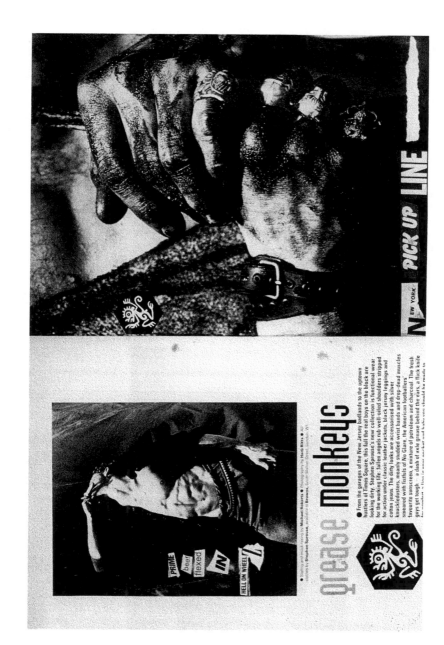

Figure 35. 'Grease Monkeys', photographer Herb Ritts, *The Face* October 1984, courtesy of *The Face*/Wagadon Ltd.

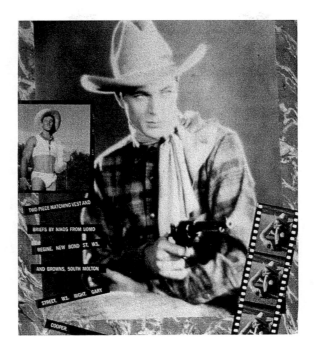

Figure 36. 'High Noon', photographer Johnny Rosza, *Unique* October/November 1986, private collection.

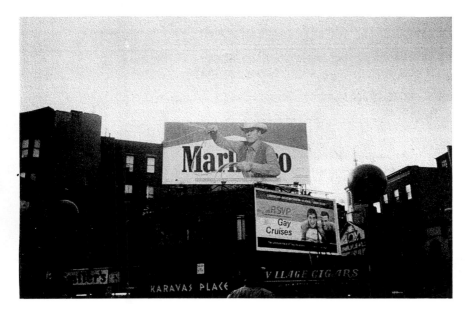

Figure 37. Advertising billboards for Marlboro and RSVP Gay Cruises, Greenwich Village, New York City, 1991, photography P. Jobling.

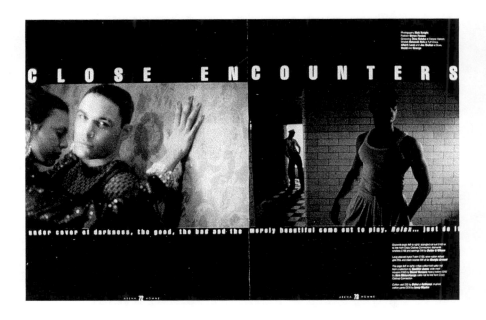

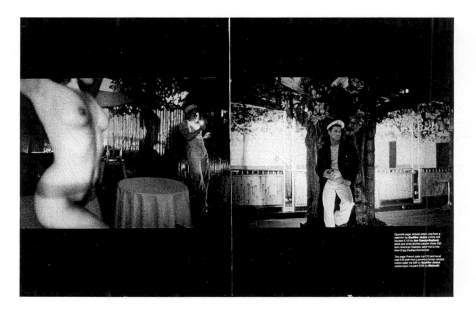

Figures 38 and 39. 'Close Encounters', photographer Nick Knight, stylist Simon Foxton, *Arena Homme Plus* Spring/Summer 1995, courtesy of *Arena*/Wagadon Ltd.

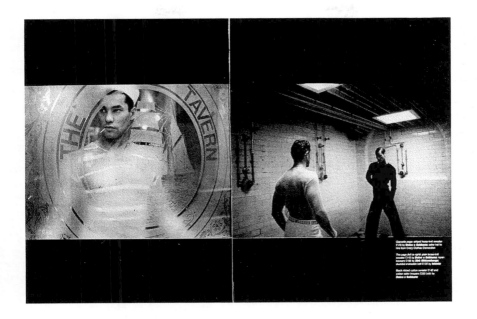

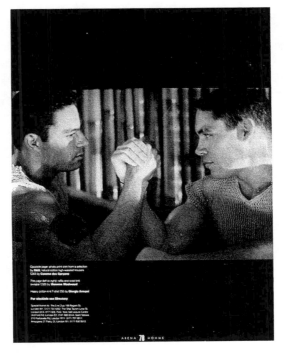

Figures 40 and 41. 'Close Encounters', photographer Nick Knight, stylist Simon Foxton, *Arena Homme Plus* Spring/Summer 1995, courtesy of *Arena*/Wagadon Ltd.

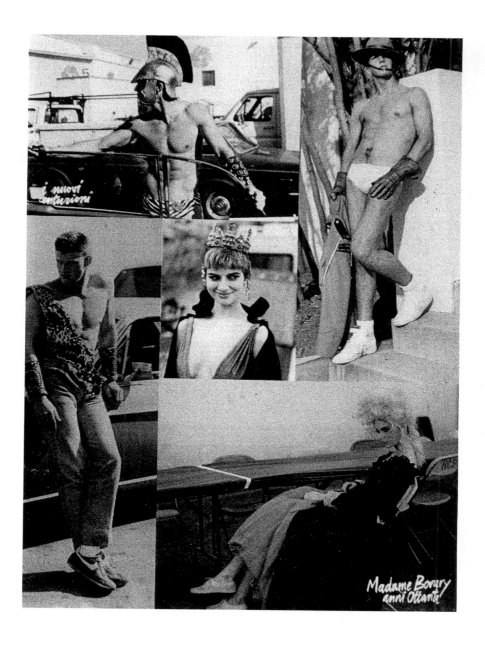

Figure 42. 'Hollywood', photographer Bruce Weber, *Per Lui* July/August 1985, courtesy of Bruce Weber.

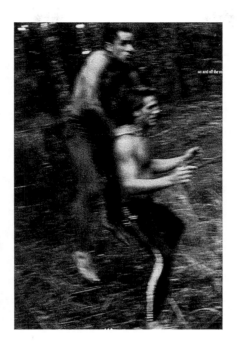

Figure 43. 'On and Off the Road', photographer Michel Haddi, stylist Debra Berkin, *Arena* December 1986/January 1987, courtesy of *Arena*/Wagadon Ltd.

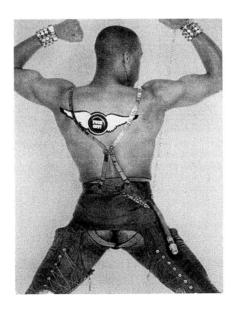

Figure 44. 'Punk', photographer Nick Knight, stylist Simon Foxton, *The Face* February 1986, courtesy of *The Face*/Wagadon Ltd.

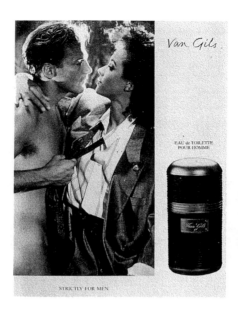

Figure 45. Advertisement for Van Gils, Strictly for Men, 1989, courtesy of the Advertising Archives.

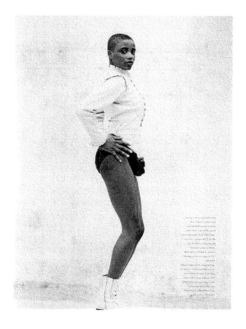

Figure 46. 'Forever Leather', photographer Marc Lebon, stylist Debbi Mason, *The Face* November 1991, courtesy of *The Face*/Wagadon Ltd.

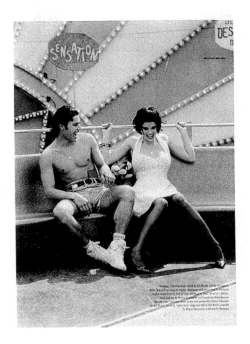

Figure 47. 'Fairground Attraction', photographer Ellen Von Unwerth, stylist Corinne Nocella, *Arena* July/August 1988, courtesy of *Arena*/Wagadon Ltd.

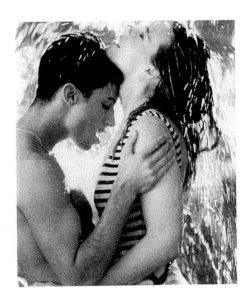

Figure 48. 'Wet', photographer Kate Garner, stylists Karl and Derick (UTO), *The Face* August 1991, courtesy of *The Face*/Wagadon Ltd.

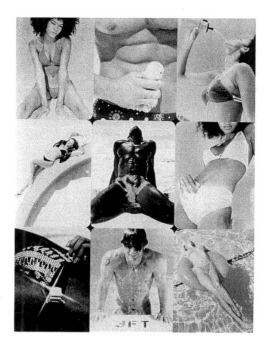

Figure 49. 'Have a nice day', photographer Christopher Griffith, stylist David Bradshaw, *Arena* July/August 1994, courtesy of *Arena*/Wagadon Ltd.

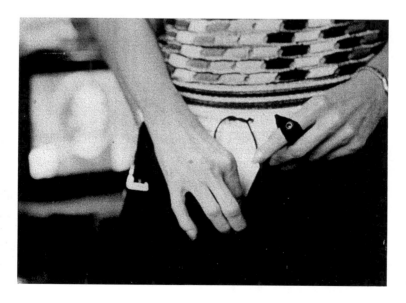

Figure 50. 'Trade', photographer Steve Callaghan, stylist Karl Templer, *The Face* June 1996, courtesy of *The Face*/Wagadon Ltd.

concerning the ontological status of photography, by implying that it is one and the same thing as reality, a spontaneous trace of what exists. Such issues are at the heart of Barthes' idea of the photographic paradox (which we have already addressed in Part II), and his exposition of denotation and connotation in 'The Photographic Message' and other writings.[10] But the notion of photographic realism/reality has a special significance in the context of this argument in so far as photographs are still more readily accepted as legal evidence than paintings or drawings.[11] By extension, they have been subject to censorship in Britain since 1959 under the regulations of the Obscene Publications Act, and, in the case of images of children under sixteen years of age (the legal age of consent in Britain for heterosexuals), the 1978 Protection of Children Act.[12] This legislation has clearly informed the policing of much recent fashion photography, but, as model Georgina Cooper attests, such concerns are often ungrounded: 'The . . . worry people have is photographers making you act sexually . . . That protectiveness goes when you reach 16 . . . They might ask you to kiss a male model, but at 16 you're allowed to have sex anyway.'[13] Indeed, those who impugned Day's representation appear to have been swayed by a hysterical or extreme rhetoric of censorship, to the extent that they seriously believed or wished Kate Moss to look as if she were both a drug addict and less than the legal age of consent (in actual fact she was 19 at the time the images were printed), something that not even Jane Kilpatrick of the Kidscape child protection charity felt to be the case.[14] A similar moral attitude was expressed by the American Family Association in 1995 when it accused an advertising campaign for CK Jeans that clearly depicted mature teenagers of lapsing into child porn.[15]

Certainly, the visual rhetoric of both 'Under Exposure' and 'Alex Eats' seems to stray into the territory of pornography, or at least of erotic art: the former in the way that it appears to mobilise a keyhole aesthetic; and the latter in the way that it fetishes the relationship between the body, underwear and food, a point that I discuss in more detail later on. But the form and content of these fashion images are also more aesthetically subtle, and the sexual codes in them more elliptically connoted than those in most pornography, as a glance through the prurient and crudely composed split-beaver shots in any obscene magazine will testify. A sense of proportion is wanting here, therefore, concerning the aesthetic or commercial intentions of the producer and the imputed realism of the fashion iconography under discussion, which we can regain by comparing it with some other similar images.

There are some shoots by Day, for instance, such as 'England's Dreaming' (*The Face*, August 1993), in which the tropes of sleaze and grunge that Orbach hinted at in her criticism of 'Under Exposure' are much more in evidence, but that no one has seen fit to oppose. In one of the photographs a female model wears a heavily distressed mesh top; in another she strikes a supine pose on a grubby sofa, her shirt sleeves are rolled up and her arms lie languidly by her side, while her gaze is calm, if transfixed (Figure 13). All around her is the detritus of her laid-back lifestyle – empty coffee mugs, a discarded soda can, a cigarette lighter, a used ashtray, a discarded newspaper, a remote control, and several pieces of scrunched-up paper. Yet for all this, the girl's milieu and pose do not necessarily mean that she does drugs, and, as with the images of Moss, there is not really a clear-cut case for stating that she is a junkie. Likewise, the alleged paedophilic content of 'Under Exposure' is thrown into sharper relief if we compare the image of Moss lying on her back with that of the blatantly prepubescent and provocatively blindfolded girl in an advertisement for Puiforcat watches that was banned from publication in Britain by the Advertising Standards Authority in 1991.[16]

But to argue in favour of banning even this image returns us to the initial dilemma concerning the tension between reality and photographic representation, and the vexed issue of freedom of speech. For by which standards are we realistically to judge what constitutes child pornography? The answer to this is not easy to find, and the issue has been obscured both by tendentious arguments concerning the erotic versus the pornographic,[17] and the imputed artistic value or otherwise of certain photographers' work. One thinks here, for instance, of Lewis Carroll's portraits of Victorian girls in the nude, or more recently, of the controversy surrounding Sally Mann's representations of childhood sexuality in *Immediate Family* (1992), the impounding of images of adolescents by Jock Sturges following the introduction of the appropriations bill in America in July 1989,[18] and the removal of a picture of a three-year-old nude girl by Robert Mapplethorpe from a recent retrospective at the Hayward Gallery, London.[19] Nor does the framing of the debate on moral grounds tend to resolve once and for all the conflict between those who approve of censorship and those who do not. The most that we can attempt to achieve in such cases is an objective judgement that may argue either for or against censorship and a hope that others will appreciate our point of view. Hence, for what it is worth, I openly declare myself a supporter of the anti-censorship lobby with regard to all forms of cultural production. In so doing, I take sides with the 1979 *Williams Report* in so far as it has argued that there is no scientific evidence for pornography causing harm in society, and with similar sentiments expressed by Feminists Against Censorship, who have also contended that the criminalisation of imputedly obscene imagery is politically self-defeating: 'You cannot censor sexual material without censoring feminists, because sex is what we talk about.'[20]

Perhaps a more fruitful way of negotiating the problem as it applies to 'Under Exposure' is to ask, as Patricia Holland has done, how exactly we define who is a child? And which images of female children are less innocent or more sexual than others?[21] As Holland contends, although the meaning of the terms 'child' and 'innocence' are understood in opposition to the terms 'adult' and 'experience', and as such are codified through legislation, social rules and tacit convention, in reality we do not always manage to maintain the opposition or keep the distinction intact: 'We cannot assume that there is such a thing as a child which exists independently of our knowledge of it, independently of our use of the category and the expression of that category in words and pictures.'[22] Thus the meaning of childhood is not a static or universal entity but a cultural construct – the current age of consent in Spain, for example, is 12 years old. Moreover, girls tend to be objectified from a very early age, and in such a way that 'their childish qualities cannot be expressed independently of their sexuality'.[23] We live, after all, in a culture that sanctions the portrayal of girls as young as two and a half years old as beauty queens in annual pageants like America's Royal Miss or, until very recently, the Miss Pears contest.[24] Testimony suggests that not all the finalists in these competitions are aware of the ramifications of the mimicry with which they are involved.[25] Nonetheless, the sexualisation of childhood that such contests imply, and the complicity of parents in entering their offspring to become beauty queens for the sake of financial reward, have given many critics the grounds for arguing that media images have both an impact on our consciousness and the power to inform our actions.

As a corollary, these critics have called for the stricter policing and censorship of the mass media and some, like Catherine MacKinnon, have insisted that pornography is nothing more than a patriarchal conspiracy: 'Pornography is exactly that speech of men that silences the speech of women.'[26] By this MacKinnon seems simultaneously to over-determine and to over-simplify the case. She refuses to accept that women and gays might also have an investment in pornography,[27] and postulates a causal relationship between pornography and many of society's ills, such as violence against women. But as Jennifer Wicke points out, MacKinnon's knee-jerk reaction to all kinds of sexual representation too easily appears to occupy the moral high ground, and we still seriously need to consider the idea that: '"objectification" need not be in itself a violent act'.[28] Indeed, Wicke's point is born out by recent research that suggests that the impact of the media on subversive activity is quixotically overstated. The video *Child's Play III*, for instance, was invoked as a motivating factor in the murder of James Bulger from Liverpool in 1993, even though there was no firm evidence to prove that his killers Jon Venables and Robert Thompson had ever seen it. Further research by Ann Hugell and Tim Newburn has also revealed that the viewing habits of young offenders in Britain is much the same as it is for their non-offending counterparts, and that sometimes they are less frequent consumers of the mass media.[29]

I do not intend to deny that paedophilia exists as a real and disturbing threat in society or to detract from those who struggle against it. Yet at the same time I feel that it would be myopic, if not erroneous, to claim a one-to-one relationship between fashion publishing, or advertising for that matter, and the actual incidence of child pornography. And if such a correlation between fashion photography and child pornography can indeed be seen to exist, then not only must it be regarded as being inclusive but also gauged in terms of its cumulative impact. As waitress Tara Bartlett responded incisively when she was asked if she thought the *Vogue* shoot was offensive: 'You can see little girls in their knickers any day in catalogues and no-one's bothered by that. I should think a potential child-abuser would be more likely to read catalogues than *Vogue*.'[30] By the same token, we could argue that fashion shoots like 'Alex Eats', and 'The Baby Sitter', photographed by Bertrand Marignac for *The Face* in March 1994 (Figure 32), which included intimate scenes of an adult female bathing and caressing her ward, should be subject to the same moral surveillance as 'Under Exposure'. And not only this; for the representation of ephebic male bodies in fashion photography would be seen to raise similar problems. Shoots like Michel Haddi's 'Kid Gloves', for example, depicting child boxers in Thailand for *Arena* (September/October 1988), would need to be scrutinised for their possible portrayal of the youthful male body from a sexually ambiguous perspective.

Although photographers may initially produce fashion images for purely aesthetic or commercial considerations, at the same time it must be realised that their work can take on other discursive connotations, over which they do not necessarily have any control, as soon as it is viewed in contexts such as paedophilia. Nevertheless, as Susan Edwards points out, the question still remains whether: 'pictures have the power to obliterate the values taught by other institutions in our culture'.[31] And, if they do, would the censorship of images that either represent children in the nude or deal with childhood sexuality have any real power in curbing the incidence of the sexual abuse of children? Or in compensating those who have been the victims of such abuse? Sadly, as Edwards also testifies, the evidence to date suggests otherwise: 'None of the efforts to censor art photographers who make photographs of children nude has made any difference in the lives of the genuine victims of child abuse.'[32]

Objectification, Mimicry and the Female Photographer

By extension, the accusations of pornography and fetishism that were levelled against Day's images are probably more what we have come to expect to hear concerning the objectification of the female body by male photographers; Helmut Newton's work, as we have already noted, was constantly prone to opposition during the 1970s for its imputed sexist and pornographic intentions. In complete contrast, Gordon's work failed to stir up any appreciable groundswell of hostility, although in effect it is much more graphically extreme than 'Under Exposure' in its fetishistic objectification of the female body (indeed in a subsequent shoot called 'Alex Works' for *The Face* (September 1988), the photographer claimed somewhat proprietorially that: 'Alex is an Anthony Gordon production'). The production and consumption of such images are revealing, therefore, of the tensions that arise not just when a photographer moves from one channel of circulation to another, but when women attempt to have or do things their own way. As the fashion journalist Lisa Armstrong contended:

> The pictures show a reality that is closer to home than the usual overstyled fashion icons . . . If Moss, Day and Shulman are happy with the pictures then why the fuss? It seems that pictures of a well-endowed woman in lacy underwear are more acceptable than images of a flat-chested one in a vest . . . It seems that women still cannot win, whichever way they portray themselves'.[33]

The kind of patriarchal 'overstyled fashion icons' to which Armstrong indirectly refers include, for example, John Stember's 'Soft Understatements' for British *Vogue* (November 1980), in which we observe a female model in fetishistic see-through underwear lying face down on a bed. Indeed, Alexandra Shulman, the editor of British *Vogue*, had openly stated that her intention in publishing 'Under Exposure' was to undermine this type of sexist objectification, and to break the mould of the male photographer 'shooting a female model wearing black, lace lingerie at hotel dressing table'.[34] Corinne Day had also envisaged her photographs as humorous and, given the *mise-en-scène* of Moss's apartment, the mixture of designer and high-street undergarments she wears, and their circulation in *Vogue*, as making a deliberate statement against high fashion and the artificiality of studio photography. She insisted that the storyline was intended to deal with 'a sixteen year old discovering her sexuality, playing around with lacy knickers the way young girls do' (a point born out by the naïf rhetoric of the subtitle: 'What to wear beneath effort-free clothes? Barely-there underwear, naturally'), and protested that:

The remarks were very annoying. These people have reacted in such a negative way, I feel, and have totally lost touch with their youth . . . I do think it's good to see things like this in such an élite magazine, it has raised a lot of questions . . . I want people to look at the pictures and feel that they want to know them, that they're not just of another model glowering from the page.[35]

Here, we seem to encounter a difference in intention between Day and a female photographer like Ellen Von Unwerth, whose work, often modelled on Helmut Newton's style, harps on the normative idea of woman as the glamorous and passive object of male desire.[36] This much is evident in both 'Idle Kitsch' (*Arena*, March/April 1993; Figure 33) and 'Bodyline' (British *Vogue*, January 1991). In the latter, for example, she represents a nubile female model wearing various items of black lingerie. Furthermore, one of the photographs in the spread depicts a man shaving while a model wearing a black body holds up a mirror in front of his face; as he shaves we can clearly see that he is not looking at his own reflection, and instead his gaze wanders off to the right where she is standing.

Although Von Unwerth's iconography appears to be more stereotypically superficial in its objectification of the female body than Day's, nonetheless it could be argued that the work of both photographers appears to elaborate the strategy of mimicry that is discussed by Luce Irigaray in *This Sex Which Is Not One* (1985 [1977]). Here, Irigaray insists that, until such time as men and women are regarded as being truly equal, women should deliberately sequestrate their feminine role and emphasise or exaggerate it so as to parody and destabilise patriarchal stereotypes and men's phantasies of what a woman should be or do. The basis of Irigaray's argument, therefore, concerned women's reclamation of some form of power from men that would at least put them in control of their own self-image: 'One must assume the feminine role deliberately. Which means already to convert a form of subordination into an affirmation, and thus begin to thwart it . . . It also means "to unveil" the fact that, if women are such good mimics, it is because they are not simply resorbed in this function. They remain elsewhere.'[37]

Such an act of textual mimicry, and the aims and objectives of producers, of course, find no place in the arguments of those critics intent on opposing Day's portrayal of Moss for what they regard as its pornographic connotations. Indeed, their criticisms are a sobering reminder of the way that certain acts of mimicry can backfire on themselves or be misunderstood. To put this in slightly more political terms, the case against 'Under Exposure' reveals a gulf in material existence between men and women that seems to operate on the level of the differend, a concept that Lyotard uses in discussing the univocalism of the judicial system: 'I would like to call a differend the case where the plaintiff is divested of the means to argue and becomes for that reason a victim.'[38] Thus it can be argued that the experiences of women are inappropriately accounted for or represented in words that are not of their own making, in phrases that issue from patriarchal language, and that when used by women they consequently appear to naturalise their own subordination. That is to say, even though Day has attempted to break with this language by representing Moss from a personal perspective, her contribution has nevertheless been misconstrued and framed in patriarchal terms by those who regard her work as either exploitative or pornographic. We can detect a similar patriarchal message concerning the transgressive nature of mimicry and power in Irvin Kersher's film *The Eyes of Laura Mars* (1978), in which Faye Dunaway portrays the eponymous female fashion photographer. Consequently, I feel it would be useful and instructive at this point in my discussion to draw a parallel between the way the role of the female producer is represented in the film and the reception of Day's work for *Vogue*.

Like Ellen Von Unwerth, Mars' work stylistically appears to mimic Helmut Newton's in its fetishistic display of sex and violence. In one scene, for example, we see her photographing a simulated car crash involving two female models in underwear and fur coats, who feign to tear out each other's hair. But Laura's images are not simply the same as Newton's, for her photographs of death and violence are not only intended to undermine the tension between pornography and fashion but are also previsualised inasmuch as they are based on her paranormal experiences. Moreover, as the plot unfolds, reality and representation appear to collapse into each other in a complex *mise-en-abyme*, since her psychic visions turn out to be premonitions of the murders that actually take place in the film, and that both she and we, as spectators, experience from the point of view of the killer. Here, the film differs in a significant respect from Antonioni's rather more shapeless vehicle *Blow-Up* (1966), which centres on an anonymous male and archetypally sexist fashion photographer played by David Hemmings.[39] The plot of *Blow-Up* also hinges on a murder mystery; but, unlike Mars, Hemmings' character inadvertently photographs a death scene as he aimlessly wanders through a park looking for inspiration, and he only becomes aware of the fact retrospectively when he repeatedly blows up a detail in one of the images he has taken. His own vision is limited, and it is by virtue of using photographic technology that he sees the bigger picture. Thus when Hemmings arrogantly asserts to his agent that he has seen a man being killed this morning, more accurately he should state that it is his camera that witnessed the murder. Finally, the murder that takes place in *Blow-Up* is coincidental to and eclipses the film's fashion plot. Indeed it seems to be deployed in such a way as to enhance the photographer's status as a producer of more 'serious' work; he is planning, for example, to publish a book of documentary images.[40]

By contrast, the very motive for assassination in *Laura Mars* is the killer's psychotic relationship to fashion photography and, particularly, the way that it seems to trouble his own sexual identity and desires. Each of the murderer's five victims is involved in the fashion business, having either sponsored or worked with Laura, and four of them are women. The fifth victim is male, although tellingly he is a portrayed as an effeminate gay, and when he is killed he is wearing Laura's clothes. All of these characters, however, meet the same cruel and dramatically ironic death by having their eyes poked out by police lieutenant John Neville (played by Tommy Lee Jones), the very person who is supposed to be helping the photographer trace the killer, and with whom she has a brief affair. Thus not only is Laura's paranormal scopophilic drive portrayed as a transgressive force, but also as one that leaves her powerless to help save any of the victims' lives. In fact, Neville has intended all along that she will be his final victim, a point both she and we remain blind to until the closing scene of the drama when, his cover having been blown, he implores her to shoot him with the gun that he originally trained her to use in self-defence. On either side of the camera, whether as subject or object, women – and by analogy gays – are ultimately portrayed in the film as unsuccessful or impotent when they are seen to challenge a phallogocentric view of the world; something that is clearly underscored when Laura's ostensible mimicking of Helmut Newton's sado-masochistic imagery literally backfires on her. As is the case concerning the dynamics of production and representation in 'Under Exposure', therefore, *The Eyes of Laura Mars* implies that the fate of women is to be the ultimate victims of a patriarchal view of the fashion world.

Female Spectatorship and Pleasure

The Eyes of Laura Mars is also pivotal to this assessment of the objectification of the female body in fashion photography, since it implies that visual pleasure in such instances is the province of men, and in particular of the pervert, a point that the criticisms levelled at 'Under Exposure' also seem to maintain. Both Hume's contention that we are invited 'to stare at the crotch and breasts of a child', and Orbach's framing of the work in the context of paedophilia, for example, assume that spectatorial pleasure is a monolithic process. Thus the assumption is made that the potential consumer or spectator of the work will be exclusively heterosexual and male. The majority of British *Vogue*'s readers, however, are female – in 1987, for example, 80 per cent of its readers were women, predominantly in the age category of 15 to 44 years old[41] – and not all of them, as Reina Lewis and Katrina Rolley have demonstrated, should be regarded as being straight.[42] A propos 'Under Exposure', we witness the rehearsal of a well-worn debate that locates the gaze squarely in a psychoanalytical context. But this also reduces Lacan's original concept of the phallic gaze, assessed in *Four Fundamental Concepts* (1978) as a transcendental and 'unapprehensible' ideal, which issues 'from all sides' and to which we are all subjected, into something that the active male 'does' to the passive female in order to resolve his castration anxiety.[43]

Laura Mulvey's 'Visual Pleasure and Narrative Cinema' is the *locus classicus* of such arguments; and in it she attempts to demonstrate a strict correlation between masculinity and voyeurism, and femininity and exhibitionism:

> In a world ordered by sexual imbalance, pleasure in looking has been split between active/male and passive/female. The determining male gaze projects its fantasy onto the female figure which is stylised accordingly. In their traditional exhibitionist role women are simultaneously looked at and displayed . . . Woman displayed as sexual object is the *leitmotif* of erotic spectacle.[44]

In a subsequent essay Mulvey does admit that women can and do take pleasure as spectators. But once again she discusses such visual pleasure with reference to the male gaze, arguing that when women become spectators they inevitably adopt a masculinized way of looking.[45]

All this serves to disavow that a particularly female or feminine mode of spectatorship is in any way possible, and the different subject positions available to women, whether straight or gay, black or white, are consequently subjugated to a totalizing idea of the dominant male gaze. But, as Ros Coward has remarked with regard to recent fashion photography: 'it is no use trying to pretend that these child-like supermodels simply pander to male fantasies of resuming control and are being imposed on a resentful womanhood'.[46] Consequently, in recent years the binarism of such thinking has been greatly contested and deconstructed by many female writers, who have postulated a multiplicity of pleasures when it comes to female spectatorship. In many respects these writers have reworked psychoanalytic theory to their own advantage, arguing that a woman's investment in looking at her own body and/or the bodies of others emanates from a primary or pre-mirror, narcissistic relationship with the mother, and not with a secondary or post-mirror identification in which the paternal phallus becomes the privileged signifier.[47] The concept of the essential or homosexual maternal finds full expression, for example in the work of two of the most influential exponents of *écriture féminine*, Julia Kristeva and Luce Irigaray.[48]

For both writers, it is the female infant's special relationship with the body of the mother that is at stake here, a bond that constitutes for Kristeva the homosexual facet of motherhood, and for Irigaray a 'secondary homo-sexuality.'[49] As Kristeva expresses it, therefore, an originary understanding and shared experience of their reproductive corporeality leads women to forge a psychosexual identity that transcends the post-Oedipal splitting into subject/object or active/passive positions:

> Such an excursion to the limits of primal regression can be phantasmatically experienced as the reunion of a woman-mother with the body of *her* mother . . . one toward which women aspire all the more passionately simply because it lacks a penis: that body cannot penetrate her as can a man when possessing a wife. By giving birth, the woman enters into contact with the mother; she becomes, she is her own mother; they are the same continuity differentiating self. She thus actualizes the homosexual facet of motherhood, through which a woman is simultaneously closer to her instinctual memory, more open to her own psychosis, and consequently, more negatory of the social, symbolic bond.[50]

But primary narcissism between women is not just literally born out of their capacity for reproduction, for, as Kristeva further argues, it is also by identifying with the mother's face, in effect the first mirror image any child perceives, that the female subject is ineluctably grounded in a fundamental form of homosexuality. In a similar fashion, Irigaray postulates a primary corporeal bond between women, though one that is not necessarily tied to reproduction, and that exceeds the law of the phallic father:

> In that connection, given that the first body they have any dealings with is a woman's body, that the first love they share is mother love, it is important to remember that women always stand in an archaic and primal relationship with what is known as homosexuality . . . This love is necessary if we are not to remain the servants of the phallic cult, objects to be used and exchanged between men, rival objects on the market . . . there is a relationship with *jouissance* other than that which functions in accordance with the phallic model.[51]

The ramifications of the homosexual/lesbian gaze elaborated by Kristeva and Irigaray have not been lost on feminist and gay writers who have subsequently attempted to account for the diverse pleasures that women take in looking at images of other women in advertisements and fashion photography. Few contemporary fashion shoots have dealt directly with lesbian desire, that is, not until certain photographers began to emulate the work of Helmut Newton during the 1990s (Figure 34 is a striking example, as is 'For Your Pleasure', *The Face*, June 1995, photographed by Inez Van

Lamsweerde and styled by Vinoodh Matadin). Reina Lewis and Katrina Rolley have nonetheless attempted to explain what is at stake for lesbians as spectators of fashion photography in general. Thus, rather than simply assuming that there is one type of lesbian, and as a corollary one type of spectatorship, Lewis and Rolley propound that the pleasure lesbians take in viewing images in *Vogue* and other mainstream fashion magazines is 'multi-coded', and pose the question: 'how for example, would a self-consciously butch lesbian react to the prospect of being the glamorous model?'[52]

In part, the question is answered by Diana Fuss in her essay 'Fashion and the homospectatorial look' (1992) where, mobilising Kristeva, she analyses the prevalence of the close-up in fashion photography in terms of the female's desire to recuperate the primary, scopic love object that is the mother's face.[53] But Fuss also builds imaginatively on Kristeva's ideal of the maternal homo-sexual facet by contending that such forms of identification are vampiric. Here she argues that female spectatorship is not just an act of consumption, that is, as Freud expresses it, a way of satisfying the ego's desire to have or become the other through 'the oral, cannibalistic incorporation of the other person',[54] but also a voracious 'feeding off' images that implies an act of vampiric replication, achieved through an endless supersession of female others:

> Vampirism . . . marks a third possible mode of looking, a position that demands both separation and identification, both a having and a becoming – indeed, a having through a becoming . . . Vampirism is both other-incorporating and self-reproducing; it delimits a more ambiguous space where desire and identification appear less opposed than coterminous.[55]

Consequently vampirism, as both Fuss and popular mythologies like Bram Stoker's *Dracula* demonstrate, does not just imply that the male vampire feeds off his female victims, but that the idea of incorporation and replication can involve women feeding off other women, as well as men feeding off other men, and women feeding off men.[56] The cross-gendered implications of vampiric activity are manifest, for example, in 'Fashion Vampires. The devil in me . . . the angel in you', photographed by Glen Luchford and styled by Judy Blame for *The Face*, January 1993, where the gaze of the androgyn-ously made-up male and female models beckons us into their masquerade.

As the authors discussed above profess it, therefore, the dynamics of female spectatorial pleasure are often more complex and contradictory than earlier psychoanalytic accounts of the gaze admit. Moreover, they greatly enrich our understanding of the different ways that women may respond to fashion photographs and advertisements containing other women, as well as illuminating the maternalistic tropes of both 'Under Exposure' and 'Alex Eats'. As we have already observed, for example, both shoots trade on the ideal of the woman-child, and this, combined with the models' solipsistic poses and the self-absorption they reveal in their own bodies, seems to connote the primary narcissism that Kristeva and Irigaray propound. By the same token, such ideas help us to appreciate the ambiguous sexual codes of an advertisement for Coco cologne by Chanel that appeared in the same issue of *Vogue* as 'Under Exposure' in a more imaginative and challenging way. Here another woman-child, Vanessa Paradis, appears in the guise of an exotic bird, tethered at the ankle by a red rope and clinging protectively to a giant bottle of perfume. An initial Freudian or Lacanian psycho-sexual reading of this would imply that her entrapment and relationship to the bottle signal penis-envy, or her role as the alienated love-object the man desires yet subjugates. Hence the rope to which she is attached symbolically appears to transform her into the toy or plaything that Freud argues the male subject deploys in a game of *fort/da* so as to disavow his castration anxiety and separation from the mother figure.[57] In contrast, the idea of the homosexual maternal points us in a totally different direction, and turns the logic of the *fort/da* around. The red rope attached to her foot, for example, seems to connote an umbilical cord, and together with Paradis' foetal position, suggests a deep-seated desire to return to a pristine state or site of origin and security, an indeterminate but pre-Oedipal space that Kristeva, borrowing from Plato, symbolises as the figure of the maternal/nurse or *chora*: 'The mother's body is therefore what mediates the symbolic law organizing social relations and becomes the principle of the semiotic *chora*.'[58] Likewise the perfume bottle, rather than symbolising post-Oedipal penis envy or the male phallus, now forms a sense of identification with the powerful mother, and one that accords, therefore, with Freud's argument that during the phallic stage of sexual development both male and female child still believe that the mother also has a penis.[59]

More particularly, the indeterminate sexual status of the woman-child, and Fuss's cannibalistic or vampiric spin on the female gaze, become acutely resonant when we consider both the alimentary tropes of 'Alex Eats', and the fact that Kate Moss and other supermodels have been systematically attacked for encouraging eating disorders among women.

Fashion, Food and 'The Truth Game'

Manifestly, what we are dealing with in both 'Alex Eats' and 'Under Exposure' are not the bodies of actual children but rather those of ectomorphic or purposefully underdeveloped adults, a somatic ideal that more often than not has provoked extreme and not always insightful criticism. In June 1993, for example, New York's *Daily News* called Moss a 'skin-and-bones model . . . who looks like she should be tied down and intravenously fed'.[60] Such a patriarchal response is particularly inept when we consider the fetishistic relationship between model and food portrayed in 'Alex Eats', with its patent connotations of anorexia and bulimia. Instead, this kind of iconography represents, as Susan Bordo has argued: 'the cultural reality that for most women today – whatever their racial or ethnic identity, and increasingly across class and sexual-orientation differences as well – free and easy relations with food are at best a relic of the past.'[61] Not only does the ectomorphic ideal to which Bordo refers here cross racial and class barriers (witness 'Cherry Drops and Jelly Babes', *The Face*, March 1994; and 'Yard Times', *The Face*, April 1995), but it seems also to invoke the Foucauldian idea of the 'truth game', the belief of every overweight or unhappy person, for example, that there is a thinner and happier individual on the inside waiting to be released.[62] As Foucault also contends, however, this is a contest that can never be won, a point which is reinforced by the final tagline of 'Alex Eats' (Figure 31), advising us that the piece is 'continued on page 64', which command, however, ironically returns us to the opening page of the feature. Clearly, the fashion model has a part to play in perpetrating thinness as an ideal, given that the 'average model . . . is thinner than 95 per cent of the female population'.[63] But this does not necessarily mean, to borrow a term from Caputi, that the 'vocational anorexia' of the fashion world is unquestioningly and unreservedly transported into the lives of other women.[64] It can be argued, therefore, that the nexus between fashion photography and society's attitudes towards body size and sexuality is as intricate to unravel as its alleged relationship to paedophilia. Consequently, in analysing such a connection here I want to adopt a methodology similar to the one we took in assessing the accusations of child pornography that were made against 'Under Exposure', and to eschew any overt moralising. That is, I do not wish to detract from the seriousness of eating disorders or to diminish their complex aetiologies. But nor is it my intention to maintain that a simple correlation between the portrayal of the female body in fashion photography and the actual incidence of anorexia and bulimia in terms of cause and effect exists.[65] In this respect it is salutary to note the comments made by Alan Lavender, who was working at the time in the psychological laboratory at the University of St Andrews in Scotland, in a letter published in *The Face*. Although Lavender clearly disliked 'Alex Eats', he argued not that the piece would universally encourage its female readers to develop eating disorders, but that the editors of the magazine had been extremely insensitive to the actual predicament of those already suffering from them: 'In presenting binge eating as obscene, the creators of this feature might self-righteously think they are terribly right-on but . . . do they really think that anorexics would pick up on the pastiche before the pastry, and remain unaffected by such an over-the-top portrayal of food as sin?'[66] Lavender's comments here seem to echo Dick Hebdige's reservations concerning the danger of merely regarding the deployment of the simulacral image in *The Face* as a form of depoliticised, postmodern irony that leaves us in a world in which advertising copywriters and image consultants create, 'a reality as thin as the paper it is printed on'.[67] At the same time, however, he appeared to appreciate how the shoot symbolised the overlap between psychical and physical development: 'the expressions and postures of the model . . . attribute psychological traits to her role/character that an anorexic is most likely to identify with, thus turning the images even more into a family-size overbaked guilt pie'.[68] Let us, therefore, pursue things from Lavender's perspective to ask how accurate the shoot might be in representing the real conditions and experiences of women suffering from eating disorders, and what the psychosexual implications of such a portrayal could be.

Coming Out to Dine

In the first instance, the type of junk food that we observe Alex eating and the commercial spheres in which she eats it appear to pinpoint the fact that anorexia and bulimia are symptomatic manifestations of a particular paradox in affluent, consumer culture, and one that has intensified around the world since the 1980s. That is, we live at a time when we are simultaneously encouraged to take care of our bodies through dieting or exercise while we are offered the opportunity for uninterrupted consumption through fast-food multinationals like MacDonalds and late-night supermarkets.[69] Now, as Donald Lowe argues: 'Capital accumulation and the body constitute the new binary opposition: the body acts as the other to late-capitalist development.'[70] Moreover, the range and quantity of foodstuffs that Alex is portrayed as eating also appear to be a realistic depiction of what the prototypical bulimic would consume during any particular binge. This, for example, is how Tracy, one of the correspondents consulted by Morag MacSween in her study of anorexia nervosa, describes her personal experiences of food bingeing:

> I drink gallons of milkshake, I eat ice-cream, cakes, pastries, pork pies, chips, sweets, chocolates, bread, roast potatoes. I can eat half a loaf of bread, 15 fish fingers, 6 fried eggs, platefuls of chips, 4 doughnuts, 6 chocolate cakes, 2 large

bars of chocolate, 10 bars of Mars bar, etc., 1 litre of ice-cream, and probably more . . . Like a maniac that hasn't eaten in years! I ram one food after another into my mouth, hardly having time to butter the next slice of bread beforehand.[71]

Yet while Alex is represented guzzling everything from hamburgers, fries and milkshakes to potato chips and yogurt, the alimentary and clothing tropes in the fashion spread appear to connote the spatial experience of anorexia/bulimia in significantly ambiguous terms, blurring the distinction between what is public and private and interior and exterior with regard to both physical and mental states of being. Hence, the model dons underwear, literally, as outerwear, or items of clothing outside their expected context – for example, she wears a bustier and panty girdle in a bagel factory and a swimming cap in a fish and chips restaurant (a convergence of the public and private that is also evident in the way that Kate Moss performs the wearing of underwear in 'Under Exposure'). Furthermore, Alex's prandial activities seem to constitute, as Mikhail Bakhtin has argued, 'an extremely dense atmosphere of the body as a whole',[72] through which mealtimes become not a private concern but a social event: 'Man's encounter with the world in the act of eating is joyful, triumphant; he triumphs over the world, devours it without being devoured himself. The limits between man and the world are erased, to man's advantage.'[73]

For the majority of women with eating disorders the possibility of being 'caught in the act', however, has deep-seated, psychological meanings associated with shame and guilt – 'no one must see me swallow'.[74] This form of alienation is connoted by the way the model has been portrayed in total isolation or self-absorption. In three of her encounters with food her eyes are shut; and even in the picture in Smithfields Meat Market with the male worker on her left, neither subject acknowledges the existence of the other: she stares longingly at the dead turkeys above her head, while he sits intently reading. In stark contrast, we have to take note of the fact that, in all but one instance, we observe Alex consummating her desire for food in the public arena, most notably in the messy scenes set in Ed's Easy Diner, Evering's Beigels and Star Food. Furthermore, in five of the pictures her gaze is aimed directly at us as she voraciously attacks her food in such a way as to transgress the inconspicuousness the anorexic would typically desire by beckoning the spectator into the act. At one and the same time, therefore, the spread appears to trade on myth and reality, paradoxically maintaining and disavowing the privacy and invisibility the anorexic craves by turning consumption into a mostly public affair while portraying the model as an isolated and abject individual. By extension, the ideas of incorporation and excess, inclusion and exclusion with which the spread deals can also be seen to operate on another level in which the relationship between oral pleasure and the disciplined female body symbolises the precarious emergence and maintenance of a fully-formed sexual identity.

The Abject Body

In *Powers of Horror* (1982 [1980]), Julia Kristeva explores the meaning of abjection and the tension between the clean and dirty body in the context of the Lacanian symbolic order. Thus she argues that the formation of stable subject identities is continually threatened by modes of corporeality that are considered excessive, unclean or anti-social. As such she compounds Lacan's idea that certain of the body's organs – the mouth, eyes, ears, genitals, anus – in so far as they can both receive and expel objects exist at the interface between the inside and outside of the body, forming the erotogenic *rim* between interior and exterior surfaces. For Kristeva, then, the abject body is configured as a kind of metaphorical threshold, a being somewhere between subject or object, an abyss into which we can all fall, since it holds Symbolic identity in suspension while appearing to return us to an earlier (pre-Oedipal) state of existence:

> We may call it a border: abjection is above all ambiguity. Because, while releasing a hold, it does not radically cut off the subject from what treatens [*sic*] it – on the contrary, abjection acknowledges it to be in perpetual danger. But also because abjection itself is a composite of judgment and affect, of condemnation and yearning, of signs and drives. Abjection preserves what existed in the archaism of pre-objectal relationship, in the immemorial violence with which a body becomes separated from another body in order to be – maintaining that night in which the outline of the signified thing vanishes and where only the imponderable affect is carried out.[75]

Thus in abject states any fixed ideas concerning our core identity are undone; we confront the limits of our bodies' solid boundaries and glimpse the possibility of ourselves as Other.

The ingestion and excretion of food have a particular part to play in such a process of abjection, and Kristeva speaks of food loathing in highly visceral terms. Invoking a dislike of coming into contact with the skin of milk, for example, she writes: 'I experience a gagging sensation and, still farther down, spasms in the stomach, the belly; and all the organs shrivel up the body, provoke tears and bile, increase heartbeat, cause forehead and hands to perspire.'[76] We find a similar extreme form of disgust expressed in the sentiments of anorexics themselves – 'When I eat and have food in my mouth

I feel dirty, guilty and fat'[77] – and such abject feelings are also graphically portrayed by the poses struck in Figures 27–9 and 31 of 'Alex Eats'. As the fashion spread suggests, therefore, not only does the anorexic-bulimic have an extreme relationship to food as a source of pleasure, but in continuously ingesting and expelling food, identity itself becomes a form of abjection, a matter of negotiating subject positions with respect to both inside and outside the body itself. But not only this, for the kind of junk food that we observe the model toying with in several of the photographs suggests another form of contamination – that is, the political defilement of the body through its contact with the 'unclean' products of certain forms of capitalist food production such as hamburgers and coke.

Meat is Murder

Moreover, as Kristeva assesses it, hatred of food involves not just a physical response, but it also signals the psychical refusal of parental love: '*nausea* makes me balk at that milk cream, separates me from the mother and father who proffer it. "I" want none of that element, sign of their desire.'[78] The two photographs of Alex modelling a corset dress in Smithfields Meat Market are particularly replete with this idea of abjection (Figure 30). Here the model demonstrates a fetishistic interest in raw flesh that seems to verge on cannibalism – in one image she stares longingly at a host of dead turkeys that hang on meat hooks above her head, while in another she lifts up the flesh of a carcass and bares her teeth ferally as if to suggest she is just about to devour it. Initially these details remind us of the rotation into primitive baseness (*bassesse*) that Bataille raises in two of his essays in the Surrealist journal *Documents*, 'The Big Toe' and 'Mouth'.[79] Here Bataille conflates the idea that the mouth is a civilising tool through which human beings speak with the idea that it is also a symbol of carnivorous barbarism, used for killing and ingesting prey, and he therefore maintains that in the greatest moments of pleasure and pain, the human mouth is not spiritual but that of a predatory animal. In a similar vein, they also seem to evoke Freud's *Totem and Taboo* (1913), where he allegorises the relationship between identity formation and cannibalisation with reference to the myth of the brothers who killed and devoured their despotic father. The story of the totem meal becomes significant in Freud's telling not just because it re-enacts the primordial drama of the 'Oedipus complex', in which every male child is in love with his mother and jealous of his father, but also for the way that it deals with identification in terms of violence and oral incorporation so as to justify patriarchal authority. For Freud the totem meal takes on psychological momentum, since it symbolises identification with the paternal figure as a case of love/hate, simultaneously allowing the brothers to expiate their guilt for having killed him and to commemorate their stake in patriarchal power by 'cannibalising' him or wanting to be like him:

> The violent primal father had doubtless been the feared and envied model of each one of the company of brothers: and in the act of devouring him they accomplished their identification with him, and each one of them acquired a portion of his strength. The totem meal, which is perhaps mankind's earliest festival, would thus be a repetition and a commemoration of this memorable and criminal deed, which was the beginning of so many things – of social organization, of moral restrictions and of religion.[80]

But how are we to square Freud's symbolisation of parricide and power with the depiction of Alex in Smithfields Meat Market? That is, are we necessarily to assume that the totemic animal flesh she desires stands in for the father's body? Is cannibalisation of the father's body by the daughter a possibility, and if so, at what cost? And would not such an interpretation contradict the maternal identification that I have already argued the tropes of the spread represent? While Freud does not entirely provide answers to these questions, he does, of course, pave the way to an understanding that oral incorporation and identification are not just to do with the fulfilment of male desires. Indeed, in 'The Ego and the Id' (1923) Freud contends that in the pre-Oedipal phase of development the child's identity is inextricably bound up with the mother's body through breast feeding and other forms of oral gratification: 'At the very beginning, in the individual's primitive oral phase, object-cathexis and identification are no doubt indistinguishable from each other.'[81] And in 'Group Psychology and the Analysis of the Ego' (1922), although he argues that identification and desire 'subsist side by side',[82] he nonetheless portrays identification as an ambivalent process that can 'turn into an expression of tenderness as easily as into a wish for someone's removal'.[83]

Indeed, there is a complex triangulation in the image of Alex with the turkeys that seems to portray identity as something that is similarly *en procès*, that is, as Kristeva puts it, something that is simultaneously 'in process' and 'on trial'.[84] For here, not only do we observe the female model and the dead birds, but on the left of the picture a seated male figure wearing a white coat. As I have already assessed it, the uninterested poses of the male and female figures and role of the gaze in this photograph are strategic in connoting the sense of isolation that the anorexic craves in the act of bingeing. But, decoded in the context of the tension between identification and oral gratification, could not the male presence now also serve to symbolise the abjection of paternal authority by the 'daughter', while the animal flesh at which the model intently stares like a stealthy cat transfixed by her prey and that she seemingly wishes to incorporate, stands in for the 'primitive', maternal love object that we either try to recuperate or try to escape from without success? Perhaps Kristeva brings us closer to the dualities of such an interpretation when she speaks of abjection as a state that 'strays on the territories of *animal*', and describes the desire 'to release the hold of *maternal* identity' as 'a violent, clumsy breaking away, with the constant risk of falling back under the sway of a power as securing as it is stifling'.[85]

'Glutton Dressed as Glam'

Finally, as Kristeva also expresses it, an abject relationship to food is not just a case of rejecting one's parents but a concomitant revulsion from the self: 'But since the food is not an "other" for "me", who am only in their desire, I expel *myself*, I spit *myself* out, I abject *myself* within the same motion through which "I" claim to establish myself.'[86] Here Kristeva seems to nod in the direction of a third form of abjection that is achieved through the resolution of the Oedipal Complex and the emergence of the individuated ego in the Symbolic order, and that manifests itself bodily in signs of sexual difference such as menstruation and giving birth: 'Menstrual blood . . . stands for the danger issuing from within the identity (social or sexual); it threatens the relationship between the sexes within a social aggregate and, through internalization, the identity of each sex in the face of sexual difference.'[87] This stage of sexual development is, therefore, of particular physiological and psychological significance to women, since it not only marks them off or objectifies them as what is outside or Other to the male subject but as the Other of the self as well. Thus the liminal identity of an ego in crisis that this kind of abjection implies is evidenced in the ostensible blurring between adult and adolescent bodies throughout both 'Under Exposure' and 'Alex Eats'. But is given a more pronounced psychosexual spin in one of the pictures from the latter spread representing the model sitting in disarray on a toilet at Maison Bertaux, Soho, wearing a vest, bloomers and a wig, and looking as if she has just been caught up in some transgressive act (Figure 29).

The picture is redolent of a photograph of a model sitting on a toilet with her tights rolled down taken by Jeanloup Sieff for *Nova* (March 1972), and, indeed, Gordon may even have been influenced by him. Both images are clearly disconcerting, and although Sieff's image was published 'despite the management's reservations', it is also much less ambiguous than Gordon's, and its self-referential status as a fashion photograph is connoted by the way the model has been posed looking at the portfolio of *Vogue* tearsheets at her feet.[88] In contrast, in Figure 29 the floor is littered with discarded potato chip packets, and the model's face is besmirched with what appears to be cream, an ambiguous detail that alludes to the fact that she is situated in the toilet of a popular patisserie and that, at first, seems to symbolise the fact that she has just thrown up. But the tousled wig she is seen readjusting, her stunned expression and the location of the toilet in London's red light district also evoke prostitution and, more particularly, the cream around her mouth seems to connote the proverbial male money shot that is commonly enacted in hard-core movies, an idea that is additionally compounded in the final, 'climactic' picture of the fashion spread in which Alex dribbles yogurt all over her clothing.[89] In both instances, therefore, we seem to witness the abject body, with its fixation on oral and anal forms of pleasure, in the guise of the melancholic who transmutes her failure to grieve for the lost (maternal) love object and inability to transfer her desires elsewhere into adverse behaviour and self-debasement that lead to 'an impoverishment of the ego on a grand scale'.[90]

The picture of Alex in Maison Bertaux is also significant, however, in the way that the masquerade we observe seems to evoke the tension between being both self and other that Lacan argues is enacted in the mirror phase. For it is as if Alex becomes a fully-fledged Magdalen by virtue of having to play the part; and even then, unconvincingly. On the one hand, the wig she wears seems to dissemble the innocent persona of the girl that her cropped hairstyle in the other images symbolises. But on the other, her startled demeanour and the way that she awkwardly adjusts the tousled tresses of the wig to ensure a perfect fit, suggest that this is a sexual identity that is provisional and under threat of being unmasked. Here the tables have been turned, and the imaginary ego, rather than guaranteeing the vision of a more complete and desirable identity, returns to us the grotesque, the body in pieces. Thus, as Kristeva contends: 'Abjection ... is a precondition of narcissism. It is coexistent with it and causes it to be permanently brittle. The more or less beautiful image in which I behold or recognize myself rests upon an abjection that sunders it as soon as repression, the constant watchman, is relaxed.'[91]

Conclusion

What I have tried to argue in this chapter, in keeping with Susan Sontag, is the idea that, 'fashion photography is much more than the photography of fashion'.[92] Consequently, as we have seen, any serious analysis of the iconography of fashion must take into account not only the complex intersection of concerns and interests relating to both producers and consumers, but also the ways in which it generates meanings for the body with respect to sex, gender and identity. The polemic concerning the imputed pornography and paedophilia of Day's imagery, for example, clearly raises important issues concerning reality and representation by circumscribing the body as a crucial site for the exercise and regulation of pleasure and power. However, as I have attempted to assess it here, the discursive body can be accounted for from several other meaningful perspectives rather than being mired exclusively in debates around the binarism of pornography and erotica. Hence a more productive way of framing both the work of Day and Gordon, I feel, has been to discuss them in the context of female spectatorship, and the ideal of the underdeveloped or abject adult female body and the psychosexual identities that this implies.

There are, of course, obvious differences concerning the production and circulation of the two pieces of work – one representing a highly publicised supermodel, the other a relatively unknown subject (Alex Arts, an American model, who had previously appeared in 'Beached bums – or sex and the shingle girl', also photographed by Anthony Gordon and styled by Simon Foxton for *The Face*, December 1987); one executed by a male, the other by a female photographer; and one circulated in a vehicle for youth culture, the other in a high-fashion magazine. Nonetheless, they can also be seen to be linked in terms of content and instrumentality. Both spreads, for example, are indicative of the disruptive or transgressive potential that fashion photography displays in its representation of young female bodies in various states of undress and sexualised poses. At the same time, as we have assessed them here, these images seem to connote the erosion between private and public spheres of experience and visibility; Kate Moss is seen trying on different types of underwear in the intimacy of her own home, while Alex Arts is represented wearing hers as she proceeds through various establishments in London like some kind of proto-bulimic in search of the ultimate alimentary fix. In both spreads, therefore, identity is represented as a case of not totally belonging to one's cultural context, or at least to what passes as the real world, but to some degree being out of place in it. Finally, it is as if the disjunction between interior and exterior spaces and the activities that take place in them has been unified by the scopophilic gaze of both models and the conflation of their desire to be both the looker/*voyeur* and the looked at/ *surveillée*. Thus, we can observe fashion photography play with our own desires and fears and appreciate how the discursive body appears, as Barthes expresses it in *The Fashion System*, to represent the fundamental dilemma of all human existence, 'Who Am I?'[93]

Notes

1. Ann K. Clark, 'The Girl: a rhetoric of desire', *Cultural Studies*, 1:2 (May 1987), pp. 195, 197 and 202.

2. Unfortunately it has not been possible to clear copyright either with British *Vogue* or Corinne Day to reproduce 'Under Exposure'.

3. M. Hume, 'When fashion is no excuse at all', *The Independent* (26 May 1993), p. 22.

4. L. Alford, 'Don't get your knickers in a twist over fashion', *The Observer* (30 May 1993), p. 52.

5. V. Williams, 'Agenda benders', *The Guardian Weekend* (4 September 1993), p. 21.

6. *The Face* (May 1988), p. 10. D. Brown, Manchester, England complained: 'What has happened to the fashion photography in your magazine? Once the reader got clear, full length photos of models in smart, attractive clothes . . . Instead we are given soft focus images of turkeys, or cream cakes and models with toothache.' In fact, after 1983 *The Face* rarely printed full-length photos of models of the type that Brown refers to, as my research has revealed. The second reader's letter, entitled 'A boffin explains', is discussed more fully in the main text.

7. Interview with Amy Raphael, *The Face* (August 1993), p. 38.

8. *The Observer* (30 May 1993), p. 52.

9. D. Hebdige, *Subculture: The Meaning of Style* (London, 1979), p. 17, argues that incorporation involves: 'a struggle for the possession of the sign which extends to even the most mundane areas of everyday life'. See also pp. 92–9 for a fuller assessment of incorporation and Punk during the late 1970s, and P. Jobling and D. Crowley, *Graphic Design: Reproduction and Representation Since 1800* (Manchester and New York, 1996), Chapter 7, pp. 237–40, which examines incorporation in the context of the underground press.

10. R. Barthes, 'The Photographic Message', in S. Sontag (ed.) *Barthes: Selected Writings* (London, 1983), pp. 194–210. See also Parts I and II of this work for a fuller exposition of Barthes' writing on photography.

11. See K. Walton, 'Transparent pictures: on the nature of photographic realism', *Critical Inquiry*, 11 (1984), p. 255.

12. See 'Siding With Rosie', *New Statesman* (20 September 1996), p. 5.

13. E. Mills, 'Kittens on the catwalk', *The Observer* (12 May 1996), p. 5.

14. 'Are these photographs offensive?', *Independent on Sunday* (30 May 1993), p. 22. Jane Kilpatrick is quoted as saying: 'The pictures don't strike me as offensive: I just looked at them and thought "That's Kate Moss." I definitely think she looks over 16, and our concern is when under-16s are used for sexual purposes to reinforce the idea of the child as a valid sexual being. Women have been portrayed in vulnerable positions before and I would count her as a young woman.' Kilpatrick was among 12 correspondents whose opinions on 'Under Exposure' were solicited.

15. 'Jeans ads dropped after protestors see blue', *The Guardian* (29 August 1985), pp. 1 and 2.

16. See T. Timblick, 'Ads on the Offensive', *Observer Magazine* (7 June 1992), pp. 24–6.

17. Two useful discussions concerning the nature of pornography and erotica are to be found in Part III of L. Nead, *The Female Nude: Art, Obscenity and Sexuality* (London and New York, 1992), and K. Myers, 'Fashion 'n' passion', *Screen*, 23:3–4 (1982).

18. The US Senate passed its appropriations bill (HR 2788) on 26 July 1989; this contained the Helms amendment forbidding the NEA 'to promote, disseminate or produce' any obscene or indecent materials depicting 'sadomasochism, homo-eroticism, the exploitation of children or individuals engaged in sex acts'. See J. Tannenbaum, 'Robert Mapplethorpe: The Philadelphia Story', *Art Journal*, 50:4 (1991), p. 76.

19. See: M. N. Cohen, *Lewis Carroll's Photograph's of Nude Children* (Phila-delphia, 1978); Susan H. Edwards, 'Pretty Babies – Art, Erotica or Kiddie Porn?', *History of Photography*, 18:1 (Spring 1994), pp. 38–46; K. Dieckmann, 'Immediate family', *The Village Voice Literary Supplement* (November 1992), p. 15; M. Bywater, 'If Mapplethorpe made me a pervert, then there's always Esther Rantzen to save me', *New Statesman* (20 September 1996), pp. 38–9; and A. Ginsberg and J. Richey, 'The Right to Depict Children in the Nude', pp. 42–5, and Edward de Grazia, 'The Big Chill: Censorship and the Law', p. 50 in *The Body in Question* (New York, 1990).

20. *Report of the Committee on Obscenity and Film Censorship*, Chairman, Bernard Williams (London, 1979), Cmnd. 7772. The Williams Report sought to restrict the *public* display of pornography in the interests of those who might find it offensive; Avedon Carol quoted in M. El-Faizy, 'The naked and the deadly', *The Guardian Media* (6 December, 1993), p. 11. FAC also believe that the attention paid to pornography is a distraction from the real, social problems, such as low pay and childcare, that many women have to face in patriarchal culture.

21. P. Holland, 'What Is A Child?', in P. Holland, J. Spence and S. Watney (eds), *Photography/Politics Two* (London, 1986).

22. Ibid., p. 43.

23. Ibid., p. 44.

24. The Miss Pears competition ran in Britain between 1958 and 1997. In 1997 Lever Brothers, the company who manufacture Pears soap, decided to reposition the brand as a 'grown-up' product aimed at the 20-to-30 age group.

25. The winner of the final Miss Pears title, 'Ella from the West Country', was only three years old and, apparently, an unwilling participant in the contest. N. Gerrard, 'Little girls lost', *The Observer Review* (31 August 1997), p. 5 records that: 'She didn't want to be here, in a big hall surrounded by strangers . . . She wanted her mummy but her mummy wasn't there.'

26. L. Williams, 'Second Thoughts on *Hard Core*, American Obscenity Law and the Scapegoating of Deviance', in Pamela Church Gibson and Roma Gibson (eds), *Dirty Looks, Women. Pornography. Power* (London, 1993), p. 48.

27. See, for example, N. Strossen, *Defending Pornography, Free Speech, Sex and the Fight for Women's Rights* (Abacus, 1996) and F. V. Hoover III, *Beefcake: The*

Muscle Magazines of America 1950–1970 (Cologne, 1995). Strossen's central thesis is that censorship laws work against women's rights, and she records that 40 per cent of porn video rental in the US is attributed to women.

28. J. Wicke, 'Through a Gaze Darkly, Pornography's Academic Market', in *Dirty Looks* (1993), p. 79.

29. See David Edgar, 'Shocking Entertainment?', *The Guardian Media* (1 March 1997), p. 3.

30. *Independent on Sunday* (30 May 1993), p. 22.

31. S. Edwards, *History of Photography* (Spring 1994), p. 45.

32. Ibid., p. 45.

33. L. Alford, *The Observer* (30 May 1993), p. 52.

34. M. Hume, *The Independent* (26 May 1993), p. 22.

35. L. Horsburgh, 'Seize the Day', *British Journal of Photography* (8 July 1993), p. 17.

36. See K. Flett, 'sex, success and the single girl . . . exposed', *Arena* (July/August 1992), pp. 88–95) in which Von Unwerth 'cites Helmut Newton as an influence', (p. 89).

37. L. Irigaray, 'The Power of Discourse and the Subordination of the Feminine', in *This Sex Which Is Not One*, trans. Catherine Porter (Ithaca, NY, 1985), p. 124.

38. J. F. Lyotard, *The Differend: Phrases in Dispute*, trans George Van Den Abeele (Minneapolis, 1988), p. 9.

39. The film is based on a short story by Julio Cortazar. The character Hemmings plays treats fashion models like mindless zombies; in one of the most notorious sequences in the movie he is represented straddling the supine model Veruschka as if he is 'making love' to her with his camera.

40. In the opening scenes from the film, Hemmings is seen leaving a dosshouse in the east end of London where he has been taking documentary photographs for his forthcoming book.

41. D. O'Donaghue, *Lifestyles and Psychographics* (London, 1989), p. 64.

42. Reina Lewis and Katrina Rolley, 'Ad(dressing) the dyke. Lesbian looks and lesbian looking', in P. Horne and R. Lewis (eds), *Outlooks – Lesbian and Gay Sexualities and Visual Cultures* (London and New York, 1996), pp. 178–90.

43. J. Lacan, *The Four Fundamental Concepts of Psychoanalysis*, trans. Alan Sheridan (New York, 1978), pp. 84 and 83.

44. L. Mulvey, 'Visual Pleasure and Narrative Cinema', in idem, *Visual and Other Pleasures* (Basingstoke, 1989), p. 19.

45. 'Afterthoughts on "Visual Pleasure and Narrative Cinema"', ibid., pp. 29–38.

46. R. Coward, 'Innocence made ripe for the plucking', *The Observer* (26 September 1993), p. 21.

47. See J. Lacan, 'The Meaning of the Phallus' (1958) in *Écrits, A Selection*, trans. A. Sheridan (New York, 1977).

48. The role of maternal identification also finds expression in the work of Nancy Chodorow, 'Family structure and feminine personality' in M. Z. Rosaldo and L.

Lamphere (eds), *Women, Culture and Society* (Stanford, CA, 1974), pp. 49–66 and Eugénie Lemoine-Luccioni, *Partage des femmes* (Paris: Éditions du Seuil, 1976). Sections of the latter are translated into English in S. Heath, 'Difference', *Screen*, 19:13 (1978).

49. Julia Kristeva, *Desire in Language: A Semiotic Approach to Literature and Art*, ed. L. S. Roudiez (New York, 1980), p. 239; L. Irigaray, 'The Bodily Encounter With The Mother', *Sexe et Parentes*, trans. D. Macey in M. Whitford (ed.), *The Irigaray Reader* (Oxford, 1991), pp. 44–5.

50. Kristeva, *Desire in Language*, p. 239.

51. Whitford, *The Irigaray Reader*, pp. 44–5.

52. Horne and Lewis, *Outlooks*, p. 183.

53. D. Fuss, 'Fashion and the homospectatorial look', *Critical Inquiry*, 18:4 (Summer 1992), pp. 721–8.

54. S. Freud, *New Introductory Lectures on Psycho-analysis* (1932), in J. Strachey (ed.), *The Standard Edition, Vol. 22* (London, 1964), p. 63.

55. Fuss, *Critical Inquiry*, p. 730.

56. See L. Wolf (ed.), *The Essential Dracula* (New York and London, 1993). André Gide in his autobiography *Si Le Grain Ne Meurt* (*If It Die . . .*, 1950 [1920]), offers an interesting perspective on the idea of the homosexual vampire. Describing his visit to a disreputable bar in Algiers with his companion Daniel B. and Arab catamite Mohammed, and the former's subsequent buggering of the latter, he writes: 'As he bent over the little body he was covering, he was like a huge vampire feasting on a corpse. I could have screamed with horror. . . I was horrified both by Daniel's behaviour and by Mohammed's complacent submission to it.' See, A. Gide, *If It Die . . .*, trans. D. Bussy (London, 1950), pp. 284–5.

57. S. Freud, 'Beyond the Pleasure Principle' (1920) in J. Strachey (ed.), *The Standard Edition, Vol. 18* (1955), pp. 1–64. In this essay Freud discusses both the idea of repetition in the *fort/da* game (p. 15), which he extrapolated was the child's way of compensating for the absence of his mother, and the compulsion of the ego instincts, which he associated with the body, towards infirmity and death. This is how he describes the *fort/da* game he observed: 'The child had a wooden reel with a piece of string tied round it ... What he did was to hold the reel by the string and very skilfully throw it over the edge of his curtained cot, so that it disappeared into it . . . He then pulled the reel out of the cot again by the string and hailed its reappearance with a joyful "*da*" ("There"). This, then, was the complete game – disappearance and return.'

58. Julia Kristeva, *Revolution in Poetic Language*, trans. M. Waller (New York, 1984), p. 27.

59. In a footnote to 'Three Essays on Sexuality' [1905], which he added in 1920, Freud observes, 'We are justified in speaking of a castration complex in women as well. Both male and female children form a theory that women no less than men originally had a penis, but that they have lost it by castration.' See, Freud, *On Sexuality*, trans. J. Strachey, ed. A. Richards (Harmondsworth, 1977), p. 113, n. 2. The idea of the maternal penis is also raised in the following essays in *On Sexuality*:

'The Sexual Theories of Children' [1908], p. 196; 'Fetishism' [1927], p. 352; and 'The Infantile Genital Organization' [1923], p. 311, n.2. This last reference is based on one of his case studies and portrays attachment to the female penis more specifically as a form of pathological neurosis: 'I learnt from the analysis of a young married woman who had no father but several aunts that she clung, until quite far on in the latency period, to the belief that her mother and her aunts had a penis.'

60. M. Gross, *Model, The Ugly Business of Beautiful Women* (London, 1995) p. 420.

61. S. Bordo, *Unbearable Weight, Feminism, Western Culture and the Body* (Berkeley, CA. 1993), p. 103. An interesting discussion of bulimia as a form of female fetishism can also be found in L. Gamman and M. Makinen, *Female Fetishism: A New Look* (London, 1994).

62. See Arthur W. Frank, 'For a Sociology of the Body: An Analytical Review', in M. Featherstone, M. Hepworth and B. S. Turner (eds), *The Body – Social Process and Cultural Theory* (London, 1991), pp. 56–7.

63. N. Wolf, *The Beauty Myth* (London, 1991), p. 185.

64. J. Caputi, 'One Size Does Not Fit All: Being Beautiful, Thin and Female in America', in C. Geist and J. Nachbar (eds), *The Popular Culture Reader* (Bowling Green, Ohio, 1983), p. 195.

65. For a fuller discussion of eating disorders see J. Brumberg, *Fasting Girls: The Emergence of Anorexia Nervosa as a Modern Disease* (Cambridge, MA, 1988); Bordo, *Unbearable Weight*; Wolf, *The Beauty Myth*; and Morag MacSween, *Anorexic Bodies – A Feminist and Sociological Perspective on Anorexia Nervosa* (London and New York, 1993).

66. *The Face* (May 1988), p. 10. See also Note 6. Psychologist Iain Williams of Huddersfield University proposes a similar point of view to Lavender, contending: 'it's like saying girls with anorexia want to look like supermodels. It makes them seem passive, without looking at the fact that their diet might be the only thing in their life over which they feel they have control.' See C. Hammond, 'Thin end of the Reg', *The Guardian G2* (16 September 1997), p. 13.

67. D. Hebdige, 'The bottom line on Planet One – Squaring up to THE FACE', *Ten.8*, No.19 (1985), p. 41.

68. Lavender, *The Face* (May 1988).

69. See J. Brumberg, *Fasting Girls*.

70. D. M. Lowe, *The Body in Late-Capitalist USA* (Durham, NC, 1995), p. 174.

71. MacSween, *Anorexic Bodies*, pp. 231 and 233.

72. M. Bakhtin, *Rabelais and His World* (Cambridge, MA, 1968), p. 226.

73. Ibid., p. 281.

74. MacSween, *Anorexic Bodies*, p. 235.

75. Julia Kristeva, *Powers of Horror: An Essay in Abjection*, trans. L. S. Roudiez (New York, 1982, [1980]), pp. 9–10.

76. Ibid., pp. 2–3.

77. MacSween, *Anorexic Bodies*, p. 235.

78. Kristeva, *Powers of Horror*, p. 3.

79. See G. Bataille, 'The Big Toe', *Documents*, Vol. 1, No.6 (1929) and 'Mouth', *Documents*, Vol. 2, No.5 (1930).

80. Freud, 'Totem and Taboo' (1913), in J. Strachey (ed.), *The Standard Edition*, Vol.13, pp. 141–2.

81. See S. Freud, *On Metapsychology* (Harmondsworth, 1984), p. 368.

82. See S. Freud, *Civilization, Society and Religion* (Harmondworth, 1985), p. 134.

83. Ibid., p. 134.

84. J. Kristeva, *Revolution In Poetic Language* (1974), trans. M. Waller (1984); see T. Moi (ed.), *The Kristeva Reader* (Oxford, 1986), p. 91.

85. Kristeva, *Powers of Horror*, pp. 12–13.

86. Ibid., p. 3.

87. Ibid., p. 71.

88. See D. Gibbs (ed.), *Nova 1965–1975 – THE Style Bible of the 60s and 70s* (London, 1993), pp. 132–3.

89. The money shot is the term used to describe the way that the male sex worker ejaculates on the female body to demonstrate that orgasm has taken place. The gender implications of this practice and the way that the male's climax is taken to stand in for that of both partners are discussed by L. Williams in *Hard Core: Power, Pleasure and the "Frenzy of the Visible"*, (Berkeley, 1989). Williams regards the money shot as 'the very limit of the visual representation of sexual pleasure' (p. 101).

90. Freud, 'Mourning and Melancholia' (1917) in *On Metapsychology*, p. 254.

91. Kristeva, *Powers of Horror*, p. 13.

92. S. Sontag, 'The Avedon Eye', British *Vogue* (December 1978), pp. 104–7.

93. R. Barthes, *The Fashion System*, trans. M. Ward and R. Howard (Berkeley, 1990), p. 257.

7

'Statue Men': The Phallic Body, Identity and Ambiguity in Fashion Photography

He reached Q. Very people in the whole of England ever reach Q . . . But after Q? . . . Z is only reached once by one man in a generation. Still, if he could reach R it would be something.

Virginia Woolf, *To the Lighthouse*, 1926.

Introduction: Active or Passive?

Although men had been represented in fashion imagery in Britain before the 1980s in magazines such as *Vogue* and *About Town*, it was not until the launch of titles like *The Face*, *Blitz* and *i.D.* in 1980 that their presence at least became more common, and the concept of an unproblematic, normative masculinity began to be contested.[1] It is not for nothing, therefore, that many feminist writers, including Ros Coward, Julia Kristeva, and Hélène Cixous, have commented on the way that patriarchy has been concerned with keeping men out of the picture. Coward, for example, writing in *Female Desires* (1985), remarked: 'Somewhere along the line, men have managed to keep out of the glare, escaping from the relentless activity of sexual definitions. In spite of the ideology which would have us believe that women's sexuality is an enigma, it is in reality men's bodies, men's sexuality which is the true "dark continent" of this society'.[2]

In a similar vein, Kristeva has argued that self-representation for men is always potentially 'something to be scared of',[3] while Cixous has contested that: 'men still have everything to say about their sexuality, and everything to write'.[4] Such criticisms are certainly valid; but, I feel, they are also prone to some qualification. More accurately, what seems to be the motive behind them is the idea, not that men have been entirely absent from representation, but that the myth of an active and patriarchal masculinity has tended to predominate. Until the homoerotic work of photographers like Bruce Weber and Herb Ritts began to appear in fashion and advertising during the 1980s, for example, the norm in fashion photography had been to connote masculinity in exclusively heterosexual terms. This is evident in the way that men appeared either as a partner to the female model, as in 'Amoureuse' (*Elle*, 16 June 1958), or, if represented with other men or on their own, in stereotypically male poses, activities and milieux.[5] Even if a male model was known to be gay, as was the case with Horst during the 1930s,[6] or there had been some blurring at the edges of strict gender positioning, as occurred during the 1960s with the impact of mod culture and the reinsurgence of the male peacock,[7] men were keen to portray themselves, at least in terms of their bodily desires, as being unequivocally straight. Consequently, Marc Bolan could comment that, 'Mod was mentally a very homosexual thing, though not in any physical sense.'[8] And in 1971, actor-singer Ken Rodway was reluctant to admit that he sometimes worked as a model in case people thought he was 'a bit soft'.[9] Much of this chauvinist posturing still remains intact today, with many male fashion models protesting their heterosexuality in a culture in which narcissism or creativity are often equated with being gay. The American male supermodel, Hoyt Richards, for example, has testified to the way that the fashion industry forced both him and his family to confront their own, latent homophobia.[10]

In recent years, however, there have also been some interesting developments in the representation of gender and sexuality in fashion iconography, and men have been depicted unashamedly as narcissists, preening and showing off their well-honed bodies. As we have just mentioned, this has tended towards a patently homoerotic photographic style that can be attributed to Weber and Ritts (Figures 35 and 42). But it also finds expression in the work of many other photographers and stylists, including Michel Haddi, Nick Knight, and Jamie Morgan and Ray Petri (Figures 9, 16–17 and 38–41). Moreover, with the advent of so-called androgynous models like Nick Moss (brother of Kate Moss), and the wraith-like appearance of grunge models such as Keith Martin and Jerome during the early 1990s, an alternative and more indeterminate vision of the types of bodies that 'real' men are supposed to inhabit appeared to be on the agenda. While few of this new generation appear to be as muscle-bound as most other male models, nor are the majority of them exactly diminutive, however. Martin, for example, standing at over six feet tall with a 40-inch chest, is comparable in stature to Joel West, whose rippling muscles have been clearly displayed in advertisements for Calvin Klein underwear and Escape Cologne. It is often by virtue of the way that they have been photographed and the fashions they are seen modelling, therefore, that male models like Moss and Martin appear vulnerable or languid (Figure 10).[11] Consequently, in examining how masculinity has been represented in fashion photography between 1980 and 1995, my intention in this chapter is to unpack one of its most persistent tropes – the ideal of the muscular or phallic body – and to expand on some of the ambiguities in the objectification of sexuality and ethnicity that this implies.

Lacan argued in 'The Mirror Stage' that the erect, phallic body may be regarded as a petrified, immobile form, a 'statue in which man projects himself'.[12] Certainly, the iconography of muscular men in many fashion spreads and advertisements seems to trade on an ideal of rigidity and solidity, as demonstrated in 'grease monkeys', for example (Figure 35). But by no means should their taut bodies and flexed poses lead us to believe that masculine identities are either perpetually uniform or immutable. For, as I discuss in more detail in this chapter, the intertexuality of word and image in 'grease monkeys' also demonstrates that the muscular body may be represented as being hard and soft, or active and passive, at one and the same time. What I am arguing here, therefore, is that the ideal of the hard statue provides only the illusion of a stable and permanently frozen ego. Consequently, in explicating how the masculine body is constructed as a site of power and pleasure in the discourse of fashion publishing, my intention is to queer the pitch somewhat by drawing on certain aspects of psychoanalytic theory and the concept of gender as performativity. By extension, in suggesting that there is often an imbrication or tension between active and passive gender identities, and straight and gay sexualities, in terms of both the production and consumption of such imagery, this examination of male bodies serves to parallel the analysis of femininities pursued in my discussion of 'Alex Eats' and 'Under Exposure' in the last chapter.

The Advent of New Man

If it is at all possible to identify an exact point in time when we can discern the objectification of masculinities beginning to be queered in fashion photography, then the advent of new man, *circa* 1984, is probably as close as we get. Thus, as we have already assessed it in Part II, new man became common currency in media circles, if not in society at large, to describe the consumerist ethos of a certain constituency of British males (arguably, white-collar professionals, aged 18–35 years old). The term itself, however, was somewhat ambiguous and loosely-defined, and was gradually used to sum up several different masculine typologies, from style leaders in fashion to the more emotionally-centred, caring, sharing partner or father figure.[13] Furthermore, new man was something of a cliché by the mid-1980s, and we can find several earlier examples of the prototype before this time. As early as 1829, for example, the social and political reformer William Cobbett (1763–1835) had encouraged men to get in touch with the emotional and caring side of their personalities. Although he could scarcely be regarded as a supporter of feminism, in his treatise on family life, *Advice to Young Men*, he nonetheless acknowledged that the husband should contribute to domestic tasks and chores so as to maintain a virtuous household.[14] Between 1880 and 1910, debates on sexuality and the rise of the feminist movement once more led to the rhetoric of the new man,[15] and in 1919 a pamphlet entitled *New Man* was published by C. J. Welton, containing subjects that, as the anonymous author put it: 'no other writer in England has ever dared to broach' (the subjects being impotency, courting and the mysteries of married life).[16]

The new man of the 1980s, therefore, has to be placed in the wider historical context of debates on gender and sexuality, although we should be wary of simply regarding him as of a piece with his antecedents, not least in terms of his attitude towards narcissism and style culture. By 1994, for instance, the male beauty industry was worth £469 millions in Britain, an increase of 26 per cent in value terms since 1985.[17] Indeed, for many commentators it is precisely on account of such consumerist values that the epiphany of new man during the 1980s can be explained away as nothing more than a fiction or case of media hype that had but little impact on patriarchal power structures, or the way that the average male treated his body. Style guru Peter York called him an advertiser's invention, who was driven by 'greed, corruption and treachery',[18] and Judith Williamson concurred, stating: 'the key fact about the new man is that he doesn't exist'.[19] This perspective on new man is born out by findings in Mintel's *Men 2000* report, published in 1993, in which only 18 per cent of those consulted admitted that men were contributing to domestic chores and matters of child-raising.[20] It is in this regard that we seem to be dealing with new man as a form of popular mythology or, more specifically, a type of ideal body effected by process of what Barthes has called inoculation. For, as he argues, it is through such acts of inoculation, which admit only a controlled amount of change or subversive activity to take place, that society immunises 'the contents of the collective imagination', and thereby maintains its original hegemonic order.[21] But even if this is the case, we would still have to make sense of new man as a cultural construct, however limited that may be, and to argue whether and to what extent we are dealing with the redefinition of masculinities, if not in reality, then idealistically in media texts like advertising and periodicals intended for fashionable male readers such as *The Face* (founded 1980), *Unique* (July 1986–December 1987), *Arena* (founded November 1986), *FHM* (founded 1987), and the British edition of

GQ (founded 1988). An instructive way of approaching this set of problems is to deconstruct one of the most common new man figures to be found in the iconography of fashion since the early 1980s, that is, the muscular or phallic body.

Between Straight and Gay: Whose Hard Body is it Anyway?

Like new man, this type of body in itself was hardly new in either cinematic discourse or that of advertising, although it was not really until after 1980 that men were photographed ingenuously displaying their muscles in fashion magazines. It is not surprising, therefore, to find that several critics have drawn historical parallels between the classical, statue men of contemporary fashion photography and earlier manifestations of muscularity in terms of what has come to be commonly known as body fascism. Alan Klein, for instance, has argued that narcissism and fascism are isologous concepts in bodybuilding culture,[22] while E. Roger Denson has called the iconography of Weber and Ritts: 'the restitution of Nazi metaphors and the perverse recharge of their power as sexual and emotional fetishes'.[23] Here, Denson appears to compound an idea that Susan Sontag had expressed in her critical review of an exhibition of Nazi art in Frankfurt in 1974: 'Nazism fascinates in a way other iconography ... does not ... For those born after the early 1940s, bludgeoned by a lifetime's palaver, pro and con, about communism, it is Fascism – the great conversation piece of their parents' generation – which represents the exotic, the unknown.'[24] Born in 1946 and 1952 respectively, Weber and Ritts were clearly old enough to be members of the generation that, as Sontag puts it, has been 'fascinated by fascism'. With regard to form and content many of their images of muscular male subjects certainly bear more than a passing resemblance to the athletic bodies portrayed by Leni Riefenstahl in her film *Olympiad* (1938).[25]

In many ways, however, this is to miss the point about such imagery, and as Baudrillard suggests: 'it is naive to conclude that the evocation of fascism signals a current renewal of fascism (it is precisely because one is no longer there, because one is in something else, which is less amusing, it is for this reason that fascism can again become fascinating in its filtered cruelty, aestheticized by retro)'.[26] Although the phallic body is a symbol of power, therefore, it would be wrong to think of it purely and simply in terms of its relationship to Nazism or, indeed, as an exclusively heterosexual phenomenon, as the popularity of bodybuilding with both straight and gay men since the early 1980s demonstrates.[27] What is more, the traduction between straight and gay identities that muscularity implies also became evident after 1984 in a wide range of fashion shoots in style magazines intended to appeal to both straight and gay male readers.

One of the earliest, and certainly the most egregious, examples of such sexual double-coding, is 'grease monkeys', which appeared as a five-page spread in *The Face* in October 1984. Here, a series of high-contrast photographs by Herb Ritts of a male model wearing clothes by the cult American designer Stephen Sprouse have been laid out in an eclectic, Neo-Dada cut-and-paste style, with typography by Neville Brody and snippets of text from other sources. In many respects we are once again on the familiar territory of the simulacral fashion masquerade, as written clothing and image-clothing converge to portray both work and working dress as nothing more than an essay in style. But the masquerade also seems to deconstruct a whole series of oppositions: between legitimate and anomic forms of labour; between hard and soft masculinities; and between straight and gay sexualities. This much is established by the introductory editorial that sets the subversive tone and mood for the entire piece:

> From the garages of the New Jersey badlands to the uptown hustlers of Times Square, this fall the real boys on the block are looking dirty. Stephen Sprouse's new collection is functional wear for the working life: fallen angels rub well-oiled shoulders stripped for action under classic and leather jackets, black jersey leggings and cotton jeans. The dirty looks are accessorised with silver knuckle-dusters, meanly studded wrist bands and drop-dead muscles smeared with fistfuls of No Glare, the American footballers' favourite sunscreen, a mixture of petroleum and charcoal. The fresh guys get tough – a dash of axle grease behind the ears, a flick knife for comfort, a lion in your pocket and baby you should be ready to roar.

Here, then, mechanics and hustlers literally rub 'well-oiled shoulders' and 'drop-dead muscles' together in the name of fashion. At the same time, the sweat and grime of real toil are portrayed as nothing more than fashion accessories, and 'dirty looks' can be achieved through the mere application of 'No Glare' sunscreen. Such sexual and social ambiguities are compounded further in the photographs and collaged fragments of text with their *double-entendres*. Thus the bodies and professional roles of the car mechanic and the sex worker are fetishistically conflated in the words and images of one of the layouts from the piece (Figure 35). The first comprises a photograph of the model flexing his muscles while he adopts a somewhat camp pose. He protectively crosses an outstretched, greased hand over his chest, which is juxtaposed with torn-out periodical headlines referring to 'gang violations' and the fact that 'He Works Hard For Your Money'. The second represents a close-up of his hands, which are again greased and decked out with knuckledusters, and clenched as if he were ready to throw a punch like a boxer – a point that is also connoted by the tight leather band around his wrist, on to which the words 'New York Pick Up Line' have been grafted. The confused verbal and visual codes of the piece seem, therefore, to contest the distinction in cause and effect that D. A. Miller, in his highly imaginative essay, *Bringing Out Roland Barthes*, suggests exists between straight and gay men in their mutual pursuit of the mesomorphic ideal. In alluding to the centrality of macho body-image, for example, he maintains:

> Only those who can't tell elbow from ass will confuse the different priorities of the macho straight male body and the so-called gym-body of gay male culture. The first deploys its heft as a *tool* (for work, for its potential and actual intimidation of other, weaker men or of women) – as both an armoured body and a body wholly given over to utility . . . whereas the second displays its muscle primarily in terms of an *image* openly appealing to, and deliberately courting the possibility of being shivered by, someone else's desire.[28]

Certainly, as Alan Klein has demonstrated, the gym is a border territory that permits a kind of institutionalised homosexual 'hustling' and the potentiality of sexual transgression.[29] Yet the difference between the body as *tool* and the body as narcissistic *image* are not necessarily as easy to distinguish in the way that Miller describes. This indeterminacy is evident in the homo-erotic tropes of 'grease monkeys'. But it is also conveyed in several other fashion spreads that problematise the meaning of normative masculinities through the deployment of camp postures, and the reworking of cultural stereotypes such as the cowboy and stud.

In this respect, the role of the cinema appears to be an instrumental factor in the way that many fashion shoots have redefined the boundary between active and passive identities. In 'High Noon' (*Unique*, October/November 1986), for example, images of well-known stars of Westerns such as Clint Eastwood, Charlton Heston and Gary Cooper have been juxtaposed with photographs by Johnny Rosza of male models cavorting in their underwear (Figure 36). Along with the biker, the mechanic and the construction worker, the cowboy is one of several archetypal males whose overt machismo has been subverted and parodied within gay culture since the 1970s. As I have already mentioned in my discussion of *Arena* in Part I, the oscillation between straight and gay identities has, of course, led many manufacturers to tap into the economic power of the pink pound. In the context of my current argument, for example, it is probably worth noting that Marlboro cigarettes realised the sales potential of masquerading its iconic cowboy high on a billboard in New York's Greenwich Village next to another advertisement for gay cruises (Figure 37). But, as Pumphrey has also argued, acts of mimicry like this have not led *tout court* to straight men moving away from such styles and images; rather, dress can be regarded as the prime motivator for a kind of homosocial resistance that affords 'new ways in which . . . men can relate to each other'.[30] This form of masquerade is further exemplified, for instance, by the manufactured, marginal sexual status of the American pop band The Village People. In 1978 they shot to fame with the ambiguously phrased hit single 'YMCA', which was played in both straight and gay discos. Likewise, their eclectic dress code, incorporating the personae of the biker, construction worker, cowboy, red indian and sailor, was a deliberately knowing attempt to exploit a contemporaneous gay style without alienating a straight audience.[31]

The blurring of distinct straight and gay identities that dressing up in uniform engenders, and to which 'High Noon' alludes, is foregrounded further in spreads like 'Close Encounters' (Figures 38–41, to which I shall return later), and 'NYC–Urban Cowboy' (*Arena*, September/October 1987; photographer, Norman Watson; stylist Ray Petri), as well as in the work of Bruce Weber. Like Rosza, Weber traded on the sexual ambiguities of the film industry in his extended photo-essay 'Album. Phototour', produced for the Italian men's fashion magazine *Per Lui* (July/August 1985), and loosely based on a Hollywood film set (Figure 42). At the same time, however, the layout and visual codes of the fashion spread are redolent of the type of imagery to be found in physical culture magazines such as *Physique Pictorial*. Launched in America in 1950 by photographer Bob Mizer, *Physique Pictorial* was one of several titles aimed at a gay readership that managed to circumvent the strict censorship of the McCarthy era by masquerading as bodybuilding or health magazines, and eschewing the use of picture and editorial credits and gay terminology.[32] In its heyday *Physique Pictorial* had a circulation of 40,000 copies, and by the end of 1952 was widely available across both America and Europe.[33] F. Valentine Hooven, III, in his study of post-war bodybuilding magazines, remarked that *Physique Pictorial* 'celebrated the male body with a directness that had not been seen since the collapse of the Roman Empire', and we can see this kind of heroic masculinity literally encoded in the pictures of centurions included in 'Hollywood'.[34]

But while many of Weber's pictures are similar to the homoerotic poses to be discerned in the photographic collages in *Physique Pictorial*, the inclusion of female models (in this instance one dressed as a Roman empress, the other as Madame Bovary, '80s style') transcends the more overt homosociality, if not homosexuality, of the bodybuilding spreads. Moreover, in its simultaneous evocation of both the style and imagery of the physical culture magazines and the way that the narrative structure references a Hollywood film set, the fashion shoot returns us once more to Weber's involvement with post-modern simulation that I discussed in Part 1 with regard to his contribution to British *Vogue*.

A somewhat parallel border-crossing between straight and gay masculinities can also be discerned in 'Throw Back', photographed by Michel Haddi and styled by Debra Berkin for *Arena* (January/February 1988). Here, much as in Weber's 'Phototour', the filming of a movie by director Paul Morrisey, based on the story of a young Brooklyn boy who falls disastrously in love with a Puerto Rican girl, provides an opportunity for a behind-the-scenes fashion shoot featuring several of the film's actors. Although the film's narrative seems to be based exclusively on a heterosexual romance, however, several of Haddi's images portray its male stars adopting more ambivalent poses and gestures that disrupt the conventional masculine codes of the male pin-up Richard Dyer has identified. As Dyer describes it, the male pin-up is never supine and, if not represented directly in action, then his body is always tensed as if to suggest action. In addition, his look must connote self-assurance and confidence; it is direct and staring and never coy or flirtatious in the manner of his female counterpart: 'images of men must disavow this element of passivity if they are to be kept in line with dominant ideas of masculinity-as-activity.'[35] In 'Throw Back', however, one of the male characters has been photographed lying languidly on his back, and as he looks at us he also breaks an inviting and mischievous smile in such a manner as to evoke the idea that he is on the director's casting couch (Figure 16). Thus reference seems to be made here to the closet gay culture of major Hollywood stars, something that was common even after Rock Hudson admitted that he was HIV-positive in 1984. Indeed, Hudson was one of many 1950s and 1960s idols, including James Dean, Montgomery Clift and Sal Mineo, who complied with the film industry's code of silence concerning homosexuality in order to maintain their box-office appeal.[36] The covert or latent homosexuality of the film industry is also connoted in another picture from 'Throw Back' that includes a pair of male bodies; one represented in silhouette and seen from behind, the other bare-chested and looking out of the picture (Figure 17). At first glance, it could be that they are one and the same person: that this is an image of Paul Dillon the actor who is identified at the top of the photograph, staring at himself in the mirror. But the shallow, tenebrous space, the proximity of the male forms and the shadow which is cast behind Dillon lead us to another understanding of the image – that it is, in fact, one representing two men gazing at each other in desire.

Non-white Phallic Bodies

At the same time, nor should the phallic body be regarded as an exclusively white, masculine ideal – see, for example, Figure 24 from 'once upon a time', and 'Hard Edged', photographed by James Martin and styled by David Bradshaw for *Arena* (March/April 1993), which depict the muscular body as the province of both black and white men. It must also be stated at the outset, however, that the frequency of fashion spreads including non-white models is extremely meagre in comparison to those featuring white ones. Of all the spreads listed in Appendix 1, for example, just over 8 per cent represent men and women from more than one race, and of these just over half represent models of one race only, most prevalently Japanese, Afro-Caribbeans and African-Americans. These figures clearly unmask the covert racism of the fashion industry, where just the use of a black face on the cover of a magazine can set sales plummeting by 20 per cent,[37] and in which a mere handful of non-white models seem to have made the grade. In 1990, only six of the 75 models registered with the agency Models One were black, and as Irene Shelley, editor of *Black Beauty and Hair*, attests: 'Most agencies can take only one or two on their books at a time, so the majority of black models end up working part-time at other jobs.'[38] Supermodel Naomi Campbell is probably the most well-known black female working in the fashion business today; but even she admits to losing out to white colleagues when it comes to landing big advertising accounts: 'You've got to understand, this business is about selling, and blonde and blue-eyed girls are what sells.'[39] A similarly restrictive situation seems to pertain for male black models. In 1969, David Mainman established a British modelling agency called Blackboys to help both male and female black models to find work more easily; but since then things have scarcely improved.[40] Of the 92 male models who were represented by Boss in 1996, for example, only four were non-white – Gary Dourdan, Robbie Brooks, Asio and Rod Foster.[41] American Tyson Beckford, who has been modelling since 1993, is perhaps the most high-profile of contemporary black male models, and has appeared regularly in advertisements for Ralph Lauren Polo Sport. But while his distinctive looks are easily recognisable, like most male models he is hardly a household name, and his earning power is also considerably less than that of his black female counterpart Naomi Campbell.[42]

I have already identified two examples of the way that fashion magazines deal with race and ethnicity at the level of what Barthes calls poetic significa-tion in Part 2 of this study (Figure 25). But in the context of the current argument we still need to examine how they come to terms with the phallic body as a non-white entity, and to ask whether there are any significant differences between the representations of white and non-white muscularities. On the surface, the answer to this question in many instances appears to be negative, since black models are represented adopting the same stereotypical, macho poses as white ones – compare the models in Figure 24, for instance – or performing similar heterosexual acts of flirtation, witness Figures 11 and 47. But the aggressive stance of the black male can also be a political one, a point that is amply illustrated by the verbal and visual elements of 'Malcolm X', which appeared in *The Face* in November 1992. Here the photographs, shot on location in Harlem by Albert Watson, and styled by Karl and Derick, appear like stills from Spike Lee's eponymous biopic. At the same time, Malcolm X's reputation for violence is recast in the light of his activities as a scholar and educationalist. Thus we are told:

> The popular image of minister Malcolm X is of a man who preached hate and violence, but there are other, less-publicised images. There was the man of learning who turned a jail cell into his university, copying out every word in the dictionary to improve his handwriting and vocabulary, then devouring books in the prison library. Books remained his passion, and education the core of his message to fellow African-Americans.[43]

Fashion also was a source of inspiration to him in his political activism. The editorial relates how, 'The sober dress code of America's black Muslims reflected their message of self-respect', and the fact that he taught his younger brother to dress well, since 'in order to get something, you had to look as though you already had something'.[44] Consequently, the spread concentrates on the merging of fashion and politics, representing 'Malcolm X' as a stylish demiurge, dressed in sharp suits and designer glasses as he delivers one of his speeches in the name of Islam (Figure 19). It would be misguided to conclude, however, that fashion really can unite subjects from disparate ethnic backgrounds, or transcend racism. Fashionable dress notwithstanding, Malcolm X himself was assassinated while speaking at a public meeting in the Audubon Ballroom in Harlem on 21 February 1965, an incident that is recalled in the final shot of the sequence, depicting one of his nattily-dressed followers carrying a bunch of flowers outside the venue. Moreover, it must be born in mind that the investment of the black male in looking good and in muscularity does not necessarily signify racial equality, but rather racial difference: 'not only must the black man be black; he must be black in relation to the white man'.[45]

In popular white mythology, the identity of the black man has long been bound up with his body, and more particularly with an idea of phallic power that resides in an over-sized penis. As Kobena Mercer puts it: 'the fantasy of the big black willy – that black male sexuality is not only 'different', but somehow 'more' – is a fantasy that many people, black and white, men and women, gay and straight, continue to cling on to'.[46] While Frantz Fanon has argued a similar point, contending, 'the negro is eclipsed. He is turned into a penis. He *is* a penis',[47] for him phallic power connotes not simply the sexuality of the black male but, more significantly, his thirst for freedom. Thus he propounds that the muscular body is a central fantasy for subjects who have been colonised or held in a position of subordination; a symbol of white power and domination that could be turned against itself through a process of mimicry, and that would enable the oppressed black native to attain his independence:

> This is why the dreams of the native are always of muscular prowess; his dreams are of action and of aggression. I dream, I am jumping, swimming, running, climbing; I dream that I burst out laughing, that I span a river in one stride, or that I am followed by a flood of motor-cars which never catch up with me. During the period of colonization, the native never stops achieving his freedom from nine in the evening until six in the morning.[48]

Such a tension between white power and black powerlessness is evident in several of the images included in 'On and Off the Road', photographed by Michel Haddi, and styled by Debra Berkin for the very first issue of *Arena* in 1986, where we observe white and black models cavorting with each other in the woods. In Figure 43, for example, the suggestion is made that the black male is just about to overpower the white one as he springs upon him from behind. But there is also an ambiguity connoted by this image that leaves us pondering whether the act is performed with a sexual motive in mind. This idea is underscored by two more pictures from the spread: in one of them, a black and a white man are seen jubilantly embracing each other, while in the other, two male models perform a double handstand that involves the groin of one pressing against the buttocks of the other. Moreover, 'On and Off the Road' is not exclusive in the way that it mobilises homoeroticism in the context of black masculinities. We find similar images of bonding amongst black men in several other fashion spreads: see for instance, 'Wide Boys Awake', photographed by Martin Brading and styled by Ray Petri for *Arena* (July/August 1988).

Steven Maynard, in his assessment of the white symbolism of advertisements for Calvin Klein men's underwear, contends that 'homoeroticism comes to be defined as white'. But what images like these clearly reveal (as much as Robert Mapplethorpe's photographic studies of priapic black men) is that it can also be coloured non-white.[49] Equally as much, these images contest –

or at least problematise – Fanon's assertion that homosexuality is culturally a white pathology, and something that black men would only ever imitate temporarily as a 'means to a livelihood'.[50] Indeed, the cult of muscularity in the context of post-colonialism leads us to question whether there is still sufficient space between white and non-white phallic bodies for us to agree with Fanon's one-sided view of mimicry as a politically and socially empowering strategy. For, as Homi Bhabha contends, 'mimicry emerges as one of the most elusive and effective strategies of colonial power and knowledge'.[51] That is, while mimicry may initially set out to be a disruptive strategy, it can also end up subtending the colonial system of power it seeks to depose (as represented in the case of 'Malcolm X') and vice versa. Moreover, one must also take into consideration the idea that the cultivation of muscles, rather than necessarily dividing white and non-white male subjects, could unite them in a shared cultural tendency or dialectic of power. For, as I assess it below, since the early 1980s the phallic body has become for many men, whether straight or gay, white or non-white, a way of asserting some kind of self-worth and authority. Now muscles can be seen to signify the transcendence of men's social and political emasculation by feminism and unemployment, as well as appearing to be a defence mechanism against the threat of HIV/ AIDS.

Probably the most extreme and contradictory objectification of transgressive sexuality and racial subordination to be found in any fashion spread since 1980, however, is Nick Knight's image of a muscular, black male model, photographed from behind, and wearing a pair of bottomless aeronaut trousers, which was published to illustrate an article on Punk culture in *The Face*, February 1986 (Figure 44). Mapplethorpe's stylistic influence is not so far away here. But we also encounter a signification of otherness that conflates power and powerlessness in a complex double-coding, and that appears to emasculate the phallic black male subject on two levels. First, he becomes a symbol of a central paradox within the Punk movement; of the way that it appeared, on the one hand, to break with racism and nationalism by espousing reggae music and combating the rise of the National Front, while on the other, it colonised or subjugated black culture in the name of style so as to forge a musical identity that, as Dick Hebdige puts it: 'was emphatically white and even more emphatically British'.[52] Thus, like any self-respecting white punk, we observe him wearing bondage trousers and an emblematic leather eagle stating 'Fuck Off!' (a truncated version of the punk anthem, 'If You Don't Want To Fuck Me, Fuck Off') in an act of anarchic rebellion. But, dress code aside, his pose suggests that he is still under the cultural sway of the 'white master', still tethered by the chains he wears. And not only this, for the mythic sexuality of the black man is also much on display in this photograph, connoted not just by his phallic body but also by the flame-red background of the image. This serves to distinguish him as the hot, exotic Other who inhabits what Sir Richard Burton called the 'Sotadic Zone', that is the sultriest areas of the world close to the equator, where sodomy and sexual licentiousness were allegedly endemic.[53] Although he has been represented as a sex object in this spread, then, it is in a way that runs counter to the priapic stereotype of the oversexed 'black male rapist'.[54] Thus, instead of being equated with his penis, the model has been represented 'from the other side', as it were, and we are given a tantalising glimpse of his buttocks, fetishistically displayed through the gap in his pants. But this is a disquieting detail, inasmuch as it seems simultaneously to harp on the dual nature of Bataille's 'solar anus', which is a site of both pleasure and shame,[55] and to evince the double register of desire and fear that Stuart Hall argues is operative in the representation of black sexualities: 'Just as masculinity always constructs femininity as double – simultaneously Madonna and Whore – so racism constructs the black subject: noble savage and violent avenger. And in the doubling, fear and desire double for one another and play across the structures of otherness, complicating its politics.'[56]

Thus on the one hand, the black punk's spreadeagled pose, bondage trousers, jock strap and chains mark him out as a gay man, or at least the sexually passive sex-slave or object of desire for another man, while on the other, although his identity appears to have been reduced to nothing more than a corporeal one, it is not entirely clear whether he accepts the role of passive love object willingly. Accordingly, as Bhabha argues, the mimicry of subjugation can unexpectedly give rise to opportunities for subversion: 'in occupying two places at once ... the depersonalized, dislocated colonial subject can become an incalculable object, quite literally, difficult to place. The demand of authority cannot unify its messages nor simply identify its subjects.'[57] His pose, for instance, could also suggest an act of resistance: his arms are raised, his fists are clenched, and his taut body is active rather than passive, as if he is just about to break his chains apart. This is a body to be feared and reckoned with, and that admonishes us, literally to 'fuck off!'. Rather than simply accepting his status as the inferior or perverse Other of the white man's gaze, therefore, the black punk we observe here also appears to defy such colonisation. His aggressive pose resists the idea that his own sexuality is docile, that it must always conform to or be imposed on him by the mythology of his own white Other. Consequently, as Hall contends, contemporary representations of the black male body, such as those by Mapplethorpe or fashion images like this, problematise the traditional Manichaean binaries of black/white, straight/gay and active/passive by revealing: 'the unwelcome fact that a great deal of black politics, constructed, addressed and developed in relation to questions of race and ethnicity, has been predicated on the assumption that the categories of gender and sexuality would stay the same and remain fixed and secured'.[58]

Phallogocentrism and Muscularity

In attempting to analyse the ideal of the phallic body within the discourse of fashion photography since the mid-1980s, then, we are confronted by an extremely polysemous entity that seems to symbolise both sublimated desire and fear. It is Mikkel Borch-Jakobsen who probably brings us closer to understanding the psychosexual implications of this type of masculinity when he states in Lacanian terms that the phallic body is a symbolic form of the ego's 'optical erection'.[59] In the classic, phallogocentric economy Lacan posits the phallus as the transcendental signifier of power relations between the sexes in the post-mirror phase of psychosexual development, arguing that there is an overlap beween sexual difference and the acquisition and use of language (or the Symbolic) in the formation of masculine and feminine identities.[60] In other words, he posited a version of psychosexuality based on linguistics or the law of the father, maintaining that once the child is separated from the maternal love object, having lost it to the father figure, he/she becomes both a sexual and a social body, who begins to symbolise and to compensate for the lost object of desire in language and other forms of representation. For Lacan (as for Freud before him), this Oedipal scenario sets up an economy of restraint and prohibition, organised around the threat of castration and the phallic signifier. It is the phallus, which he links to the father figure, that is the central or primary signifier for all forms of desires and repressions, but one that also, in the individual's enacting of the law of the 'name of the father', remains veiled in the unconscious.[61]

This phallogocentric economy implies a perpetual sense of incompleteness or searching for both male and female subjects, since it postulates that the phallus is nothing more than a signifier, an entity without specific meaning in itself that can only open the way to a system of metaphors, a chain of arbitrary and unstable meanings. The power of the phallus, therefore, can be seen to be essentially bogus. But the implications of such powerlessness are nonetheless not the same for both sexes, and the phallus establishes a particular dynamic between them based on 'having' and 'lacking' that leads to the construction of masculinity as active and femininity as passive. One significant way of connoting the power of the male subject is to exaggerate or idealise dominant masculinity in the form of the sturdy, pillar-like body, so that, as Richard Dyer contends: 'When not actually caught in the act, the male image still promises activity by the way the body is posed.'[62] And, of course, this kind of muscular prowess has been a recurring motif in much fashion photography, and is evident, for example, in the hard symbolism of Buffalo Boy (Figure 9), the mythical self-made workers in 'once upon a time' (Figure 24), and the fake militarism of 'Who's Shooting Who?' (Figure 18). However, most of the hard, muscular bodies represented in contemporary fashion and advertising photography appear to be erect by default, even though it takes a lot of time and effort to cultivate muscles. Male stripper Greg Callaghan, for instance, contends that bodybuilders 'go to hell and back to win their Adonis-like physiques', working out in the gym for at least two hours, six days a week.[63] We do not catch so much as a glimpse of such activity in fashion photography, and rarely do we see men actually at work. If we do, work as it is depicted in Figure 35, 'grease monkeys', and in shoots like 'high tension, no-nonsense sportswear working as hard as it plays . . .' in *Arena* (March/April 1994; photographer Christopher Griffiths, stylist David Bradshaw), appears to be nothing more than a form of spectacle, something that, as Barthes argues in *Système de la Mode*, is performed exclusively in the service of being fashionable.[64] This still seems to invite the question: how did these bodies become hard? And, equally as much, we are still left pondering whether all such muscular bodies could be regarded as being unequivocally straight – whether the perverse sexual charge of this overt form of masculinity parallels that of the dandy, who first emerged in the eighteenth century and whose ambiguous eroticism and narcissism reached their apogee in the aestheticism of the late nineteenth century.[65]

Consequently, although the male subject by virtue of his body may be argued 'to have' a phallus, this is a misrecognition of the possession of power. He is, therefore, compelled to compensate for this lack in his domination of the Other who appears less powerful still, that is, woman. Within this framework, woman is cast in the role of the already castrated object who appears to be no more than a passive victim, and who can only attain some sense of recognition, or obtain a phallus, by symbolically 'being' a phallus: that is, by appearing to be the alienated love object that man desires, an act she performs in masquerade.[66]

The Phallic Woman

An interesting spin on such phallogocentrism and the role of the masquerade is discernible in the way that woman is represented as the penis/phallus in fashion photography and advertising. At this point in my discussion, therefore, I feel it will be illuminating to examine how the phallic woman in such contexts can be seen to symbolise another kind of reckoning with the law of the father. Nowhere is this more evident than in those images associated with Surrealism, which, since the 1920s, has proved to be one of the most persistent of the many stylistic options to be found in fashion photography. This much is due in part to the theatricality of fashion itself, which lends itself, to an otherworldly beauty and the possibility of dynamic identity transformation through dress.[67] But it must also be explained in the way that both fashion designers and surrealist artists and writers have tended particularly to fetishise the woman's body. Thus it is hardly surprising to find that there were close links between several fashion designers and members of the surrealist movement during the 1930s. Chanel colloborated with Salvador Dalí, for instance, and Elsa Schiaparelli with Dalí, Jean Cocteau, Cecil Beaton and Horst. Similarly, Molly Fordham, who was editor of British *Vogue* at the same time, discussed the aims and objectives of Surrealism with her readers.[68]

After visiting Max Ernst's Fatagaga exhibition in 1922, which had included a large number of photo-montages, André Breton, leader of the original surrealist movement in France, began to promote the transformative potential of photography. He realised, for instance, that both the camera and the photograph could have a pivotal position in developing automatism, which centred on ideas of the mechanical and transcendence.[69] The chief aesthetic underpinning surrealist practice was the role of the marvellous and Breton's concept that 'Beauty should be convulsive', by which he meant that every being, thing or idea had the propensity for being transformed into something else through representation.[70] There were, moreover, three separate ways of representing convulsive beauty, namely: the *érotique voilée* (veiled erotic); the *explosante-fixe* (fixed explosion); and *magique circonstantielle* (circumstantial magic). The first of these describes a kind of superimposition through which two distinct objects may be signified in the same form, one becoming a metaphor for the other. Man Ray's photograph the *Violon d'Ingres* (1924) exemplifies this approach. Here, a woman wearing a turban has been represented from behind so that she appears like a nude odalisque from a painting by Ingres. At the same time the serpentine outline of her back resembles closely the shape of a violin, and this signification has been underlined by the marking of two symmetrical f-holes on her skin. The second term deals with the capturing of an arrested motion or second of time through which the person or object represented takes on the aspect of another form. This can be discerned in Man Ray's photograph *Explosante-Fixe* (1934), where a woman dancing is suddenly transfixed into the shape of an exotic flower. The final term is perhaps the most complex of the three, since to a certain extent it is based on a more subjective interpretation. This can involve the manipulation of an object not only through visual representation – the strangely paranoic world in Dalí's painting *The Persistence of Memory* (1931), for example, where solid masses appear to liquify into soft forms – but also through totemic hallucination. Hence a chance encounter with a *trouvaille* or found-object can set into action a chain of subconscious associations. In the Spring of 1934, for example, Breton stumbled on a wooden spoon with an intriguing tiny shoe at the tip of its handle in a flea market in Paris, which triggered him to suggest: 'it symbolized for me a woman *unique and unknown*'.[71] On either level, however, the association takes on a personal significance, since the forms that appear to be in a state of transubstantiation do so precisely in order to become obscure or fetishistic objects of desire.

The role of convulsive beauty must also be understood, therefore, in psychosexual terms and through its inevitable relationship to Freudian and Lacanian theory. Between 1916 and 1917, Breton had been employed as a military psychiatrist. Through this experience he initially became aware of the clinical use of Freudian theories of free association, although it must also be said that his deployment of such thinking was both desultory and eclectic. He met Freud briefly in Vienna in 1921, for example, but recorded that he was somewhat disappointed by the encounter.[72] Moreover, it was not until after 1925 that he would have been able to read key Freudian texts in translation – *The Interpretation of Dreams* (1900) was published in French in 1926; *Beyond the Pleasure Principle* (1920) and *The Ego and The Id* (1923) appeared in the *Essais de Psychanalyse* in 1927; and *The Uncanny* (1919) in *Essais de Psychanalyse appliqué* in 1933.

It is probably in *Mad Love*, (*L'Amour Fou*, 1937), that we find Breton articulating his intense interest in the Freudian subconscious and the inter-dependence of identity and psychosexuality to its most marked and poetic effect. The role of the *trouvaille* is of particular significance here, since it acts as an external sign of an internal impulse: 'Chance is the form of manifestation of an exterior necessity as it opens a path in the human unconscious.'[73] Thus, in encountering a *trouvaille*, the subject is prompted to repeat a traumatic experience, real or imaginary, that he he/she has repressed and does not ordinarily recall. In his hallucinatory encounter with the wooden spoon, for example, Breton is reminded of a '*waking sentence*' he had conjured up some time before, 'the Cinderella ash-tray' (*Le cendrier cendrillon*), and how, on the strength of this, he had invited Giacometti to sculpt for him a tiny glass slipper that he could use as an ash-tray.[74] The object never materialised, and in turn, this set up the memory of an unfulfilled childhood desire for Breton: 'The *lack* of this slipper, which I really felt, caused me to have a rather long daydream, of which there was already a trace in my childhood'.[75] In referring back to the repressed psychic loss of his childhood, Breton also appears to invoke Freud's theory of infantile sexuality and the way that he links breast feeding with the first stirring of sexual desire.[76] Separation from the mother's breast is inevitable in order that the child can become a subject in its own right, but this sense of loss also sets up a desire to repeat pleasure and to find the lost love object elsewhere. But the chain of associations does not end there, for Breton had also symbolised the spoon in terms of sexual difference and the sublimation or fear of another form of lack – castration. Consequently, he states in *Mad Love*: 'So it became clear, in these conditions, that the whole movement of my thought before this had as its starting point the objective equation: slipper = spoon = penis = the perfect mold of this penis.'[77]

Additionally, the imbrication of symbols that Breton articulates through the totemic spoon sets up another equation. For, as we have already mentioned, he also enunciates how the slipper evokes the image of 'a woman, *unique and unknown*'. In which case we could now argue that the slipper = spoon = penis = woman. The convulsive transformation of woman into a penis also became one of the central motifs in surrealist painting and photography, and was achieved in various ways. In Brassaï's 'Untitled' (1933), for example, a female nude has been photographed from behind and lying in a horizontal position so that her torso takes on the appearance of a penis and her buttocks double up as a scrotum. While in Man Ray's photograph 'Anatomies' (*c.* 1930), the female model tilts her head back as far as it will go, so that her neck and chin take on the aspect of an erect penis, as if viewed from below. Indeed, it was Man Ray who, during the 1930s, was responsible for elaborating a similar psychosexual identity in fashion photography. Thus, in describing the images he produced for the American monthly *BAZAAR*, he professed in true Bretonian style that it was not his concern to portray accurately the garments themselves: 'Inspiration, not information, is the force that binds all creative acts.'[78] In 'Augustabernard's new line' (*BAZAAR*, October 1934), for example, we can see how the fabric and details of the garment have been depicted as secondary to body form, and that with regard to the latter, the female body has been convulsed into a phallic silhouette. For the Surrealists, therefore, steeped in the Freudian tradition of psychoanalytical theory, the representation of the phallic woman was principally a way of configuring male castration anxiety. As Breton's commentary reveals, the equation between woman and penis raises the spectre of woman as castrating bitch, someone who is determined to have the symbol of power that she lacks. It is this trauma that is symbolised in Brassaï's and Man Ray's photographs, where not only is the female body transformed into a phallic shape, but body parts are also represented in close-up or in isolation, as if anatomically dismembered.

During the late 1980s, several fashion photographers began to latch on to the transformative aesthetic potential of Surrealism, including Lee Jenkins, Jean Baptiste Mondino, Marc Roger and Stephane Sednaoui. In particular, Man Ray's fashion vision seemed to undergo something of a revival with the likes of Alan David-Tu and Andrew Bettles, and we can detect a similar treatment of the female figure in their work. Both of these contemporary practitioners have deployed various devices and techniques, such as distortion through the use of unfocused lenses and double exposure, to achieve an idea of convulsive beauty in their images. In Figure 14, for example, the female body appears to be dissolving before our very eyes, and in doing so she takes on a Bretonian aspect of woman as penis that is also redolent of Man Ray's 'New Line'. United by a common style, however, the two photographers and periods are also divided by a theoretical gulf. The practitioners of the 1930s were clearly aware of the implications of the Freudian unconscious and theories of psychosexuality, and channelled this through the idea of convulsive beauty. In contrast, photographers during the 1980s tended to treat Surrealism in postmodern terms as an interesting aesthetic style, rather than using it to demonstrate their involvement with the intricacies of Freudian or Lacanian theory. When asked what was the intention behind his work, for example, David-Tu replied that he wanted 'the image to stand as an image' and nothing more.[79] Thus, as Derrida comments in 'The Double Session', texts do not have to be linked in terms of direct influence, but may be linked together instead through 'structural' necessity.[80] It is in this regard, then, we seem to be dealing with an idea of 'Surrealism without the subconscious' in contemporary fashion photography.[81]

Yet whether we view them in terms of style or sexual politics, these images of phallic women, of the body in pieces, are highly fetishised, and hardly a positive or empowering portrayal of femininity. The reversal of gender roles and the transgressive play on power and identity that the phallic woman implies, however, does not necessarily have to result in negative images of women. Moreover, the phallic woman is not the exclusive province of surrealist art, and nor does she have to be symbolised in the form of a castrated penis. An alternative and more ambiguous objectification of the woman as phallus, for example, can be found in a 1989 advertisement for Val Gils men's cologne (Figure 45). The act or masquerade we witness here seems to return us at once to the territory of Lacanian psychosexuality and fetishism on two interconnected levels. First, with regard to the mirror stage and the sedimentation of the bodily ego, and second, with regard to the idea of woman as phallus, as object of man's own desire. As Lacan expressed it in his *Seminar II*: 'What did I try to get across with the mirror stage? . . . The image of (man's) body is the principle of every unity he perceives in objects . . . all the objects of his world are always structured around the wandering shadow of his own ego.'[82] For Lacan, therefore, the mirror stage is not just to do with the way that the male subject perceives himself, but also the way that he sees himself objectified in others, and others objectified in him. This idea is also compounded by Irigaray in her essay *Speculum of the Other Woman* (1974), where she enlists woman as the silvered backing of the mirror that when functioning properly – that is passively and objectively – returns to man an image of his own desire. Thus woman ('she'): 'must be no more than the path, the method, the theory, *the mirror* for the subject that leads back, via a process of a repetition, to re-cognition of the unity of (his) origin . . . a glass for the "subject" to gaze upon himself and re-produce himself in his reflection.'[83]

But for Irigaray the question still remains – what happens when the mirror is recalcitrant? What happens when woman steps outside the frame and no longer reflects man back to himself unproblematically as the phallic ideal? It is this very disruption or reversal of the specular logic of the 'masculine imaginary' that the Van Gils advertisement appears to foreground in its ambiguous treatment of sex, gender and race. Clearly, the man and the woman in the image seem desirous of each other, but a doubt remains as to who is active and who is passive. This confusion is symbolised by the conflicting tropes of power that the ad portrays. On the one hand, the man appears naked and thus vulnerable, while the woman is clothed and seen wearing a – presumably his – suit and tie. But on the other, each of them seems to be caught up in a struggle to assert authority. Both subjects, for example, appear to be staring each other out, and he has a firm hold on the tie around her neck, while she adopts a confident pose and has her right arm wrapped somewhat defensively around his neck. In turn, these symbolic details lead us to question – who is it exactly that the male nude perceives as a fetishistic reflection of his own ego/object of desire in this ad? Certainly, no longer a passive woman but an active one, and indeed in terms of her dress code, a masculinised one.

There is, moreover, another ambiguity evident here, which concerns the ethnic origin of the female. The use of shade and lighting is such that both man and woman, for instance, appear to share the same bronzed skin tone. But his blonde hair and classic physiognomy – highlighted by the halo of strong light around his profile – suggest that he is a tanned Caucasian, and her dark, frizzy hair, heavy-lidded eyes and full lips suggest that she is the exotic and indeterminate, non-Aryan Other. In other words, man looks in the mirror and encounters a whole series of 'unlivable' and 'traumatic' Others, as Judith Butler calls them,[84] who threaten to disrupt the abject borders of his ego. A powerful woman dressed as a man but who is not a man, and who is either white or non-white, and conversely a powerful woman who is a man, and again who is either white or non-white. The spectre of the non-white, phallic female and the doubling of fear that the ad raises are further symbolised in an image of a black girl wearing a leather codpiece designed by Vivienne Westwood, which was included in the spread 'Forever Leather', photographed by Mark Lebon and styled by Debbi Mason for *The Face*, November 1991 (Figure 46). Here, the leather codpiece initially appears to suggest racial identity can be reduced to body parts by harping on the common stereotype of the well-endowed black man. But not only that, for along with the assertive gaze and hip-thrusting pose of the model, it also connotes an active and transgressive female sexuality. As in the Van Gils advertisement, masculinity is represented as something that can be mimed, and thus both images signify gender as a matter of performativity, of producing one's identity in and through certain speech and body acts (a point which is explored more substantively later on in this chapter).

Furthermore, the two images seem to share similar symbolic territory in the way they trade on the fantasmic fear of patriarchal men that no longer can the hard, muscular body be regarded as sufficient defence against 'succumbing to fluidity', of being flooded by women, 'soft' men and racial inferiors.[85] Klaus Theweleit has related how this trauma was especially symptomatic amongst the German *Freikorps* during the First World War:

> If that stream reaches me, touches me, spills over me, then I will dissolve, sink, explode with nausea, disintegrate in fear, turn horrified into slime that will gum me up, mire that will suffocate me, a pulp that will swallow me like quicksand. I'll be in a state where everything is the same, inextricably mixed together, and no one will be able to tell what it is that's flowing down there.[86]

But we find similar comments concerning the tension between soft and hard expressed by Luce Irigaray in *Speculum of the Other Woman*, where she contests: 'all water must become a mirror, all seas, a glass'.[87] As we have already seen, Irigaray's specular economy is of particular relevance when it comes to decoding the play of reflections and the traducing of identities that appear to take place in the Van Gils campaign. For not only does the ad elicit the idea that in looking into the mirror the male subject could perceive himself to be simultaneously man and woman and white and non-white. But by extension, he also seems to encounter two forms of imaginary sexual identities. First, in regarding the suited woman to be nonetheless a woman, he confronts his sublimated and subconscious desire for the maternal, heterosexual love object he was obliged to renounce in the phallic stage of the Oedipal conflict. And second, in framing her as a man – a connotation reinforced by the picture caption 'Strictly for men' – he comes face-to-face with the pre-Oedipal homosexual love object, which, as Judith Butler has convincingly elaborated, has been renounced prior to the prohibition on the maternal love object by an already constituted heterosexual being: 'The Oedipal conflict presumes that heterosexual desire has already been *accomplished*, that the distinction between heterosexual and homosexual has been enforced ... in this sense, the prohibition on incest presupposes the prohibition on homosexuality, for it presumes the heterosexualization of desire.'[88]

But, as she also contends, this means that heterosexuality is a form of melancholia involving a double disavowal – 'I never loved him, I never lost him' – and as such: 'identification contains within it both the prohibition and the desire ... Masculinity will be haunted by the love it cannot grieve.'[89]

Unveiling the Phallus: Putting the Male Body in the Frame

In the Lacanian phallogocentric system, not only does the straight male subject assert whatever power or authority he feels he has by objectifying those who do not measure up to the phallic ideal as the passive objects of his gaze, but also by keeping himself out of representation. For Lacan, therefore, the phallus 'can only play its role ... when veiled',[90] since 'virile display' always feminises the phallus: 'That is why the demon of ... shame arises at the very moment when, in the ancient mysteries, the phallus is unveiled.'[91] It is this logic that appears not only to keep men's genitalia from view in fashion photography and, in particular, to prohibit the open display of the erect penis, but that also ensures that the authority of the male subject is maintained by way of the indirect gaze. This kind of 'veiled objectification' is evident, for example, in Figure 23, where we observe a male model with his back turned towards us while the reflection of his face in the picture mirror into which he looks has been photographed out of focus, seeming more like a vignette that has been inserted into the main frame. By comparison, a more complex and interesting triangulation of the veiled gaze is connoted in Figure 26. Here the gaze of both the female model, who holds centre stage, and the man reflected in the cheval mirror on the right, who watches her strip, have been obscured. As she pulls her see-through top over her head it masks her face, while the reflected male character wears dark sunglasses. Although her expression is obscured by the top, this type of masking seems to function on the level of the veiled erotic, whereby her body is represented as an alluring object of desire for a whole series of male onlookers. Clearly, within the picture frame, for the man represented in the mirror on the right, and indirectly for the man whose face appears on the television screen on the left. But also for the (presumably male) spectator of the image, who is off-scene and for whom the man reflected in the mirror seems to act as double. Indeed, the female model is the only one who is depicted as an actual, physical presence in the photograph, whereas the male subjects are connoted indirectly as surface reflections or screened presences.

The play on reflections, and the way that the framing device is used in both these images to suggest that men are somehow both within the main picture and yet, at the same time, coincidental to or even absent from it, appear, therefore, to invoke Lacan's idea of the 'veiled phallus'. But such pictorial devices also seem to play on the tension between the *ergon* (the main work) and the *parergon* (the frame or forms of ornamentation that are 'added to' the work), as it is discussed by Derrida in his book *The Truth in Painting*. Taking Kant's *Critique of Judgement* (1790) and his definition of the *parergon* as an accessory or form of ornamentation as a starting-point, Derrida deconstructs the hierarchical opposition between the *ergon* and *parergon* to ask what is inside and what is outside the system of representation, and why.[92] Thus, in analysing one of Kant's examples of ornamentation – the use of drapery in paintings of the body and on statues – he states:

> A *parergon* comes against, beside and in addition to the *ergon*, the work done (*fait*), the fact (*le fait*), the work, but it does not fall to one side, it touches and cooperates within the operation, from a certain outside. Neither simply outside nor inside . . . If any *parergon* is only added, what is it that is lacking in the representation of the body, so that the garment should come and supplement it?[93]

For Derrida, therefore, it is not so much a case that the *ergon* precedes the *parergon*, rather that they co-exist in a dialectic of supplementarity that implies that the form of the *parergon* is not purely ornamental, but central to our understanding and enjoyment of the artwork as a totality, as a work of beauty: 'The *parergon* (frame, garment, column) can augment the pleasure of taste . . . contribute to the proper and intrinsically aesthetic representation if it intervenes by its form and only by its form. If it has a "beautiful form", it forms part of the judgement of taste properly speaking or in any case intervenes directly in it.'[94]

Supplementarity does not, therefore, simply imply the reversal of roles in terms of power or identity, nor is it intended to guarantee equal status between one concept and another – 'Deconstructionism must neither reframe nor dream of the pure and simple absence of the frame.'[95] Nonetheless, Derrida's logic of supplementarity offers an alternative way of dealing with both the idea of 'having' and 'lacking' power that underpins Lacanian phallogocentrism, as well as the framing of sex and gender in much fashion iconography since the early 1960s. Now, it is no longer just a case of regarding the Fashion system as the exclusive province of women, nor a matter of objectifying the female body alone, but instead one of bringing men into the frame of representation as well. And not just as the accessory to the female subject, but sometimes also as the principal focus of attention in fashion photography – however troublesome that may be – as objects of desire.

Visibility and Desire

This leads us to address the pivotal issue concerning the somewhat ambiguous status of masculinity as a site of narcissistic or scopophilic pleasure in terms of representation and spectatorship, and the tension between active and passive identities that this seems to imply. For whose spectatorial delectation is the male body offered up, exactly? Women's or men's, or women's *and* men's? I have argued in the last chapter that the objectification of the female body in fashion photography should not be regarded as an exclusive opportunity for the pleasure of the male spectator. Equally as much, therefore, nor should we assume that the visibility of the male body is unproblematically a case of making men a spectacle of desire for women. Indeed, as we have already noted in Part I, by 1987 60 per cent of the readers of *The Face* were male, while much of the sexually-ambivalent iconography involving the phallic body appears in magazines like *Arena*, which are initially targeted at straight men. As Nick Logan, the publisher and founding editor of both magazines, has expressed it: 'Since the 1960s men have been interested in fashion and style. You can see that in everything from rockers to the New Romantics. When they reach 25 and perhaps get married, they don't suddenly stop buying clothes and music.'[96]

But the intention of appealing to a specific readership cannot ensure that only those readers will consume the product and, as a corollary, certainly cannot account for the diverse and contradictory responses that men (whether straight or gay) and women have in viewing images of men. The popularity of male strip shows like the Chippendales with women-only audiences is testimony to the changing dynamics of spectatorship that I am referring to here, although, as audience behaviour and comments reveal, it is debatable whether women take the phallic body as seriously as men do, or have the same perspective of desire on it. The restricted circulation of the much-vaunted male nude pin-up magazine *For Women* is a key indicator of such equivocation; but it is also instructive in this respect to take account of the fact that support for the narcissism of 'new man' is conspicuous by its absence in the letters submitted by female readers to *The Face* and *Arena*. Only one letter could be traced between 1980 and 1995, for example, demonstrating approval for images of nude men in *The Face*; and even then the correspondent, a certain Louise from Derby, overlooked muscle-bound models in favour of slim pop singers like Ian Brown of The Stone Roses.[97] The majority of women seem to have struck a more indifferent or deprecating attitude concerning 'new man'. Among them are Jean Cave, whose satirical letter 'Instant Arena Man' I quoted in Part I, and Tasha Fairbanks, who in a letter to *The Face* lambasted the masculinist self-referentiality of the magazine's content:

> The last issue of 1986 (FACE 81) and not a woman in sight (almost). Boys, boys, boys, and yet more boys. Working-class on-the-make and made-it boys; fey boys, pre-faded boys; self-obsessed, self-congratulatory, sell-very-well-packaged-and-doing-nicely-thank-you-boys; designer-made boys with their boy-made designs filled the page on page . . . Oh boy, don't you ever get sick of yourselves. I do.[98]

Indeed, several writers have compounded the idea that the visibility of the male body appears to be a site of pleasure more for men than for women.[99] If anything, the male body part that women seem to fetishise most is a firm stomach, as demonstrated in the preferences expressed by readers of *New Woman* in May 1997 for a close-up photograph by Deirdre O'Callaghan that emphasised the well-toned abdomen of her subject.[100] Moreover, as Kenneth R. Dutton points out: 'some psychologists have found that men tend to react more favourably . . . to muscularity than do women, many of whom find muscularity more threatening than attractive'.[101] Thus straight men like Chris Dickerson, who was Mr Olympia in 1982 and who has posed nude for photographs and videos aimed at a gay market, appear to show no resistance in offering up their bodies as objects of visual pleasure for other men, if not for women. With this in mind, it is both apposite and interesting to note here the ingenuously gnomic declaration of desire for the male model in a recent Dolce and Gabbana advertisement by one of *The Face*'s readers which stands in marked contrast to the equivocal response of female readers to male fashion models cited above. 'Have you got the name of the lad in the Dolce and Gabbana vest? Cause I want to shag him senseless'[102] inquired a certain Andy W. of Camberwell (Andrew? Andrea? the exact sex of the reader is kept in suspension by the diminutive form of the name). If Andy is in fact male, then what a comment like this seems to suggest is that the culture of male bodybuilding exceeds the process of inoculation as Barthes describes it (which we invoked earlier to make some sense of the new man phenomenon). Instead, it is located more on the level of Hebdige's idea of stylistic, if not ideological, incorporation.[103] In this way, although gay men may have pioneered an unbridled narcissism that, as Miller suggests, makes 'the male body visible to desire',[104] the cultivation of muscles offers an idealised image of masculinity that appears to transcend the norm of polarised gender positions and sexualities for both straight and gay men.

Masculinities in Crisis

There are several cogent ways of accounting for the apparent similarity or oscillation between normative and subversive masculinities in both contemporary society and media representations. On a diachronic and psychoanalytical level, for example, we could argue that these images of ideal men conform to Freud's idea that we are each of us constitutionally bisexual: 'generally speaking, every human being oscillates between heterosexual and homosexual feelings'.[105] That is to say, given that masculine and feminine currents co-exist in everyone, there also exist multiple possibilities for pleasure in every human being. In contrast, Foucault's idea of the discursive body, whose identity and status is prone to shifts in the exercise of power and knowledge, leads us to a more specific and synchronic understanding of such iconography. Thus, although the cultivation of the phallic body during the 1980s and 1990s is something that can be seen to have transcended barriers of age, class and race, it must not be regarded simply as a token of confident masculinity, but conversely as a sign of masculinity in crisis, a way of coming to terms with male insecurities that speaks of both desire and lack: 'In a world where things seem so out of control ... it's nice to have control of one's body.'[106] As Barry Glassner has argued, muscularity unites men in a 'passionate battle against their own sense of vulnerability',[107] and as former bodybuilder Sam Fussell has testified, pumping iron became for him an escape route from the demands of the real world:

> The gym was the one place I had control. I didn't have to speak, I didn't have to listen. I just had to push or pull. It was so much simpler, so much more satisying than life outside. I regulated everything ... It beat the street. It beat my girlfriend. It beat my family. I didn't have to think. I didn't have to care. I didn't have to feel. I simply had to lift.[108]

Consequently, the cultivation of muscles is one important symbolic way for both straight and gay males to reclaim some kind of personal or individual control and self-respect. This should not just be taken, however, as a response to the challenge of feminist politics, of 'beating one's girlfriend'. More particularly, since the early 1980s, working out can be seen to symbolise the way that men have sought to come to terms with specific social and political developments. These include high unemployment in heavy industries and the concomitant shift to sedentary occupations, as well as the threat of HIV/AIDS.[109] Indeed, the iconography of many campaigns dealing with the latter mobilises the phallic body as an object of desire in ways that are not totally dissimilar to promotions for clothing and perfume, witness advertisements for the Health Education Authority photographed by Herb Ritts and Jean Baptiste Mondino in 1991.[110] But while Elizabeth Wilson has suggested that, 'Versace man is impenetrable man – a body for an age of AIDS',[111] sometimes not even the carapace of the phallic body can provide immunity from such life-threatening epidemics. This point is neatly crystallised in the contrasting verbal and visual rhetoric of recent campaigns in America for HIV home testing kits that juxtapose images of contemplative, muscular sportsmen with captions like 'You used to worry you'd never have sex. Now you worry when you do.' By extension, if I may slightly modify the thesis propounded by Horkheimer in his essay 'The End of Reason' (1941) that fascism is a pre-condition for the overturning of paternal authority,[112] then body fascism, or the cult of the phallic body, as evidenced in an 1990s advertisement for Chanel Egoïste, can be seen to signal the disruption of the bond with the post-Oedipal superego that Freud postulates is 'the representative of our relation to our parents . . . the representative of the internal world'.[113] Thus, 'Conflicts between the ego and the ideal will . . . ultimately reflect the contrast between what is real and what is psychical, between the external world and the internal world.'[114] In this advertisement, then, we observe the very personification of the struggle between the inner and outer worlds that Freud describes, as the male body shadow boxes not with itself but with the Other, that is a putative father-figure, in order to wrest from him the symbol of power, in this instance connoted as a perfume bottle, that he lacks.

Gender, Identity and Performativity

The struggle between external and internal forms of experience that Freud elaborated with regard to the formation of identity in writings such as 'The Ego and the Id' (1923) has been subject to re-evaluation in recent years. In particular, this leads us to consider both the ambiguity of the phallic body and the portrayal of gender in much recent fashion photography as transitional or liminal concepts in the context of Butler's complex theory of gender performativity. I propose this for two significant and interdependent reasons: first, in so far as performativity appears to reconcile the psychoanalytic and the social, which is to say the mind and the body, into a more discursive and proactive whole; and second, because it allows us to regard gender and sexuality as dynamic and polymorphous phenomena. At the outset, Butler repudiates the idea that gender identity is simply the result of one's sex. Nor does she believe that identities are simply embodied in appearances and the donning and discarding of an appropriate mask or look. Accordingly, she contests the concept of the superficial masquerade as expressed earlier by Barthes in *The Fashion System*.[115] Rather, Butler expands on the Lacanian idea that for men as well as women, the status of one's sexual identity is not just provisional but also prone to the perpetual threat of dissolution.[116]

As she frames it, the norm of sex and gender can only emerge and be maintained in the reiterated performance of a series of culturally assigned or engendered speech and body acts, which 'produce the effect of an internal core or substance'.[117] Moreover, performativity is not just a 'ritualized production' but one that is: 'reiterated under and through constraint, under and through the force of prohibition and taboo, with the threat of ostracism and even death controlling and compelling the shape of the production.'[118] Thus the sedimentation of gender identity is not merely realised in the act of dressing up, nor is it attained in a single or ephemeral performance, but accrued in the *'stylized repetition of acts'*: 'The effect of gender is produced through the stylization of the body and, hence, must be understood as the mundane way in which bodily gestures, movements, and styles of various kinds constitute the illusion of an abiding gendered self.'[119] According to Butler, therefore, the formation of one's identity always turns on a central paradox. That is, it is materialised in and through the ritual of a pre-ordained gender performance, yet its status remains volatile, precisely because the performance needs to be repeated in order to maintain authority. Hence she concludes that gender is:

a complexity whose totality is permanently deferred an 'act' as it were, that is open to splittings, self-parody, self-criticism, and those hyperbolic exhibitions of the 'natural' that, in their very exaggeration, reveal its fundamentally phantasmatic status . . . because gender is not a fact, the various acts of gender create the idea of gender, and without those acts, there would be no gender at all.[120]

It is in this way, for example, that a man is expected 'to be' an autocratic manager at work, and a woman 'to be' his subservient housekeeper, both acts illustrating the function of performative gender roles to reinforce sexual and power differences in patriarchal society. Likewise, in fashion photography, the phallic body can be seen to be continuously reiterated so as to sediment patriarchal ideas of masculinity and, by extension, femininity. This much is evident, for example, in the play on male domination and female subordination in spreads such as 'South of the Border', photographed by Norman Watson and styled by Ray Petri in *Arena*, November/December 1987; 'Fairground Attraction', photographed by Ellen Von Unwerth and styled by Corinnne Nocella in *Arena*, July/August 1988; 'Wet', photographed by Kate Garner and styled by Karl and Derick in *The Face*, August 1991; and 'Have a nice day', photographed by Christopher Griffiths and styled by David Bradshaw in *Arena*, July/August 1994 (Figures 47–9).[121]

Initially, Butler postulates that in the repeated performing of speech and body acts we substantiate and conform to the paradigm of normative gender identities that serve to authorise the hegemony of straight society. As she also suggests, however, through performativity we may contest and sublate this ideal, negotiating alternative or recalcitrant types of femininities and masculinities in the process. It is worth restating here, therefore, that the idea of performativity produces only the illusion of a cohesive heterosexual identity, for, as Butler contends:

> sex is both produced and destabilised in the course of (this) reiteration . . . its power to establish what qualifies as "being" . . . works not only through reiteration, but through exclusion as well. And in the case of bodies, those exclusions haunt signification as its abject borders or as that which is strictly foreclosed: the unlivable, the non-narrativizable, the traumatic.[122]

The idea of haunting that Butler raises here as an integral aspect of gender performativity has been intelligently amplified by Anoop Nayak and Mary Kehily in their social examination of homophobia in co-educational secondary schools in the West Midlands.[123] In this study, the authors identified a series of 'silences and absences' concerning homosexuality, and the fact that the schoolchildren consulted would repeatedly use abusive language, jokes and gestures, as a kind of defence mechanism to convince both themselves and others that they were not gay. Especially significant was the fear of homosexual contagion that boys would ward off by making a crucifix sign with their fingers.[124] This last act seems to conform with Freud's argument in *Group Psychology* that a point of identification can be performed involuntarily, 'under the influence of the pathogenic situation', and thus unite those (white and black males, for instance) who might otherwise have little or nothing in common in a mutual desire or fear:

It would be wrong to suppose that they take on the symptom out of sympathy. On the contrary, the sympathy only arises out of the identification, and this is proved by the fact that infection or imitation of this kind takes place in circumstances where even less pre-existing sympathy is to be assumed than usually exists between friends in a . . . school.[125]

'Close Encounters': A Case Study in Gender Performativity

Conversely, it can be argued that when we reiterate gendered acts oppositionally and against the grain, we effect not only a radical reorientation of our psychic personalities but one that also enables us to contest/transgress patriarchy. Numerous examples of fashion spreads which queer gender and sexuality on these terms have been cited already in this chapter. But in conclusion I would like to concentrate on the performative sexual and racial ambiguities of the shoot 'Close Encounters', photographed by Nick Knight, and styled by Simon Foxton for the Spring/Summer 1995 issue of *Arena Homme Plus*. The set of seven images have been framed at top and bottom by black borders and laid out as if they are pillar-box stills from a movie, although they have not been sequenced to unfold a continuous narrative. Rather, each of the atmospheric, shadowy images appears to represent a fragmentary idyll in time and space that illustrates the central theme of the piece: 'under cover of darkness, the good, the bad and the merely beautiful come out to play. Relax . . . just do it.'

In many respects, the mood and tone of the pictures, as well as the obvious maritime dress codes and underworld milieux, appear to reference not only the performative homoeroticism of Jean Genet's picaresque novel concerning murder and passion, *Querelle de Brest* (1953), but also Fassbinder's film adaptation of it in 1982. Both texts have already been alluded to in the Introduction to this study in my discussion of *The Face*'s fashion spread 'Guys N Dolls' (Figure 2). The narrative structure of 'Close Encounters', however, invites a more in-depth analysis of the performative nature of Genet's text, and its incorporation into fashion photography.

Although Genet states that, 'neither Mario nor any of the chief characters in this book (with the exception of Lieutenant Seblon, but then Seblon is not *in* the book) is a real homosexual',[126] as the plot of the novel loosely unfolds most of the male characters either flirt with the idea of going with another man or indeed, Querelle included, actually do so. Querelle is desired by both Nono and Seblon, for instance, and in turn is desirous of Gil, Roger and Mario; while Roger flirts with Gil and is infatuated with Querelle and Robert.[127] Thus normative masculinity is persistently under siege in the work, and, as the following passages concerning the policeman Mario's seduction of Querelle close to a railway cutting demonstrate, so-called straight men are also only too willing to be 'shivered by someone else's desire':[128]

> They kept up the pretence of innocence – one as much as the other – though both were well aware of the game they were playing. They were afraid of dashing forward too precipitously to meet the truth and take their pleasure in the unveiled symbol of their mutually accepted excitement . . . Querelle was in the clutches of so powerful a feeling of abandon that he allowed Mario to do what he liked. The train sped on into the night with unmitigated desperation. It was speeding towards the serene, peaceful, and terrestrial unknown, to something so long denied to the matelot . . . At the very moment that the train plunged into the tunnel before entering the station, the policeman's prick, as if fated, plunged deep into his mouth.[129]

We do not encounter such an explicit scene of lovemaking as this in any of the pictures from 'Close Encounters', but the overall sexual deviancy and the transgressive undertow of Genet's writing is amplified throughout the entire piece. The layout of the photographs, therefore, does not correspond point for point with the sequencing of events or scenes as they crop up in the novel. Nonetheless, the spread does appear to condense the general flow of the storyline, and to conflate several of the speech and body acts that Genet deploys in his subversive treatment of sexuality and desire. Five of the photographs, for instance, seem to reference the bar/brothel 'La Féria', that is 'decorated with purple and gold' (Figures 38–41),[130] while the two remaining images appear to represent the homosocial/homosexual underworld that Genet depicts taking place in urinals, close to railway cuttings and against ramparts (Figures 38 and 40). With this general schema in mind, I want now to analyse the exchanges and/or parallels that take place between the form and content of the original text and the fashion images, and to see how they both appear to reiterate a similar point concerning the instability of gender identities.

In each of the openings from the spread we encounter scenes evoking activities that take place in the novel either in or around 'La Féria', the bar/brothel owned by Nono and presided over by his wife, Madame Lysiane. Lysiane, 'rounded, rich and polished', and who 'moulded by the passing of time . . . was beautiful',[131] was also the lover of Querelle's brother Robert, and by turns desirous of Querelle himself. Genet relates how, 'To start with, Querelle had paid but half-hearted heed to the Madam's advances', and in the closing passages of the novel we learn that he only sleeps with her in retaliation against Robert.[132] This sense of *ennui* and distance is connoted by the gaze of the male subject in the first picture of the shoot (Figure 38), who stares directly out towards us as a female prostitute presses him against the wall. His mind appears to be on other things, and we are directed to what this might possibly be in the photograph on the facing page. At this point we encounter two male figures in a shady, compartmentalised subterranean setting. The walls are tiled, suggesting that this could be a gentlemen's lavatory or some kind of gymnasium dressing/shower room. One of the men stands in the foreground, facing the spectator and wearing a figure-hugging vest. The other, who wears a sailor's outfit and hat, is back-lit in the doorway at the rear left of the picture. His right hand appears to be stroking his penis, while his left hand is tucked into his pocket, a gesture which is echoed by the man in the vest. Here, the ostensible chance encounter of two men in an enclosed, homosocial space appears to echo the scene in *Querelle* where Seblon visits a urinal in search of sexual trade: 'He undid his flybuttons and, after a careful survey of the other occupants, he wrote out his first message: 'Young man passing through Brest would like to meet sailor with big prick.'[133] In the course of the novel, this act of desire is reiterated by Seblon's obsession with Querelle, as much as it is by Querelle's knowing game of cat and mouse with the Lieutenant and his eventual seduction of him:

> Querelle . . . gave a slight swing to his hips, narrow as they were, and this sent a gentle ripple along the tops of his trousers where they were overlapped by his white underpants . . . He had, of course, with his usual cunning, not failed to notice the Lieutenant's gaze often wandered down to this part of his body, just as he knew instinctively the most effectual seductive points about himself.[134]

Are we to understand, then, that this image could parallel the sexual tension between Querelle and Seblon? Yes, in so far as the distance between the two male figures seems to connote the way that the Lieutenant struggles to keep the sailor, and by implication his desire to have him, sublimated or at bay. Throughout the narrative, for example, his relationship with Querelle is represented as an inner monologue or series of meditations: 'He wanted to take Querelle with him on this ceremonial adventure . . . What secret thought, what dazzling confession, what exciting new light lay concealed beneath this pair of trousers . . . ? What shadowy phallus hung enshrouded there, its sooty stem pendulous among withered moss?'[135] But, along with Figure 40, which is set in the same underground milieu, the image could also serve to encapsulate the general sublimation of homosexual desire by several of the straight protagonists that forms the leitmotiv of Genet's text. In this respect the play of hands in Figure 38, whether inside or outside of pockets, to symbolize sexual arousal is particularly illuminating, and appears to conflate two other idyllic moments from the novel in which homosexual urges overwhelm heterosexual identity. Thus the image could also connote the scene in which Genet describes how Gil's desire to make love to his girlfriend Paulette is breached by the close presence of her brother, Roger:

> Gil put his hand on the lad's shoulder and let it rest there . . . [he] removed his hand to thrust it in his trousers pockets again . . . All the same, in the act of removing it, Gil could not help pressing harder on the lad's shoulder as he let go his hold: it was as if some sort of regret at taking it away added to its weight. All of a sudden, Gil got a hard on.[136]

By the same token, the image also seems to evoke Querelle's desire for Gil, and the sexual encounter with him that Genet relates toward the end of the work: 'He loved Gil. He forced himself to love him . . . He took Gil's arm and forced his hand to touch his penis . . . For the first time in Querelle's life, a man was feeling him. He crushed his mouth against Gil's ear . . . Gil squeezed the throbbing penis all the harder.'[137]

Although Querelle and Gil fall in love with each other, however, theirs is a passion that appears to have been forged out of a shared sense of guilt. As such, their relationship functions more on the level of atonement for the calculated *Lustmorde* (sex murders) of two of the avowed homosexuals, Joachim and Theo, who desire them. Moreover, the coupling of gender ambiguities and psychopathic guilt that Genet deals with, and that is suggested by the opening sequence of 'Close Encounters', is repeated in the following two pairs of photographs from the spread (Figures 39–40). In the first of these, a photograph with a female nude in the foreground and an uninterested sailor lighting up a cigarette behind her on the right has been juxtaposed with an image of another sailor, on his own and leaning against a fake tree trunk. Once more, these images appear to reference Querelle's confused sexual appetite for both men and women. For they form a parallel with the scene in the novel where, shortly after he has slit the throat of the sailor Vic, his accomplice in crime, for resisting his advances – 'Tell me, aren't I as good as Mario?'[138] – he brushes up against the branches of a tree shrouded in the fog that remind him of 'the soft light on a woman's breasts'.[139]

In the next sequence of images we encounter a photograph of a sailor staring through the frosted glass window of a tavern, juxtaposed with another of two men confronting each other in the tiled and tenebrous 'underworld' of homosocial/homosexual activities (Figure 40). Here, the first image seems to symbolise Querelle's return to 'La Féria', just after he has killed Vic, while the second seems to portend the fate he met there, that is, his subsequent sacrificial buggering by Nono: 'He was going to his doom with despair in his soul, but at the same time with the inner certitude, still unexpressed, that this form of execution was vitally necessary to him . . . To his despair . . . was added the comforting certainty that this execution would wash him clean of the murder.'[140]

As these passages reveal, Querelle remains a complex and elusive object of desire, but equally as much he appears well aware of the transgressive nature of his own gender performativity. Genet writes of him, for instance: 'Only in this way will you be able to appreciate the apparent – and real – beauty of his body, his attitudes, his exploits, and their slow disintegration.'[141] In the final analysis, therefore, we cannot ever really ascertain whether his sexuality, and by extension that of all men, regardless of age, class or ethnic background, is either permanent or provisional. This much also appears to be compounded in 'Close Encounters', where we observe the white and non-white male models hover on the brink of indecision and indeterminacy between straight and gay consciousness. Consequently, it is fitting in this respect that the final image of the fashion shoot should represent the idea of masculine identities as a contest (Figure 41). Here, the two muscular models represented closely resemble each other in such a way as to invoke the common beauty Madame Lysiane perceives in Querelle and his brother Robert, which almost drives her mad with indecision as to whom she desires the most.[142] But, as we observe the two models arm wrestling, the outcome as to who will be the winner – sanguine and ostensibly stable 'Robert,' or mutable and sexually deviant 'Querelle' – remains in the balance.

Conclusion

My discussion of performativity in the representation of sex, gender and race in 'Close Encounters', and the way that the spread seems to reference Genet's novel *Querelle de Brest*, brings us full circle in this study of the construction of the body in word and image in fashion photography. As my analysis demonstrates, even when images appear to be autonomous entities and written clothing is kept to a bare minimum, the fashion spread can nonetheless trade on an idea of intertextuality through the poetics of clothing. Now, without having to specify the cultural models it mobilises – literature, the cinema, art – 'the signified of connotation', as Barthes puts it, 'is literally hidden',[143] and accordingly the rhetorical code of fashion articulates a metalanguage of its own making, oscillating between meaning and form.

Furthermore, the idea of performativity constitutes one of the most troubling but cogent challenges to how we understand and negotiate the meaning of sex, gender and race. Hence, it echoes Kristeva's idea of abjection by propounding that identities are provisional and the concept of a stable, unitary subject is bogus. Yet, as Butler argues, it also has a distinct momentum of its own in so far as it maintains that the construction of one's individual identity in the real world is crystallised in a kind of ritualistic and continual role-playing. Of course, this is not to deny that distinctly straight and gay subjects, be they white or non-white, exist. As we have already seen in this chapter and in earlier sections of the study, there are very many instances of fashion spreads that repeat heterosexuality as the norm for men and women. But equally as much, there are very many spreads which blur and undermine sexual and gender differences, particularly between straight and gay masculinities. In the iterative spirit of performativity and by way of conclusion, therefore, it is probably worth reaffirming this point with reference to the fashion spread 'Trade' (photographer, Steve Callaghan; stylist, Karl Templer), which was published in *The Face* in June 1996.

The spread ostensibly plays on gay hustling and male prostitution, a message that is underscored by the subtitle, 'Love and passion, back in fashion. At a price', and the various scenes of men attempting to pick up other men included in it. It opens, for example, with a photograph of two boys flirting in a club, and progresses to an opening that juxtaposes an image of a younger man being cruised by an older man in a toilet, with a picture of the same young lad riding the London Underground. But the spread simultaneously deals with the idea of hustling and the status of sexual identities in a highly ambivalent and ambiguous way. In the final opening, we encounter another picture of two men in a club, placed opposite a closely-cropped picture of what appears, at first glance, to be a man unzipping his trousers (Figure 50). The juxtaposition of the two photographs and the focus on the pelvic area of the person in the final shot leads us to conclude that the two men have scored, and are just about to have sex at home. If we investigate the details in the last image more closely, however, the slender, manicured hands appear to be those of a female, who stands behind the man as she undoes his flies. The possibility that there is a female present in the room is further connoted by the woman's head on the television screen in the background of the image. 'Trade' ends, therefore, in such a way as to confound our expectations. But through a subtle double-coding it illuminates once again the central leitmotiv of this chapter, that is, the way that many contemporary fashion photographers, either consciously or unconsciously, have represented sexuality and the male body in more ambiguous or queer terms as a site of power and pleasure for men as well as women.

In some respects this is achieved through parody and pastiche, in which the macho posturing of the straight, phallic body is undermined on its own terms. This much is evident in Figures 35–36 and 42, and since late 1994 also in those fashion spreads that depict camp, ectomorphic and androgynous male bodies, such as 'Army Dreamers' (*The Face*, November 1994; photographer, Donald Milne; stylist Nancy Rohde); 'Brute 33' (*The Face*, June 1995; photographer, Anette Aurell; styling Annett Monheim), and 'Performance' (*The Face*, December 1995; photographer Steven Klein; styling, Nancy Rohde). Conversely, it is also realised by figuring the abject or unlivable Others that Butler mentions – women, gays, non-whites (and sometimes individuals are at least two, if not all, of these things at once) – as powerful subjects in their own right who resist the normalizing judgement of the heterosexual, white, male gaze, witness Figures 38–41 and 44–46. But the transgressive potential of performing sex and gender against the grain, and the polymorphous identities that result do not end here in fashion photography. For, as recent spreads such as 'Simplex Concordia' (*The Face*, July 1996) illustrate, through image-manipulating computer systems like Quantel Paintbox and Barco, female and male bodies can mutate into each other, and thereby both biology and gender can be transcended.[144] In Figure 22, for instance, the potential of the simplex cell not only to replicate but also to transform itself genetically is amplified both by the image and the caption, 'Jason with Ketuta's head, Ketuta with Jason's head'. A similar transsexuality is connoted in Inez Van Lamsweerde's photographic project, *The Forest* (1995), in which she uses computer technology to mix and match male and female bodies to form uncanny hybrids.[145] Of course, as cross-dressing, plastic surgery and genetic engineering all make demonstrably clear, sex and gender reassignment can also become a social and physical reality rather than being merely a matter for representation.

But, as I have argued throughout this chapter and, indeed this study in general, reality and representation do not always have distinct aims and objectives. In both spheres, identity is a question of mind and body, and the performative indeterminacies of sex and gender that are connoted in much recent fashion photography are a significant reminder that the potential for real change exists. At the very least, therefore, performativity, whether in life or in images, opens the way to the more radical sex and gender utopia that Barthes portended would be necessary before the categories of powerful and powerless are able to be undone:

> *Virile/non-virile*: this famous pair, which rules over the entire *Doxa*, sums up all the ploys of alternation: the paradigmatic play of meaning and the sexual game of ostentation . . . the purest paradigm imaginable, that of *active/passive*, of *possessor/possessed*, *buggerer/buggeree* . . . Nonetheless, once the alternative is rejected (once the paradigm is blurred) utopia begins: meaning and sex become the object of a free play, at the heart of which the (polysemant) forms and the (sensual) practices, liberated from the binary prison, will achieve a state of infinite expansion.[146]

Notes

1. As we have seen in Part 1, *Vogue* had included men in fashion images since the late 1920s, while *Man About Town*, which was launched in 1953 and was latterly known as *About Town* and *Town* during the 1960s, featured fashion photographs with men represented in isolation or with other men.

2. R. Coward, *Female Desires: How They Are Sought, Bought and Packaged* (New York, 1985), p. 227.

3. Julia Kristeva, Powers of Horror: *An Essay in Abjection*, trans. L. S. Roudiez (New York, 1982 [1980]), p. 32.

4. H. Cixous, 'The Laugh of the Medusa', in E. Marks and I. de Courtivron (eds), *New French Feminisms*, (New York, 1981), p. 247.

5. G. O'Brien, 'Pink Thoughts', in *The Idealizing Vision: The Art of Fashion Photography* (New York, 1991), p. 78.

6. M. Gross, *Model: The Ugly Business of Beautiful Women* (London and New York, 1995), pp. 45–7.

7. See E. Wilson, *Adorned in Dreams: Fashion and Modernity* (London, 1985), Chapter 9. Of the dandy she writes: 'The role of the dandy implied an intense preoccupation with self and self presentation; image was everything, and the dandy a man who often had no family, no calling, apparently no sexual life, no visible means of financial support. He was the very archetype of the new urban man who came from nowhere, and for whom appearance was reality. His devotion to an ideal of dress that sanctified understatement inaugurated an epoch not of no fashions for men, but of fashions that put cut and fit before ornament, colour and display. The skin-tight breeches of the dandy were highly erotic; so was his new, unpainted masculinity. The dandy was a narcissist. He did not abandon the pursuit of beauty; he changed the kind of beauty that was admired' (p. 180).

8. M. Bolan quoted by N. Cohn, 'Ready, steady, gone', *The Observer Magazine* (27 August 1967), p. 12.

9. 'Ken Rodway, A Sort of Male Model' in *Look-In Fashion Model Annual* (London, Independent Television Publications Ltd., 1971), pp. 17–22.

10. B. D'Silva, 'Some like it Hoyt', *FHM* (September 1993), p. 112.

11. See S. Garratt interview with Nick Moss in *The Face* (August 1993), p .60; A. Heath, 'Sonic boom boy', *The Face* (April 1994), pp. 80–5; N. Compton, 'Likely Lads', *The Face* (August 1995), pp. 40–51; and *Male Super Models: The Men of Boss Models* (New York, 1996), p. 32.

12. J. Lacan, 'The Mirror Stage as formative of the function of the I' (1949) in *Écrits: A Selection*, trans. A. Sheridan (New York, 1977), p. 2.

13. These typologies were foregrounded in McCann-Erickson's 'ManStudy Report', which was presented by Colin Bowring at the Institute of Practitioners in Advertising on 18 June 1984, and subsequently promoted by Marplan. See S. Marquis, 'The publishing conundrum: How to reach the "New Man"', *Campaign* (26 July 1985), p. 39.

14. Cobbett was a prolific polemicist, between 1802 and 1835 publishing *Cobbett's*

Weekly Political Register. In *Advice to Young Men And (Incidentally) to Young Women in the Middle and Higher Ranks of Life* (London, 1829), p. 167, he writes: 'I began my young marriage days in and near Philadelphia . . . I had business to occupy the whole of my time . . . but I used to make time to assist [my wife] in the taking care of her baby, and in all sorts of things; get up, light the fire, boil the tea-kettle, carry her up warm water in cold weather, take the child while she dressed herself and got breakfast ready, then breakfast, get her in water and wood for the day, then dress myself neatly and sally forth to business.'

15. See J. Paoletti, 'Ridicule and role models as factors in American men's fashion change 1900–1910', *Costume*, No. 29 (1985), pp. 121–34. During this period the term 'new man' was used as a pendant to the term 'new woman', which during the 1890s became common currency in both Britain and France to describe those women who began to agitate for female emancipation and for equal social, judicial and political rights. In the 1898 preface to his *Plays Unpleasant*, for example, George Bernard Shaw says that the 'New Woman' debate was at its height in 1893, when he wrote *The Philanderer* (ibid. p.14), and is inclined to date this whole train of thought back to the London production of *A Doll's House* in 1889; see G. B. Shaw, *Plays Unpleasant* (Harmondsworth, 1946), pp. 132–3. In France the first International Congress on Women's Rights was held at the 1889 Paris Exhibition and between 1889–1900, twenty-one feminist periodicals were published in France; see Karen Offen, 'Depopulation, nationalism and Feminism in fin-de-siècle France', *American Historical Review*, 89 (1984), p. 654.

16. *The New Man* (Nottingham, C. J. Welton, 1919).

17. See L. O'Kelly, 'Body talk', *Observer Life* (23 October 1994), p. 32, and R. Stengel, 'Men as sex objects', M (July 1992), pp. 72–9.

18. Peter York quoted by C. Bowen-Jones, 'Adman finds a New Woman', *The Times* (16 March 1988), p. 26.

19. J. Williamson, 'Short circuit of the New Man', *New Statesman* (20 May 1988), p. 28.

20. Mintel, *Men 2000* (London, 1993). Mintel interviewed 1,576 men and women for their survey. More recently, research by Healey and Baker demonstrated that the number of men who did the main food shop had risen to 26 per cent during 1997. However, the increase was mainly among high-earning under-24-year-olds living in London, while only 11 per cent of men with families admitted to shopping for groceries every week. See 'Shopping new man', *The Guardian* (20 January 1998), p. 14.

21. R. Barthes, 'Myth Today', in *Mythologies*, trans. by A. Lavers, (London, 1973), p. 164.

22. A. M. Klein, 'Fear and loathing in Southern California: narcissism and fascism in bodybuilding subculture', *Journal of Psychoanalytic Anthropology* (Spring 1987), pp. 117–37.

23. E. Roger Denson, quoted in A. Ellenzweig, *The Homoerotic Photograph* (New York, 1992), p. 167. Philip Norman, 'The shock of the neo' in *The Guardian Weekend* (30–31 May 1992), pp. 4–5, proffered a similar point of view: 'Neo-Nazism is getting hip. Young people with no special interest in politics and no memory or conception

of Hitler's barbarities have latched on to the style and aesthetic that camouflaged them . . . in the 70s we had Radical Chic; in the 90s we have Fascist chic' (p. 4).

24. S. Sontag, 'Fascinating Fascism', in B. Taylor and W. van der Will (eds), *The Nazification of Art* (Winchester, 1990), p. 216.

25. See T. Downing, *Olympia* (London, 1992).

26. Baudrillard, 'History: A Retro Scenario', in *Simulacra and Simulation*, trans. Sheila Faria Glaser (Ann Arbor, 1994), p. 44.

27. L. O'Kelly stated that in 1994 500,000 British men were members of a gym – 'Body talk', *Observer Life* (23 October 1994), p. 32. For a broader discussion of the relationship of bodybuilding and gym culture to gender and sexuality since 1980 see A. M. Klein, *Little Big Men: Bodybuilding Subculture and Gender Construction* (Albany, 1993).

28. D. A. Miller, *Bringing Out Roland Barthes* (Berkeley, CA, 1992), p. 31.

29. See A. M. Klein, 'Little Big Man: Hustling, Gender Narcissism, and Body-building Culture' in M. A. Messner and D. F. Sabo (eds), *Sport, Men and the Gender Order* (Champaign, 1990), pp. 127–40.

30. M. Pumphrey, 'Why do cowboys wear hats in the bath? Style politics and the older man', *Critical Quarterly*, 31:3 (Autumn 1989), p. 97.

31. R. Dyer, 'Getting Over the Rainbow: Identity and Pleasure in Gay Cultural Politics', in G. Bridges and R. Brunt (eds), *Silver Linings: Some Strategies for the Eighties* (London, 1981), p. 61, frames Village People in similar terms, contending: 'There is a profound ambivalence in this development – which can be taken straight . . . but can also be ironic and reflexive.'

32. See F. Valentine Hoover, III, *Beefcake: The Muscle Magazines of America 1950–1970* (Cologne, 1995), p. 58.

33. Ibid., p. 46.

34. Ibid., p. 49.

35. R. Dyer, 'Don't look now – the male pin-up', *Screen*, 23: 3–4 (September/October 1982), p. 63.

36. W. Scobie, 'Pride and Prejudice', *The Observer Magazine* (12 January 1986), pp. 14–17.

37. See L. Grant, 'The old colour of money', *The Guardian G2* (15 April 1997), p. 8. Debbi Mason, former fashion director at British *Elle*, is also quoted by A. Holden in 'Any colour . . . so long as it's black', *The Guardian* (17 September 1990), p. 20, saying that, 'According to market research, black girls on covers don't sell.'

38. A. Holden, *The Guardian* (1990), p. 20.

39. B. Hugill, 'TV ads show black in the shade of white', *The Observer* (24 August 1997), p. 4. See also L. Young, interview with Tyra Banks, *The Face* (August 1993), p. 92. Banks states that fashion 'is the only industry in America that can be racist. They say to your face, "We don't want a black girl" or "Your skin is too black" or "too light" or whatever.'

40. 'Special Agents', *Look-In Fashion Model Annual* (1971), pp. 49–55.

41. *Male Super Models: The Men of Boss Models*, pp. 30–1; 96–7; 124–5; and 133.

42. See C. Leggett, 'high five', *Arena Homme Plus* (Autumn/Winter 1994), p. 15.

43. 'Malcolm X', *The Face* (November 1992), p. 60.

44. Ibid., p. 60.

45. F. Fanon, *Black Skin, White Masks*, trans. C. Lam Markmann (London, 1986 [1952]), p. 110.

46. K. Mercer, 'Reading Racial Fetishism: The Photographs of Robert Mapplethorpe', in K. Mercer, *Welcome to the Jungle: New Positions in Black Cultural Studies* (London, 1994), pp. 190–1.

47. Fanon, *Black Skin, White Masks*, p. 120.

48. F. Fanon, *The Wretched of the Earth*, trans. C. Farrington (New York, 1963), p. 40.

49. S. Maynard, 'What color is your underwear? Class, whiteness and homo-erotic advertising', *Border/Lines*, No. 32 (1994), p. 8.

50. Fanon, *Black Skin, White Masks*, p. 180, n. 44.

51. H. K. Bhabha, 'Of mimicry and man: the ambivalence of colonial discourse', *October* 28 (Spring 1984), p. 126.

52. D. Hebdige, *Subculture: The Meaning of Style* (London, 1979), p. 66.

53. R. Burton, *The Sotadic Zone* (Boston, 1973), p. 18. 'The Sotadic Zone' first appeared as the 'Terminal Essay' in Burton's translation of *The Arabian Nights* (1885).

54. See A. Davis, 'Rape, Racism and the Myth of the Black Rapist', in her *Women, Race and Class* (New York, 1981).

55. G. Bataille, *Erotism, Death and Sensuality* [1957], trans. M. Dalwood (San Francisco, 1986), p. 57.

56. S. Hall, 'New Ethnicities', in J. Donald and A. Rattansi (eds), *'Race', Culture and Difference* (Buckingham, 1993), p. 256.

57. H. K. Bhabha, 'Remembering Fanon', foreword to F. Fanon, *Black Skin, White Masks*, p. xxii.

58. Hall, 'New Ethnicities', p. 256.

59. M. Borch-Jakobsen, *Lacan: The Absolute Master*, trans. Douglas Brick (Stanford, 1991), p. 65, states that: 'the subject learns to hold itself straight, upright, by spatially identifying with the specular image'.

60. J. Lacan, 'The Signification of the Phallus', *Écrits* (1977). Similar ideas concerning phallic power were expressed during the second century AD – albeit not in a strictly psychoanalytical context – by Artemidorus in *The Interpretation of Dreams*, I, trans. R. J. White (Park Ridge, NJ; 1975), p.45, where he refers to the penis as a transcendent signifier of power that 'corresponds to speech and education' and that also 'indicates the respect that is inspired by high rank: for it is called "reverence" and "respect"'. Cited in M. Foucault, *The History of Sexuality: Vol. 3, The Care of the Self*, trans. by R. Hurley (Harmondsworth, 1986 [1984]), p. 34.

61. Lacan, *Écrits* (1977), p. 288.

62. R. Dyer, 'Don't look now', pp. 66–7.

63. G. Callaghan, 'Dropping their Daks', *Australian Women's Forum* (1:7, June 1992), p. 52. Callaghan also speaks of the painful body waxing that more hirsute bodybuilders undergo to give their muscles more definition and their skin the smooth

appearance of bronze. Cited in K. R. Dutton, *The Perfectible Body: The Western Ideal of Physical Development* (London, 1995), p. 267.

64. R. Barthes, *The Fashion System*, trans. M. Ward and R. Howard (Berkeley, CA, 1990), pp. 256–7.

65. Wilson, *Adorned in Dreams*, p. 180 (see note 7 above). A. Sinfield, *The Wilde Century: Effeminacy, Oscar Wilde and the Queer Movement* (London, 1994), Chapter 4, discusses dandyism in the context of the aestheticism and decadence of the *fin-de-siècle*. Thus of Oscar Wilde he writes: 'He is the inheritor of the effeminate and hence trivial . . . characters and preoccupations of Sterne and Sheridan. Like the rake, the dandy might debauch himself in any direction. The change is that it becomes difficult for the upper-class male to appear masculine whatever he does; so the distinction between the rake and the fop disappears' (p. 69).

66. Lacan, *Écrits* (1977), p. 280: 'it is in order to be the phallus . . . that a woman will reject an essential part of femininity, namely all her attributes in the masquerade'.

67. See R. Martin, *Fashion and Surrealism* (London and New York, 1988).

68. S. Mower, 'Surrealism in *Vogue*', British *Vogue* (May 1988), pp. 175–7 and 225.

69. Pierre Naville in his article 'Beaux-arts', for *La Révolution Surréaliste* (15 April 1925), p. 27, dismissed painting and also foregrounded photography as having a part to play in envisioning the marvellous and the spectacular.

70. The idea of convulsive beauty was advanced by Breton in three chief texts, *Nadja* (1928); *Minotaure* (1934) and *L'Amour Fou* (1937).

71. A. Breton, *Mad Love*, trans. by M. A. Caws (Lincoln and London, 1987), p. 37.

72. Breton wrote of his encounter with Freud in the surrealist journal, *Littérature* (March 1922).

73. Breton, *Mad Love*, p. 23.

74. Ibid., p. 33.

75. Ibid., p. 33.

76. See S. Freud, 'Three Essays on Sexuality' (1905) in *On Sexuality*, trans. J. Strachey, ed. A. Richards (Harmondsworth, 1977), pp. 31–169.

77. Breton, *Mad Love*, p. 36.

78. M. Ray, *Self-Portrait: Man Ray* (London, 1963), p. 244.

79. T. Baker, 'The work of Alan David-Tu', *The Face* (October 1987), p. 100. Also, 'Cindy Palmano', *The Late Show* (BBC2, 1989). Palmano calls her approach to fashion photography 'conceptual', even though she evidently seems to be working with an idea of convulsive beauty. In the programme, for example, we observe her producing an image of a model wearing an outfit designed by Georgina Godley sitting in a pod-like chair with the intention that she is meant to be a crystal breaking out of a volcanic rock.

80. See J. Derrida, 'The Double Session' (1972), in *Dissemination*, trans. B. Johnson (London, 1981), pp. 173–285.

81. This is the title of Chapter 3 in F. Jameson, *Postmodernism; or, The Cultural Logic of Late Capitalism* (London, 1991), pp. 67–96.

82. J. Lacan, *The Seminars of Jacques Lacan, Book II: The Ego in Freud's Theory and in the Technique of Psychoanalysis, 1954–1955*, trans. S. Tomaselli (Cambridge, 1988), p. 166.

83. L. Irigaray, 'Speculum of the Other Woman', trans. G. C. Gill, in M. Whitford (ed.), *The Irigaray Reader* (Oxford, 1991), pp. 65 and 66.

84. J. Butler, *Bodies that Matter: On the Discursive Limits of "Sex"* (London and New York, 1993), p. 188.

85. K. Theweleit, *Male Fantasies*, trans. S. Conway (Cambridge, 1987), p. 238.

86. Ibid., p. 429.

87. Irigaray, *The Irigaray Reader*, p. 64.

88. J. Butler, 'Melancholy Gender/Refused Identification' in M. Berger, B. Wallis and S. Watson (eds), *Constructing Masculinity* (London and New York, 1995), p. 24.

89. Ibid., pp. 25 and 26.

90. Lacan, *Écrits*, p. 288.

91. Ibid.

92. J. Derrida, *The Truth in Painting* (1978), trans. G. Bennington and I. McLeod (Chicago, 1987), pp. 15–147. Derrida uses Meredith's translation of Kant, first published in 1911. See I. Kant, *The Critique of Judgement*, trans. J. C. Meredith (Oxford, 1952).

93. Derrida, *Truth in Painting*, pp. 54, 57–8.

94. Ibid., p. 64.

95. Ibid., p. 73.

96. N. Logan quoted by A. Lycett, 'Style's in, skin's out', *The Times* (6 September 1989), p. 32.

97. *The Face* (October 1991), p. 9.

98. *The Face* (April 1987), p. 95.

99. See J. Diamond, *The Rise and Fall of the Third Chimpanzee* (London, 1991), p. 64, 'While we can agree that the human penis is an organ of display, the display is intended not for women but for fellow men', and R. Miles, *The Rites of Man: Love, Sex and Death in the Making of the Male* (London, 1991), p. 111: 'The sportsman straining for excellence, the body-builder pumping iron, is not doing it for a woman.'

100. 'Do you think I'm sexy?', *New Woman* (May 1997), pp. 64–7.

101. K. R. Dutton, *The Perfectible Body*, p. 247. Dutton is referring here to A. K Hussain's essay, 'Evaluators' Physique and Self-evaluation as Moderating Variables in Opposite-sex Physique Attraction', *Perspectives in Psychological Researches*, (April 1982), pp. 31–6.

102. *The Face* (April 1997), p. 29.

103. Hebdige, *Subculture*, p. 17. See also Note 9, p. 136.

104. D. A. Miller, *Bringing Out Roland Barthes*, p. 30.

105. S. Freud, 'Psychoanalytic Notes On An Autobiographical Account of Paranoia', in *The Standard Edition, Vol. 12*, ed. and trans. J. Strachey (London, 1958), p. 46.

106. D. Barton cited in C. Worthington, 'Time for the men to try it', *The Independent on Sunday* (September 1994), pp. 44–5.

107. B. Glassner, 'Men and Muscles', in M. S. Kimmel and M. A. Messner (eds), Men's Lives (New York, 1989), p. 315.

108. S. W. Fussell, *Muscle: Confessions of an Unlikely Bodybuilder* (New York, 1991), p. 62.

109. See R. Stengel, 'Men as sex objects', M (July 1992), pp. 72–9, and M. Baker, 'Sexual shock and the emergence of the New Man', M (February 1992), pp. 69–75.

110. P. Jobling, 'Keeping Mrs Dawson Busy: Safe Sex, Gender and Pleasure in Condom Advertising Since 1970' in M. Nava, A. Blake, I. MacRury and B. Richards (eds), *Buy This Book. Studies in Advertising and Consumption* (London and New York, 1997), pp. 157–77.

111. E. Wilson, 'Are You Man Enough?', *Independent on Sunday Review* (29 March 1992), p. 36.

112. Max Horkheimer in A. Arato and E. Gebhardt (eds), *The Essential Frankfurt School Reader* (Oxford, 1978), pp. 41–2: 'Since Freud, the relation between Father and son has been reversed. Now, the rapidly changing society which passes its judgment upon the old is represented not by the father but by the child. The child, not the father, stands for reality. The awe which the Hitler youth enjoys from his parents is but the pointed political expression of a universal state of affairs.'

113. S. Freud, 'The Ego and the Id' (1923), in *On Metapsychology*, pp. 375 and 376.

114. Ibid., p. 376.

115. Barthes, *The Fashion System*, pp. 256–7. See also J. Riviere, 'Womanliness as masquerade', *International Journal of Psychoanalysis*, Vol. 10 (1929), pp. 303–13.

116. J. Lacan, *The Four Fundamental Concepts of Psycho-Analysis*, trans. Alan Sheridan (New York, 1978) p. 49, deals with repetition as something that individuals must perform to achieve the illusion of who they are, but whose enactment also implies that ego-formation is itself somehow never totally accomplished: 'Repetition first appears in a form that is not clear, that is not self-evident, like a reproduction, or a making present *in act.*'

117. Butler, *Gender Trouble*, p. 136.

118. J. Butler, *Bodies that Matter – On the Discursive Limits of 'Sex'* (London and New York: Routledge, 1993), p. 95.

119. Butler, *Gender Trouble*, p. 140.

120. Ibid., pp. 146–7 and 140.

121. See also the following spreads listed in Appendix 1: Enrique Badulescu, 'Scratch that Itch'; Julian Broad, 'Blue Sunday'; Randall Mesdon, 'Lost In Space'; Ellen Von Unwerth, 'Idle Kitsch'; Norman Watson, 'Fatal Attraction'; Bruce Weber, 'Album Phototour', 'Greek Sun' and 'Australia'.

122. Butler, *Bodies that Matter*, pp. 10 and 188.

123. A. Nayak and M. Kehily, 'Playing it straight: masculinities, homophobias and schooling', *Journal of Gender Studies*, 5:2 (1996), pp. 211–30.

124. Ibid., pp. 216–17.

125. S. Freud, 'Group Psychology and the Analysis of the Ego' (1921), in *Standard Edition, Vol. 18*, ed. J. Strachey (London, 1955), p. 107.

126. J. Genet, *Querelle of Brest*, trans. G. Streatham (London, 1987), p. 73.

127. Ibid., pp. 16, 32, 63–70, and 75–81.

128. D. A. Miller, *Bringing Out Roland Barthes*, p. 31.

129. Genet, *Querelle*, pp. 179 and 180.

130. Ibid., p. 27.

131. Ibid., pp. 28 and 29.

132. Ibid., p. 244.

133. Ibid., p. 14.

134. Ibid., p. 77.

135. Ibid., p. 79.

136. Ibid., p. 22.

137. Ibid., p. 206.

138. Ibid., p. 57.

139. Ibid., p. 62.

140. Ibid., pp. 64 and 65.

141. Ibid., p. 21.

142. Ibid., p. 160.

143. R. Barthes, *The Fashion System*, p. 23.

144. See L. Craik, 'Pixelvision', *The Face* (March 1996), pp. 116–17.

145. See *Inez Vans Lamsweerde*, exhibition catalogue (Zürich, 1996).

146. Roland Barthes, *Roland Barthes*, trans. R. Howard (London, 1995 [1975]) p. 133.

Appendix 1

Directory of Fashion Photographers, Stylists and Magazine Features 1980–1996

1.1

The names of the photographers and stylists included in this directory have been culled from every issue of four chief periodical sources for the period 1980–1996. These are:

The Face (May 1980–December 1996);
Arena (November 1986–December 1996);
Arena Homme Plus (Spring/Summer 1994–Autumn/Winter 1996);
British *Vogue* (January 1980–December 1996).

In addition, sporadic copies of the following magazines were also consulted (*denotes USA title):

*Details**
(August 1992, September 1992, August 1993, September 1993, October 1993, September 1994, January 1995, March 1995, March 1996, April 1996, September 1996);
For Him Magazine (since 1994, *FHM*) (August/September 1990, September 1994);
GQ
(July 1992, October 1992, May 1993, December 1993, January 1994, April 1994, May 1994, July 1994, August 1994, November 1994, December 1994);
GQ, Canada (December 1995)
*GQ** (December 1991, June 1992, July 1992, September 1993, December 1995)
Mondo Uomo (July/August 1992)
Observer Life (3 July 1994, 14 January 1996)
Per Lui (July/August 1985)
Unique (March/April 1986, June/July 1986, August 1986, October/November 1986, Autumn 1987)
Vogue Hommes (April 1992, June 1992)

1.2

The content of each fashion feature by any particular photographer/stylist has been classified according to its chief themes with reference to the following codes:

A – gender (general)	K – revivalism, nostalgia
B – gender (masculinities)	L – Surrealism
C – gender (femininities)	M – photographic style
D – androgyny	N – subculture
E – race, ethnicity	O – anti-fashion
F – alien bodies	P – cinema
G – masquerade	Q – travel
H – fetishism	R – nature
I – performance	S – class
J – *fin-de-siècle*, millennium	

Photographer	Stylist	Magazine/Date	Fashion Feature and Page Numbers	Themes
John Akehurst	Polly Banks	*The Face* Sept 1996	Fancy – East of Hoxton Square (110–17)	A, E, S
Miles Aldridge	Joanna Thaw	*The Face* June 1996	Deadlier Than the Male (100–09)	A, D
Marc Alesky	Nancy Rohde	*The Face* Oct 1994	Replicant (68–77)	F
	Adam Howe	*The Face* Sept 1996	Go Westwood Young Man (174–78)	A, B
	Joanna Thaw	*The Face* Dec 1996	Abstract Poetic (108–13)	B, K
Annette Aurell		*Details* March 1996	Powder Blue	F
	Anette Monheim	*The Face* May 1993	Sunshine Playroom (66–71)	D, J
	Cathy Dixon	*The Face* Oct 1993	All Day I Dream About (72–77)	D, K
	Anette Monheim	*The Face* Jan 1994	Techno Squat (100–07)	K
	Anette Monheim	*The Face* June 1995	Brute 33 (86–90)	E
	Anette Monheim	*The Face* March 1996	Dum Dum Boy (157–65)	C, O
Enrique Badulescu		*Arena* Oct 1996	Scratch That Itch (164–71)	A, E
		The Face May 1989	Fuck Art – let's Vogue (42–9)	C, E
	Malcolm Beckford	*The Face* June 1989	Wide West (64–71)	A
	Mitzi Lorenz	*The Face* Feb 1990	Sex Pack – dirty dozen (96–101)	A, C

Appendix 1: Photographers, Stylists and Features

Photographer	Stylist	Magazine/Date	Fashion Feature and Page Numbers	Themes
Enrique Badulescu	Mitzi Lorenz	*The Face* April 1991	Motel/Hotel – holiday in hen party (68–77)	A, C
Andrew Bettles		*The Face* Aug 1987	Spellbound (38–43)	L
	Mitzi Lorenz	*The Face* Nov 1987	Vanity Dare (116–21)	L
	Paul Frecker	*The Face* May 1988	London, March 88 (52–9)	L
		The Face Oct 1988	Datelines (140–47)	L
		The Face March 1989	Striking Beauties (120–25)	L
		The Face Dec 1989	What? How? Why? (138–9)	L
Nick Baratta	William Gilchrist	*Arena* Dec 1989/ Jan 1990	After Dark – Milanese finesse (116–23)	B, P
Alan Beukers		*Arena* May 1996	The Beat Goes On (88–93)	B, O
		Arena July/Aug 1996	Marrakesh Sheltering Sky (100–09)	C
	David Bradshaw	*Arena* Sept 1996	Softlad (162–67)	D
	David Bradshaw	*Arena* Dec 1996	World's End (172–9)	B
		GQ Oct 1992	Hungary for Love (160–67)	K
		GQ May 1993	Flying Visit (86–93)	B
Hervé Biale	Beatrice Carle	*The Face* July 1989	Little Egypt (68–71)	K, Q
Joakim Blokström	Hina Dohi at Streeters	*Arena* Dec 1996	The Contender – Toby Stephens (168–71)	B
Koto Bolofo		GQ (USA) Dec 1991	Hot Around the Collar (260–3)	A
Flavio Bonetti		*Mondo Uomo*, July 1992	Fantasy Power (216–18)	M
Martin Brading	Ray Petri	*Arena* March/April 1987	Ragamuffin, Hand Me Down My Walking Cane (70–77)	B, S
	Ray Petri	*Arena* July/Aug 1988	Wide Boys Awake (90–101)	B, E, S
	David Bradshaw	*Arena* July/Aug 1991	Earth Man – easy dressing for men of the world (110–15)	B, J

Appendix 1: Photographers, Stylists and Features

Photographer	Stylist	Magazine/Date	Fashion Feature and Page Numbers	Themes
Martin Brading	David Bradshaw	*Arena* Nov 1992 *Details* Sept 1993	Nature Boy (162–7) The American Way (194–203)	B, J, R B, S
	Debbi Mason	*The Face* Sept 1984 *The Face* Nov 1984	Suit Yourself (52–55) Strapping Lasses – bon bondage (36–9)	C, D A, H
Carrie Branovan	Paul Frecker	*The Face* May 1986	Fashion-Wool (40–5)	C
Tim Bret-Day	UTO	*The Face* Feb 1994	Damaged (78–83)	B, J
Julian Broad	Debbie Mason	*Arena* May/June 1992	Lace Relations – from ballroom to boudoir (130–5)	C, N
	Christian Logan Karl and Derick	*The Face* Aug 1989 *The Face* Nov 1990	Stormy Leather (64–9) Fashion – ready, steady, go (60–7)	B, N A, E
	Malcolm Beckford	*The Face* Sept 1991	Blue Sunday (80–7)	A, I, M
Richard Burbridge		*Details* April 1996	The Real Skinny (146–51)	B,N, O
Steve Callaghan	Karl Templer	*The Face* June 1996	Trade (140–47)	B, N
Peter Calvin	Angela Hill	*The Face* Jan 1988	High Priced Anxiety! (52–9)	C, O, P
Emmanuel Carlier	Nazir	*The Face* Jan 1991	Groovy Glitterati (66–71)	A, M
Roger Charity	Ray Petri	*Arena* Sept/Oct 1988	Tuscany – burnt sienna (90–107)	B, P, Q
	Ray Petri	*Arena* Autumn/ Winter 1989	The Long Goodbye (130–37)	B
	Ray Petri	*The Face* Oct 1985	Buffalo (62–71)	B, I
Donald Christie		*Observer Life*, 14 Jan 1996	Slim Fit	B
Nick Clements		*GQ* July 1992	Olympian Ideals (104–11)	B
Elaine Constantine	Nancy Rohde	*The Face* Nov 1996	Round Our Way – the boot boy rides again (134–41)	B, Q

Appendix 1: Photographers, Stylists and Features

Photographer	Stylist	Magazine/Date	Fashion Feature and Page Numbers	Themes
Anton Corbijn		*Details* Sept 1996	New Values (208–15)	J, N
Richard Croft	Simon Foxton	*Arena* Nov/Dec 1987	Tweedy Pie (116–23)	B, N
	Angela Hill	*The Face* July 1988	Tough Guise (82–87)	C
	Tanya Gill	*The Face* Oct 1988	The Glasshouse Effect (52–7)	C, M
Monica Curtin		*FHM* Aug/Sept 1990	Streetwise	B
Kevin Davies	Christian Logan	*Arena* March/April 1989	Electric Horsemen (82–9)	B, G
	William Gilchrist	*Arena* May/June 1989	The Monochrome Set (110–15)	B, M
		The Face Nov 1988	Curves Aired (116–21)	A
Corinne Day		*The Face* March 1990	About Turn (104–11)	O
	Melanie Ward	*The Face* July 1990	The 3rd Summer of Love – the daisy age (44–51)	C, N
	Melanie Ward	*The Face* Sept 1990	Fashion (56–63)	A, K
	Melanie Ward	*The Face* May 1991	Slapheads (90–7)	A, H
	Melanie Ward	*The Face* Aug 1991	Borneo (80–7)	C, E
	Melanie Ward	*The Face* Aug 1992	Wahwah (82–9)	D
	Melanie Ward	*The Face* Aug 1993	England's Dreaming, this is the modern world (104–113)	J, N
	Cathy Kasterine	*The Face* Jan 1994	Psycho Billy (60–7)	D, J
	Karl Plewka	*Observer Life* 3 July 1994	Youth Club	J, K, N
	Cathy Kasterine	*Vogue* June 1993	Under Exposure (144–51)	C, I, O
Didier de Fays		*Unique* Oct/Nov 1986	Great Coats (59–64)	B
Horst Diekgerdes	David Bradshaw	*Arena* Sept 1996	Modern Living (152–61)	B
Warren du Preez	Jason Kelvin	*The Face* Feb 1995	Parade – military finesse gone AWOL (80–7)	D
	Jason Kelvin	*The Face* May 1996	Grease Monkey (146–51)	B
Sean Ellis	Isabella Blow	*The Face* Oct 1996	Taste of Arsenic (90–7)	C, H, J, O

Photographer	Stylist	Magazine/Date	Fashion Feature and Page Numbers	Themes
Robert Erdman	Markus von Ackermann	*Arena* July/Aug 1987	Navy and White (50–55)	D, J
	David Bradshaw	*Arena* March/April 1991	Wiseguys (70–79)	B, P
	David Bradshaw	*Arena* Nov 1991	La Dolce Vita (130–37)	B
	Caroline Baker	*The Face* Sept 1984	Role Over – and enjoy it! (20–27)	B, I
	Hamish Bowles	*The Face* Sept 1984	Another Country (48–51)	B, P
David Eustace		*GQ* Aug 1994	The Getaway (88–95)	B
Jose Manuel Ferreler	David Bradshaw	*Arena* Jan/Feb 1989	Hombre, Hombre (102–07)	B
Fabrizio Ferri	William Gilchrist	*Arena* May/June 1993	Blue Moods (114–19)	B
		GQ (USA) Sept 1993	Modern Romance (312–21)	K
Adrian Fiebig		*Unique* June/July 1986	Limelight Style (58–63)	B
Nick Fry	Yvonne Sporre	*The Face* Oct 1993	We've come to stay in the happy house (134–39)	J, N
Kate Garner	Alice Hunter	*Arena* May/June 1989	Tumbling Dice (116–23)	B, G
	Karl and Derick (UTO)	*The Face* Aug 1991	Wet (58–63)	A, H
	Kim Bowen	*The Face* April 1992	Y.w.c.a. (54–61)	C, D
	Karin Labby	*The Face* Aug 1994	Bikini Kill! (66–73)	C, M
Manfred Gestreich	Tanya Gill	*Arena* July/Aug 1989	Paris, France (98–107)	B, F, Q
	Jitt Gill	*The Face* Jan 1990	Crimes of Passion (64–73)	C
Andrea Giacobbe	Maida	*The Face* Oct 1994	Leisure Lounge (110–19)	A, F
	Maida	*The Face* March 1995	Ark Life (60–9)	F, J
	Maida	*The Face* Feb 1996	Little Earth (82–9)	F, K
	Maida	*The Face* July 1996	Simplex Concordia (90–99)	F, J
Fabrizio Gianni		*GQ* (USA) July 1992	Back to the Future (78–89)	B, K, P

Appendix 1: Photographers, Stylists and Features

Photographer	Stylist	Magazine/Date	Fashion Feature and Page Numbers	Themes
Anthony Gordon		*Details* Aug 1992	Special Delivery (114–19)	B
	Simon Foxton	*The Face* Dec 1987	Beached Bums – or sex and the shingle girl (106–113)	C, D
		The Face April 1988	Alex Eats (64–75)	C, I, O
		The Face Sept 1988	Alex Works – careering through the eighties (66–77)	C, O
Christopher Griffiths	David Bradshaw	*Arena* March/April 1994	High Tension – no-nonsense sportswear (98–107)	B
	David Bradshaw	*Arena* July/Aug 1994	Have a nice day! less is more (112–19)	A, I
	David Bradshaw	*Arena* Dec 1994/Jan 1995	Doing it yourself? (112–19)	B
	Tamara Fulton	*Arena* March 1996	This is . . . not a fashion story (12–21)	A, O
	Karl Templer	*The Face* Jan 1995	The Gents (56–65)	B, S
Guzman		*GQ* Nov 1994	Make Mine a Double (172–81)	B, E
		GQ Dec 1994	Stag Night (130–9)	B
Michel Haddi	Debra Berkin	*Arena* Dec 1986/ Jan 1987	On and Off the Road (112–19)	B
	Debra Berkin	*Arena* July/Aug 1987	Debret Pack (74–81)	B
	Debra Berkin	*Arena* Sept/Oct 1987	Riders of the Storm (116–21)	B
		Arena Jan/Feb 1988	Throwback (32–9)	B, P
	Debra Berkin	*Arena* Jan/Feb 1988	Fin de siecle (84–91)	B, J
	William Faulkner	*Arena* Sept/Oct 1988	Kid Gloves – Muay kind of Thai (58–67)	B, E
	Venetia Scott	*Arena* Sept/Oct 1989	The Back Lot (110–23)	A, P
	Christian Logan	*Arena* Dec 1989/Jan 1990	Circus Dreams (104–11)	A, I
	Venetia Scott	*Arena* March/April 1990	Flight to Tangiers (106–17)	B, E
		The Face Dec 1984	Secret Life of Arabia (28–32)	B, E
	Claude Sabbah	*The Face* Dec 1986	Hero (90–93)	B, D
	Venetia Scott	*The Face* Jan 1989	Les Yeux Dangereux – object desire (76–83)	H, L

Photographer	Stylist	Magazine/Date	Fashion Feature and Page Numbers	Themes
Michel Haddi	Venetia Scott	*The Face* April 1989	Circle of Dreams (120–27)	I, P
	Venetia Scott	*The Face* July 1989	Latin Summer (82–87)	A, P
		Vogue Jan 1991	Modern Mariners – Yasmin and Simon Lebon (122–27)	A, P
Hugh Hales-Tooke		*Details* Aug 1993	Whats in Store (76–83)	N, O
		For Him Aug/Sept 1990	Elegant Effects (122–29)	B, S
Nicolas Hidiriglou	Charlotte (TDP)	*The Face* Nov 1995	Weekenders (144–51)	A
Steve Hiett	Jennifer Elster	*The Face* Dec 1996	Neighbourhood – teen dreams and the girl next door (144–51)	C, N, P
Horst	David Bradshaw	*Arena* Dec 1994/ Jan 1995	Ground Control (128–35)	M
Seb Janiak	Gigi Lepage	*The Face* July 1995	Nu Earth – fashion style beyond the stargate (56–65)	J, P
Mikael Jansson	Karl Templer	*Arena* Dec 1996	Round Midnight (156–65)	A, M, P
Lee Jenkins	Greg Fay/ Justin Laurie	*The Face* Oct 1995	Kev's Ghost (86–95)	L
	Joanna Thaw	*The Face* May 1996	The Circus (116–25)	A, I
Jean François Julian	Christeena W	*The Face* Dec 1992	Paris Jour – country life (52–7)	K, P
Charlie Kemp		*The Face* Oct 1985	Hard Lines (36–41)	C, M
Steven Klein		*Arena Homme Plus*, Spring/Summer 1996	Morning Glory (176–81)	D
	Nancy Rohde	*The Face* Dec 1995	Performance (80–89)	A, I
	Karl and Derick (UTO)	*The Face* Oct 1991	Night Fever (70–77)	A, K, P
	Nancy Rohde	*The Face* Oct 1996	All About Eve (178–85)	C, H
Nick Knight	Marc Ascoli	*Arena* March/ April 1988	Yamamoto (78–87)	L, M

Appendix 1: Photographers, Stylists and Features

Photographer	Stylist	Magazine/Date	Fashion Feature and Page Numbers	Themes
Nick Knight	Simon Foxton	*Arena* Jan/Feb 1989	Faith (108–21)	M, R
	Simon Foxton	*Arena Homme Plus* Spring/Summer 1995	Close Encounters (72–81)	A, B, E, I, P
	Simon Foxton	*Arena Homme Plus* Autumn/Winter 1996/97	Forget Sergeant Pepper (188–95)	B, E, H
	Simon Foxton	*The Face* 1986	Fashion – Punk (42–51)	A, N, E
	Simon Foxton	*The Face* Aug 1986	Culture Clash – New England (41–9)	A, E, G
		Vogue Nov 1993	Transition Vamp (162–73)	C, D
	François Berthoud	*Vogue* Oct 1995	Couture in Colour (184–85)	M
Kim Knott	Marckus von Ackermann	*Arena* March/April 1987	Chain Reaction (88–95)	B
	Marckus von Ackermann	*Arena* Jan/Feb 1988	Unconventional Wisdom (96–103)	B
		Vogue Jan 89	Skin on Skin (108–11)	C, H
Serge Krouglikoff	Zee	*The Face* July 1987	Old Fetishes Die Hard (32–35)	C, H
Christophe Kutner	Karl Templer	*Arena* Dec/Jan 95/6	Man and Machine (140–9)	B
David Lachapelle		*Details* Sept 1996	The Smart Patrol (192–201)	A, H, M
	Arianne Phillips	*The Face* Feb 1994	Meanwhile . . . (52–9)	A, J
	Arianne Phillips	*The Face* July 1994	Glacé Girls (58–67)	A
	Arianne Phillips	*The Face* April 1995	The New Seekers (116–125)	J, R
	Arianne Phillips	*The Face* Nov 1995	The Witching Hour (86–95)	A, H
	Carrie Varoquiers	*The Face* April 1996	House of Dolls (106–13)	C, G
Marc Lebon	Ray Petri	*Arena* March/April 1987	The Boys in the Band (80–5)	B
	Ray Petri	*Arena* Jan/Feb 1989	Grooms and Gamblers (86–97)	B, D, G
	Jitt Gill	*The Face* June 1988	Paradise Lost (36–43)	K, R
	Debbi Mason	*The Face* Nov 1991	Forever Leather (64–71)	C, E, H

Photographer	Stylist	Magazine/Date	Fashion Feature and Page Numbers	Themes
Thierry Le Gouès		*Arena* July/Aug 1994	Naomi gold (96–9)	C, H
		Vogue Hommes June 1992	Mariage (118–25)	E
Trevor Leighton	David Bradshaw	*Arena* Nov 1991	The Professionals (118–29)	B
Jonathan Lennard	Helen Roberts	*The Face* July 1985	Sex . . . coming soon (56–9)	C
		The Face Aug 1985	Some like it hot! (48–51)	C, P
Mark Lewis	Finbar at Max Presents	*The Face* July 1988	Guys n Dolls (52–7)	A, I, P
	Iain R Webb	*Unique* Autumn 1987	Boys from Brazil (72–77)	B, E, Q
Peter Lindbergh	Karl Templer	*The Face* Nov 1996	South Side (96–105)	A, E
		Vogue Feb 1989	Superheroines (108–15)	C, G, P
Richard Lohr	Ray Petri	*The Face* Jan 1984	Style 2 (44–9)	A, D
Glen Luchford	Adam Howe	*Arena* Dec 1989/Jan 1990	Black on black (130–33)	A, M
	Kim Bowen	*Arena* Nov 1993	The Gripes of Roth (160–67)	B
	Judy Blame	*The Face* Feb 1992	Modern Love – three men and a babe (50–5)	A, E, P
	Dodi Greganti	*The Face* June 1992	Rising Sons – European clothes, Asian style (80–7)	D, E
	Judy Blame	*The Face* Jan 1993	Fashion Vampires (84–95)	F, J
	Dodi Greganti	*The Face* July 1993	America eats its young (90–9)	N, P
Eamonn J McCabe	Simon Foxton	Arena Sept/Oct 1987	Playing to win (106–11)	B
	Mitzi Lorenz	*The Face* April 1986	Fashion Extra (67–73)	D, I
	Stephen Linard	*The Face* Sept 1986	London Calling (44–51)	B, I
	Mitzi Lorenz	*The Face* Oct 1986	The Lady from Shanghai (84–93)	A, P
		The Face Sept 1991	Destroy! (58–65)	B
		Unique March/April 1986	Summer Fashions (54–69)	B, Q
		Unique June/July 1986	Summertime Blues (43–55)	A, Q
		Unique Oct/Nov 1986	Dentente (51–58)	M

Photographer	Stylist	Magazine/Date	Fashion Feature and Page Numbers	Themes
Eamonn J McCabe		*Unique* Oct/Nov 1986	Pravda – Revolutionary Looks (59–68)	B, G
Craig McDean	Gaby Fayol	*The Face* Dec 1992	Paris nuit – silver moon (102–07)	K
	Liz Thody	*The Face* Sept 1993	Glory Days (72–9)	C, O
	Alex White	*The Face* Nov 1994	Saturday Night, Sunday Morning (66–75)	K, P
Tony McGee		*The Face* Nov 1986	Miaow with Yasmin, feline groovy (58–61)	C
Andrew Macpherson	Mika Mizutani	*Arena* March/April 1987	Buster Keaton bounces back (58–67)	B, K, P
	Joe McKenna	*Arena* Nov/Dec 1987	Stephen Sprouse – a riot of his own (128–31)	B, D
	William Gilchrist	*Arena* Sept/Oct 1994	Phew! Rock 'n' roll . . . meet the Nancy boys (110–17)	D
		The Face Dec 1984	Apparitions (84–7)	F, J, K
		The Face Jan 1985	Veiled Threats (52–7)	J
	Cathy Kasterine	*The Face* March 1992	LA Rox – Stacey Lowe goes west (76–87)	C, M
		Vogue Hommes April 1992	Palace (90–3)	C
Robert Manzotti		*Arena* April 1996	Passeggiata (136–43)	B, Q
Bertrand Marignac	Valerie Lefevre and Camilla Serra	*The Face* March 1994	The Baby Sitter (108–13)	A, G
Kurt Markus	David Bradshaw	*Arena* Nov 1990	Comme Homme (98–107)	B, M
James Martin	David Bradshaw	*Arena* Dec 1990/ Jan 1991	Blue Mood (100–09)	B, H
	David Bradshaw	*Arena* March/April 1993	Hard Edged (124–31)	B
Wayne Maser		*GQ* (USA) Dec 1991	Acapulco bold (236–45)	A
		Vogue Sept 1995	Wild Thing (280–85)	C, H
		Vogue Oct 1995	A la Mod (166–69)	C, K
Marc Mattock	David Bradshaw	*Arena* Sept/Oct 1995	Saints and Sinners (108–11)	B

Appendix 1: Photographers, Stylists and Features

Photographer	Stylist	Magazine/Date	Fashion Feature and Page Numbers	Themes
Oliver Maxwell	Elaine Jones	*The Face* July 1986	Who's Shooting Who? (81–5)	B, E, G
Tony Meneguzzo	Marcus von Ackermann	*Arena* Sept/Oct 1987	Another Green World (96–102)	B, R
Randall Mesdon	David Bradshaw	*Arena* Sept/Oct 1991	The Last Detail (122–31)	B, P
	David Bradshaw	*Arena* March/April 1992	Class Acts – dressing in dramatic fashion (102–11)	I, K
	David Bradshaw	*Arena* July/Aug 1992	Olympians (104–15)	B
	David Bradshaw	*Arena* Nov 1992	Once upon a time (152–9)	B, K, P
	David Bradshaw	*Arena* Dec 1992/Jan 1993	Land of the BRAVE (122–31)	B
	David Bradshaw	*Arena* May/June 1993	Lost in Space (140–7)	A, M, P
	David Bradshaw	*Arena* Sept/Oct 1993	Another Country (114–23)	B, K
Donald Milne	Nancy Rohde	*Arena* May/June 1995	Undercover (122–9)	B, E
		Arena Homme Plus Spring/Summer 1996	Cul-de-sac (130–37)	B, K
	Nancy Rohde	*The Face* Nov 1994	Army Dreamers (106–13)	B, D
	Nancy Rohde	*The Face* Aug1995	An ideal for Living (120–31)	D
	Nancy Rohde	*The Face* April 1996	The Trouble with Harriet (156–63)	J, N
John Minh Nguyen		*Details* Sept 1996	Plaidness without the madness (218–23)	B
Jean Baptiste Mondino		*Arena Homme Plus* Autumn/Winter 1994	Evander Holyfield's big night in (112–19)	B, E
		Arena Homme Plus Spring/Summer 1996	The Cappuccinos (120–27)	B, D, E
	Karl Templer	*Arena Homme Plus* Autumn/Winter 1996/97	Feel the Force (141–53)	B, I
	Elisabeth Djian	*The Face* Oct 1987	Electric Lady land (90–5)	F
	Ray Petri	*The Face* Feb 1988	New Hats from London and Paris (44–49)	A, D
	Elisabeth Djian	*The Face* March 1989	Heavy Metal (86–93)	C, L

Photographer	Stylist	Magazine/Date	Fashion Feature and Page Numbers	Themes
Jean Baptiste Mondino	Judy Blame	*The Face* Aug 1993	Head Hunters – Back to the No Future (80–9)	G, H. J, K
	Brigitte Echols	*The Face* June 1994	Reality bites (68–75)	A, P
	Maida	*The Face* Sept 1994	Full Metal Jacket (66–73)	J
	Friquette Thevenet	*The Face* Jan 1996	The Usual Suspects (118–25)	P
	Joanna Thaw	*The Face* March 1996	Check Yourself (138–43)	D, L
	Friquette Thevenet	*The Face* Aug 1996	World in Lotion (76–81)	A, D
Eddie Monsoon	Adam Howe	*The Face* Dec 1988	Up from the downstroke (86–97)	A, H
Jamie Morgan		*The Face* Aug 1983	Style – summer strip (52–3)	A
		The Face Sept 1983	Style – tour de force (48–9)	B
		The Face Jan 1984	Style 2 (44–9)	A, D
	Ray Petri	*The Face* Jan 1984	Style – winter sports (28–33)	B
	Ray Petri	*The Face* May 1984	Style (26–31)	A
	Sheila Rock	*The Face* Nov 1984	Men's where? (84–91)	B, D
	Ray Petri	*The Face* March 1985	Hard (84–91)	B
	Ray Petri	*The Face* June 1985	Float like a butterfly, sting like a bee (33–41)	B
	Ray Petri	*The Face* April 1986	Buffalo (90–95)	B
	Ray Petri	*The Face* Sept 1986	Buffalo – a more serious pose (90–4)	B
	Mitzi Lorenz	*The Face* July 1990	Fashion (74–81)	C, E
Dewey Nicks		*GQ* (USA) June 1992	98° in the shade (190–7)	A
Perry Ogden		*The Face* Nov 1985	Long Day's Journey Into Night (36–41)	C
Terry O'Neill	David Bradshaw	*Arena* Nov 1993	Dirty Gary (142–51)	B
Mike Owen	Beth Shachat	*The Face* Jan 1988	Cinema scope (60–5)	A, P
Cindy Palmano	Fred Poodle	*The Face* Aug 1986	Ultra (62–5)	M
Adrian Peacock	Mike Penn	*Unique* Autumn 1987	New Classics (84–7)	B

Appendix 1: Photographers, Stylists and Features

Photographer	Stylist	Magazine/Date	Fashion Feature and Page Numbers	Themes
Mike Penn	David Bradshaw	*Arena* Dec 1991/ Jan 1992	Urban Kings – Elvis lives in London (80–5)	B, K
Stephanie Periender		*GQ* May 1993	Homme Alone (98–105)	B
Platon	Malcolm Beckford	*Arena* Dec 1995/ Jan 1996	A Family Affair (150–5)	B, E
Helen Putsman	David Bradshaw	*Arena* March/ April 1988	Seconds Out (108–11)	B
Bettina Rheims		*Details* March 1995	Detux (162–79)	D
	Joanna Thaw	*The Face* March 1996	De Lacy (94–101)	D, I
Terry Richardson	David Bradshaw	*Arena* Sept/Oct 1995	Georgie Porgie (124–31)	B, S
	David Bradshaw	*Arena* March 1996	Day Tripper (146–53)	A
		Details April 1996	The Twill of It All (124–9)	A, D
	Karl Templer	*The Face* June 1995	Mashed – liberté, egalité, par-tay (116–23)	A, C, M, N
	Andrew Richardson	*The Face* Sept 1996	Repulsion (130–7)	A, P
Herb Ritts		*The Face* Oct 1984	Grease Monkeys (69–73)	B, G, H
		Vogue July 1988	The Big Time (120–25)	C
		Vogue Feb 1989	Earthen Wear (124–28)	C, R
		Vogue March 1989	Sands of Time (296–301)	C, Q
		Vogue April 1989	Paris Couture (Kim Basinger) (163–73)	C, I, P
		Vogue June 1989	Muscle Mechanics (146–49)	C, D, G
		Vogue Oct 1989	Friends of the Earth (370–77)	C, H, R
		Vogue Oct 1989	Paris Couture – à la recherche du temps Bardot (331–41)	C, K, P
		Vogue Aug 1990	The Avenging Spirit (193–99)	C, H, K
		Vogue Sept 1990	Knight Errant (342–47)	C, D, G
		Vogue Dec 1990	Heavenly Bodies (180–87)	A, H
		Vogue Aug 1991	Molten Metallics (104–11)	C, H

Photographer	Stylist	Magazine/Date	Fashion Feature and Page Numbers	Themes
Herb Ritts		*Vogue* May 1992	A Fairy Tale ... (151–57)	C, G, K
Peter Robathan	Yvonne Sporre	*The Face* May 1993	Spook! the midsummer night's scream (98–105)	B, N
	Seta Niland	*The Face* Aug 1994	Super Nature (102–08)	E, J
	Seta Niland	*The Face* April 1995	Yard Times (64–73)	C, E
	Seta Niland	*The Face* Sept 1995	Insects Are All Around Us (130–9)	L, M
	Seta Niland	*The Face* March 1996	Tuff Metal (120–29)	D, J
	Seta Niland	*The Face* Oct 1996	The Emperor's New Clothes (118–25)	C, H
Michael Roberts		GQ (USA) June 1992	The Players (135–45)	B, I, P
Sheila Rock	Steve Bush	*The Face*, Jan 1981	Style – the Suggs Collection	B, N
		The Face Oct 1981	Style – A West Side Story	K, N
Marc Roger	Elisabeth Djian	*The Face* Dec 1987	Super Structure (100–05)	L
Aldo Rossi	Karl Templer	*Arena* Dec 1994/ Jan 1995	The Outer Limits (120–7)	B
	David Bradshaw	*Arena* March/ April 1995	Lifelines (98–107)	B, M
	David Bradshaw	*Arena* May/ June 1995	Dojo (110–21)	B
		Arena June 1996	Cadets (100–07)	B, I
Johnny Rosza		*Unique* Oct/ Nov 1986	High Noon (74–81)	B, G, J K, P
Paolo Roversi	David Bradshaw	*Arena Homme Plus* Autumn/Winter 1996/97	The Jeans That Didn't Build America (212–19)	B, M
		Vogue April 1986	New Luminaries (210–19)	B, H
		Vogue Oct 1993	Tinker Tailoring (178–87)	K
		Vogue April 1994	Out of This World (176–85)	E
		Vogue July 1994	The Beaton Track (78–86)	K, M

Appendix 1: Photographers, Stylists and Features

Photographer	Stylist	Magazine/Date	Fashion Feature and Page Numbers	Themes
Paolo Roversi		*Vogue* May 1996	Rainbow Warriors (106–17)	C, J, R
Grant Sainsbury		*Unique* Autumn 1987	Back To Business (65–71)	B
		Unique Autumn 1987	Urbane Renewal (88–95)	A, S
Hans Peter Schneider		*Details* August 1992	Café LA (82–91)	K
		GQ Jan 1994	Knowing the Score (94–101)	B
		GQ May 1994	Dress Rehearsal (124–31)	B, I
		GQ May 1994	Totally Wicket (132–41)	B, E
Schoerner	David Bradshaw	*Arena* July/Aug 1994	The Sunshine State (104–11)	B
	David Bradshaw	*Arena* Nov 1994	The Clerk (116–23)	B
		Details Jan 1995	Come as you are (88–95)	O
	Adam Howe	*The Face* Sept 1993	Suburbanites (114–21)	J, N
	Greg Fay/ Justin Laurie	*The Face* Dec 1993	Rain (66–73)	D, J
	Adam Howe	*The Face* March 1994	Cherry Drops and Jelly Babes (86–95)	C, E, N
	Adam Howe	*The Face* Sept 1994	Bad Boy Memory (90–102)	A, F, J
	Nancy Rohde	*The Face* Jan 1995	Quest for Albion (100–11)	C, H, J
	Adam Howe	*The Face* May 1995	Begging you – another girl on another planet (140–9)	F, L
	Adam Howe	*The Face* Aug 1996	Planet Waves (128–35)	J
	Joanne Yi	*The Face* Nov 1996	Sunspots (162–71)	J
Nina Schultz	Dodi Greganti	*The Face* Nov 1993	Fallout (112–17)	J, M, R
	Yvonne Sporre	*The Face* May 1994	And the little one said . . . (105–12)	A
	Seta Niland	*The Face* Feb 1995	The Birds (48–57)	C, P
	Andrew Dosunmu	*The Face* Dec 1995	Voodoo (146–53)	A, E
Stephane Sednaoui	Paul Frecker	*Arena* Nov/Dec 1988	Reflections in a Golden Eye (118–23)	L
		Details March 1996	Automotive for the People (180–89)	B
		The Face June 1988	Voici Paris (70–83)	L, M

Appendix 1: Photographers, Stylists and Features

Photographer	Stylist	Magazine/Date	Fashion Feature and Page Numbers	Themes
Stephane Sednaoui		*The Face* Jan 1989	Popeye – bonjour matelot (30–7)	A, I
	Elisabeth Djian	*The Face* March 1989	Heavy Metal (93–103)	L
	Elisabeth Djian	*The Face* Oct 1989	Showdown – the battle for planet fashion (84–109)	F, M
	Paul Frecker	*The Face* Feb 1990	Popeye – the story continues (50–7)	A, I
		The Face May 1995	Trafalgar Square (frieze pull-out)	E
Nigel Shafran		*The Face* July 1988	Faking it (40–1)	N, O
	Melanie Ward	*The Face* July 1989	Fantastic Voyage – lost in space (54–61)	F
David Sims (M.A.P.)	Melanie Ward (Opera)	*The Face* July 1991	Cowgirl in the Sand (76–85)	A, N, O
	Venetia Scott	*The Face* Feb 1993	Oh You Pretty Thing (56–63)	D, K
	Melanie Ward	*The Face* Nov 1993	Are Friends Electric (88–95)	D, K
	Nancy Rohde	*The Face* March 1995	She's in Parties (78–83)	C, N
	Nancy Rohde	*The Face* May 1995	The Warm Jets (94–101)	F, O
	Anna Cockburn	*The Face* Nov 1995	Play for Today (116–21)	C, I
	Joe McKenna	*The Face* June 1996	Wendy's House (78–87)	A
Peggy Sirota		GQ (Can) Dec 1995	Down town Racer (178–85)	B
		Vogue July 1991	The Lady Vanishes and a Star is Born Hitchcock Style	C, P
Julie Sleaford	Yvonne Sporre	*The Face* Oct 1995	The Garden Party (126–33)	J, K
Graham Smith		*The Face* Feb 1981	Style – Spandau Ballet	B, K, N
Mario Sorrenti	Camilla Nickerson	*The Face* Sept 1992	Glitter Babies (70–7)	A, D
	Cathy Dixon	*The Face* April 1993	Flesh (96–101)	B, D, H
Wayne Stambler	Marcus von Ackermann	*Arena* March/ April 1988	Kinds of Blue (102–07)	B

Appendix 1: Photographers, Stylists and Features

Photographer	Stylist	Magazine/Date	Fashion Feature and Page Numbers	Themes
Hugh Stewart	Sheena Robertson	*FHM* Sept 1994	Untamed Heart (120–27)	B
Juergen Teller	Simon Foxton	*Arena* Jan/Feb 1988	Chill Factor (104–11)	B, M
	Simon Foxton	*Arena* Sept/Oct 1988	Bodyheat (114–21)	B, E
	Venetia Scott	*Arena* May/June 1994	Liberté, egalité, fraternité (104–11)	C, D
	David Bradshaw	*Arena Homme Plus* Autumn/Winter 1996/97	More Waugh Stories (156–63)	B, S
	Tracey Jacob	*The Face* Dec 1987	Principal Boy (114–19)	C, D, I
		The Face April 1988	Victorian Principle (94–101)	K, M
		The Face May 1989	New Age – elements of style (88–97)	M
	Lorina Crosland	*The Face* Sept 1989	Eastern Promise (86–93)	C
	Judy Blame	*The Face* Dec 1990	Kinky Afro (102–11)	E
	Venetia Scott	*The Face* March 1991	Tough Kookie (98–105)	C, H
	Venetia Scott	*The Face* Feb 1992	Cuba Libre (76–81)	A, E, Q
	Venetia Scott	*The Face* April 1993	Blue Hotel (54–61)	A, P
	Venetia Scott	*The Face* Aug 1995	The Bum Deal (98–107)	A, H
	Venetia Scott	*The Face* April 1996	Skin I'm In (76–83)	C, H
		Vogue June 1996	Band Aid (130–37)	C, J, N
Mario Testino	Caroline Baker	*The Face* June 1984	Style – bodylicious: get ready for the tight fit (82–5)	A
	Michael Roberts	*The Face* July 1984	Style – styled in New York (66–9)	D
	Andrew Macpherson	*The Face* Oct 1984	Different Strokes (34–43)	M M
	Mitzi Lorenz	*The Face* Dec 1990	One Love (76–83)	C, D, E
	Adam Howe	*The Face* Aug 1995	Likely Lads (40–51)	A, D
	Carine Roitfeld	*The Face* Feb 1996	Silly Benjamin (62–7)	B, D, G
	Carine Roitfeld	*The Face* July 1996	Yves Gauche (70–9)	K, M
Christian Thompson		*The Face* Feb 1989	Laundromatic (84–91)	M
	Tracey Jacob	*The Face* June 1989	Spy – double oh trouble (80–5)	A, H
Marcus Tomlinson	Lorenzo Rieva	*Arena* July/Aug 1990	Napoli (114–21)	B
	David Bradshaw	*Arena* Nov 1995	Green Piece, Acid Reigns (144–9)	D, J, R
		Arena Oct 1996	Swingers (136–41)	B

Appendix 1: Photographers, Stylists and Features

Photographer	Stylist	Magazine/Date	Fashion Feature and Page Numbers	Themes
Marcus Tomlinson	Karl and Derick (UTO)	*The Face* Dec 1991	Cold Comforts (62)	L, M
	Kim Andreolli	*The Face* Nov 1993	Stone Rangers (132–39)	J, R
	Kim Andreolli	*The Face* July 1994	Future Shock (106–13)	A, J, M
	Kim Andreolli	*The Face* June 1995	The Secret Agent (66–73)	C, I
Alan David-Tu		*The Face* Oct 1987	Expo (100–03)	L
Max Vadukul		*Arena Homme Plus* Autumn/Winter 1994	Room Service (122–29)	A
		The Face Nov 1986	Good to Gaultier – take it to the max (80–7)	I, M
Inez Van Lamsweerde	Vinoodh Matadin	*The Face* April 1994	For Your Pleasure (60–9)	C, I, M
	Vinoodh Matadin	*The Face* Sept 1994	Global Warming TV (130–40)	J, M, R
	Vinoodh Matadin	*The Face* July 1995	Michelle ma belle (62–71)	C, G, K
	Vinoodh Matadin	*The Face* Sept 1996	L'Amour fou (84–93)	A, L
Tony Viramontes		*The Face* June 1986	Rifat Ozbek (44–51)	M
Ellen Von Unwerth	Chatounne	Arena May/June 1987	Tender is the Night (112–17)	A, K
	Corinne Nocella	*Arena* July/Aug 1988	Fairground Attraction (112–19)	A, I
	David Bradshaw	*Arena* Dec 1990/	Wildside – steppin' out after dark (84–94)	A, J, M
		Arena July/Aug 1992	... Exposed! (90–5)	C, M
		Arena March/April 1993	Idle kitsch (72–85)	A, M, P
	Camilla Nickerson	*The Face* Jan 1992	Pin ups – glamour is back (68–75)	A, M, P
	Cathy Casterine	*The Face* Aug 1993	Uptown Girl (48–59)	A, E
		The Face March 1994	Baby Doll (58–65)	C, H
	Anne Christensen	*The Face* June 1994	Night Fever (108–15)	A, P
	Derick Procope	*The Face* Nov 1994	Afro Power (118–25)	E, K
	Cathy Kasterine	*The Face* Oct 1995	Coney Island Baby (156–63)	C, K
	Venetia Scott	*The Face* Dec 1996	Philosophy in the Boudoir (128–35)	C, H, M
		Vogue Jan 1991	Bodyline (130–3)	C, H

Photographer	Stylist	Magazine/Date	Fashion Feature and Page Numbers	Themes
Ellen Von Unwerth		*Vogue* May 1992	OOH LA LA! wickedly sexy black lace lingerie (172–9)	C, H
		Vogue April 1994	Bad Girl Rising (164–9)	C, M
Troy Ward	William Gilchrist	*Arena* May/ June 1991	Italian Knights (114–17)	B, Q
Norman Watson	Ray Petri	*Arena* May/ June 1987	Dateline: Milan (64–71)	B, Q
	Ray Petri	*Arena* Sept/Oct 1987	Boys from the Bronx (58–65)	B, S
	Ray Petri	*Arena* Sept/Oct 1987	Urban Cowboy NYC (48–55)	B
	Ray Petri	*Arena* Nov/Dec 1987	South of the Border (104–11)	A, P, Q
	Bon Wee at Z	*Arena* March/ April 1988	Fatal Attraction (96–101)	A, P
	Ray Petri	*Arena* May/ June 1988	Return to Oz (38–51)	A, P
	David Bradshaw	*Arena* March/ April 1989	Café Noir (134–43)	K
	David Bradshaw	*Arena* July/ Aug 1989	Roma (84–93)	B, Q
	David Bradshaw	*Arena* May/ June 1990	Uptown – suitably New York (112–23)	B, Q
	David Bradshaw	*Arena* July/Aug 1990	Beachboys (92–7)	B
	David Bradshaw	*Arena* July/Aug 1990	Spy – cloak and dagger tactics (62–75)	A, Q
	David Bradshaw	*Arena* May/June 1991	Drifters (94–101)	B, P
	David Bradshaw	*Arena* Dec 1991/ Jan 1992	La Casa, where a man loves a woman . . . (116–27)	D, M
	Debbi Mason	*Arena* Dec 1992/ Jan 1993	Chain Reaction (132–7)	B
	David Bradshaw	*Arena* Dec 1993/ Jan 1994	Sensitive Skin, Razor-sharp Attitude (124–33)	B
		Arena Dec 1993/ Jan 1994	The Modernists (108–15)	B, K, M
	David Bradshaw	*Arena* Nov 1995	Grey Boy (152–61)	B, H, M
	Karl Templer	*Arena Homme Plus* Autumn/Winter 1996/97	The City Hall Squad (176–83)	M,K

Photographer	Stylist	Magazine/Date	Fashion Feature and Page Numbers	Themes
Norman Watson		*Details* Sept 1992	A Sharper Image (154–65)	A, K
		Details Sept 1993	The End of the Century (150–59)	J
		Details Oct 1993	Highland Thing (144–51)	F
		Details Sept 1994	Code of Honour (174–85)	J, R
		Details March 1996	Best Buys and Buttheads (132–39)	B
		Details April 1996	Blue, Period (136–43)	K
	Karl and Derick (UTO)	*The Face* June 1991	Jamaica, One Blood (80–91)	A, E
	Karl and Derick (UTO)	*The Face* Nov 1991	New Skool (98–107)	N, O
	Karl and Derick (UTO)	*The Face* Oct 1992	Traci . . . (68–77)	C
	Karl and Derick (UTO)	*The Face* Nov 1992	Malcolm X (58–71)	B, E, P
	Karl and Derick (UTO)	*The Face* June 1993	The Hit (92–103)	B, N, P
	Karl Templer	*The Face* Sept 1995	Transatlantic (74–83)	A, J
Bruce Weber		*Per Lui* July/ Aug 1985	Album Phototour (156–69)	A, P, Q
		Vogue Jan 1980	Greek Sun	A, Q
		Vogue July 1980	Australia – Coolgardie (74–86)	A, Q
		Vogue July 1980	Coastal Stripping – beauty on the beach	C, Q
		Vogue Oct 1980	Country Clothes (94–113)	C, K
		Vogue Jan 1981	On the Santa Fe Trail (72–87)	C, K
		Vogue Sept 1981	Great Classics – Margaret Howell's moving picture (226–31)	A, K
		Vogue Dec 1981	Give in to the Sensation (154)	C, H
		Vogue Jan 1982	New Morning Nebraska (74–87)	A, K, R
		Vogue Dec 1982	Under Weston Eyes (194–203)	A, K, M, R
		Vogue Nov 1983	Bodylanguage (258–63)	C, R

Appendix 1: Photographers, Stylists and Features

Photographer	Stylist	Magazine/Date	Fashion Feature and Page Numbers	Themes
Bruce Weber		*Vogue* Dec 1983	Maine Mood – fashion soft and clear (168–81)	A, M, R
		Vogue Nov 1984	A Fashion Splash (214–21)	K, M
		Vogue Dec 1984	In an English Garden (146–65)	C, K, T
		Vogue Jan 1991	Big Country (86–115)	A, Q, R
		Vogue June 1991	Great Dresses, Great Images (120–21)	A, E, M
		Vogue Oct 1995	An Irish Journey (208–25)	Q, R, S
Steven White		*Mondo Uomo* July/Aug 1992	Understatement – New York Story (284–91)	B, K
		GQ April 1994	Street Smart (152–59)	B
Pierre Winther	Greg Fay/Justine Laurie	*The Face* July 1995	Hatched – if humans came from eggs (98–107)	F, J
	Greg Fay/Justine Laurie	*The Face* Oct 1996	Swamp Rats (144–51)	A, J
Michael Wooley	Marcus Von Ackermann	*Arena* Nov/Dec 1988	The Colour of Money (124–7)	B
Zobrowski		*Unique* March/April 1986	Year of the Tiger (42–53)	B, E

Appendix 2

Photographers for British 'Vogue' 1980–1995

(*denotes that the photographer is also included in Appendix 1)

Photographer	Year
Miles Aldridge*	(1995)
Patrik Andersson	(1991–93)
Michel Arnaud	(1981, 82, 84, 89–92)
David Bailey	(1986–88, 90–92)
George Barkentin	(1980, 81)
Andrea Blanche	(1986–88, 92–94)
Eric Boman	(1980–82, 84–86, 91, 92, 94)
Martin Brading*	(1986, 88)
Nick Briggs	(1993)
Regan Cameron	(1991, 92, 94, 95)
Alex Chatelain	(1980, 82–86, 89, 90–92)
Michel Comte	(1990–92)
Anthony Crickmay	(1980–81)
Sean Cunningham	(1992)
Corinne Day*	(1993)
Patrick Demarchelier	(1980–81, 83–92)
Philip Dixon	(1990)
Terence Donovan	(1980–84, 88–91)
Sante D'Orazio	(1989–93)
Arthur Elgort	(1981, 82, 84, 86–95)
Robert Erdmann*	(1984, 86–89, 93–94)
Aldo Fallai	(1981)
Fabrizio Ferri*	(1989, 92–94)
Hans Feurer	(1985–89, 91)
Tim Geaney	(1981)
Michel Haddi*	(1985, 86, 89–92)

Pamela Hanson	(1982, 86, 88, 93–95)
Marc Hom	(1995)
Horst	(1991)
Sepp Horvath	(1981)
Marc Hispard	(1981)
Mikael Jansson*	(1992–95)
Janusz Kawa	(1986–87)
Kristian Ketteger	(1993)
Bill King	(1986)
Neil Kirk	(1980, 81, 86–95)
Kelly Klein	(1995)
Steven Klein*	(1989–91, 93, 95)
Nick Knight*	(1993–95)
Kim Knott*	(1984, 89–95)
Eddie Kohli	(1986–91)
Brigitte Lacombe	(1986)
Karl Lagerfeld	(1990–91)
Andrew Lamb	(1993)
Steve Landis	(1983–84)
Paul Lange	(1984–85, 89)
Barry Lategan	(1981, 83)
Peter Lindbergh	(1984–92)
Greg Luchford*	(1994)
Eamonn J McCabe*	(1987–91)
Tony McGee	(1981–82, 86)
Andrew Macpherson*	(1992–94)
Kurt Markus*	(1991)
Butch Martin	(1983)
Wayne Maser	(1995)
Steven Meisel	(1986, 88–93)
Sheila Metzner	(1985, 88, 90–93)
Sarah Moon	(1994)
Dewey Nicks*	(1994–95)
Jacques Olivar	(1995)
David Parfitt	(1990–92)
Manuela Pavesi	(1993)
Irving Penn	(1981)
Denis Piel	(1980, 86)
Rico Puhlman	(1986)
Alan Randall	(1981–82)
Mike Reinhardt	(1980–83)

Herb Ritts*	(1984, 85, 88–92)
Michael Roberts*	(1987–88)
Matthew Rolston	(1989, 90)
Uli Rose	(1981)
Paolo Roversi*	(1984–86, 93–94)
Lothar Schmid	(1980, 84, 86)
Hans Peter Schneider*	(1992)
Schoerner*	(1994)
David Sims*	(1995)
Peggy Sirota*	(1989–92)
Justin Smith	(1994)
Snowdon	(1982, 91)
Isabel Snyder	(1993)
John Stember	(1980, 81, 84)
Juergen Teller*	(1994–95)
Mario Testino*	(1986, 92–95)
Toscani	(1982)
Tyen	(1990–93)
Max Vadukul*	(1989, 92–94)
Javier Vallhonrat	(1989–92)
Jim Varriale	(1988)
Ellen Von Unwerth*	(1987, 91, 92, 95)
Albert Watson*	(1981–85, 93–94)
Bruce Weber*	(1980, 82–84, 90, 91, 95)
Claus Wickrath	(1986)
Lorenz Zatecky	(1980–81)

Bibliography

(i) Primary Sources

With the exception of *Elle* and *Jardin des Modes*, full details of the fashion spreads included in the following titles can be found in Appendix 1. Only those articles on fashion photography and individual photographers published in them have been cited in this bibliography.

The Face (May 1980–December 1996).
Arena (November 1986–December 1996).
Arena Homme Plus (Spring/Summer 1994–Autumn/Winter 1996).
British *Vogue* (January 1980–December 1996).
Details (August 1992, September 1992, August 1993, September 1993, October 1993, September 1994, January 1995, March 1995, March 1996, April 1996, and September 1996).
Elle (French edition; June 1958–June 1959).
For Him Magazine ; since 1994, *FHM* (August/September 1990 and September 1994).
British *GQ* (July 1992, October 1992, May 1993, December 1993, January 1994, April 1994, May 1994, July 1994, August 1994, November 1994, and December 1994).
Canadian *GQ*, (December 1995).
American *GQ* (December 1991, June 1992, July 1992, September 1993, and December 1995).
Jardin des Modes (June 1958–June 1958).
Mondo Uomo (July/August 1992).
Observer Life (3 July 1994 and 14 January 1996).
Per Lui (July/August 1985).
Unique (March/April 1986, June/July 1986, August 1986, October/November 1986, and Autumn 1987).
Vogue Hommes (April 1992 and June 1992).

(ii) Books and Chapters in Books

M. Abrams, *The Teenage Consumer* (London: London Press Exchange, 1960).
H. Aptheker (ed.), *A Documentary History of the Negro People in the United States*

1910–32 (Secausus, NJ: Citadel Press, 1973).

A. Arato and E. Gebhardt (eds), *The Essential Frankfurt School Reader* (Oxford: Blackwell, 1978).

J. Ash and E. Wilson (eds), *Chic Thrills* (London: Pandora Press, 1992).

Bad Object Choices Group, *How Do I Look?* (Seattle: Bay Press, 1991).

D. Bailey and G. Hughes, *David Bailey's Book of Photography* (London: Dent 1981).

M. Bakhtin, *Rabelais and His World* (Cambridge, MA: MIT Press, 1968).

R. Barthes, *Système de la Mode* (Paris: Éditions du Seuil, 1967).

——, *Critical Essays*, trans. R. Howard (Evanston, IL: Northwestern University Press, 1972).

——, preface to *Erté*, trans. W. Weaver (Parma: Maria Ricci, 1972).

——, *Elements of Semiology*, trans. A. Lavers and C. Smith (New York: Hill and Wang, 1973).

——, *Mythologies*, trans. A. Lavers (London: Paladin, 1973).

——, *Image, Music, Text*, trans. S. Heath (Glasgow: Fontana/Collins, 1978).

——, *The Fashion System*, trans. M. Ward and R. Howard (Berkeley, CA: University of California Press, 1990).

——, *The Pleasure of the Text*, trans. R. Miller (Oxford: Basil Blackwell, 1990).

——, *Roland Barthes* (London: Papermac, 1995).

G. Bataille, *Erotism, Death and Sensuality*, trans. M. Dalwood (San Francisco: City Light Books, 1986).

J. Baudrillard, *For A Critique of the Political Sign* (St Louis, MO: Telos Press Ltd, 1981).

——, 'The Ecstasy of Communication' in H. Foster (ed.), *Postmodern Culture* (London: Pluto Press, 1985), pp. 126–34.

——, *Simulacra and Simulation*, trans. Sheila Faria Glaser (Ann Arbor, MI: University of Michigan Press, 1994).

Benn's Newspaper Press Directory, (London: Benn, volumes for 1980 to 1996).

L. Bersani, *Homos* (Cambridge, MA: Harvard University Press, 1995).

H. K. Bhaba, *The Location of Culture* (London and New York: Routledge, 1994).

J. Blessing *et al.*, *Rrose is a Rrose is a Rrose: Gender Performance in Photography* (New York: Guggenheim Museum, 1997).

Blitz: Exposure! Young British Photographers from Blitz Magazine 1980–1987 (London: Ebury Press, 1987).

H. Bloom *et al.*, *Deconstruction and Criticism* (New York: Seabury Press, 1979).

M. Borch-Jakobsen, *Lacan: The Absolute Master*, trans. D. Brick (Stanford, CA: Stanford University Press, 1991).

S. Bordo, *Unbearable Weight: Feminism, Western Culture and the Body* (Berkeley, CA: University of California Press, 1993).

——, *Twilight Zones: the Hidden Life of Cultural Images from Plato to O.J.* (Berkeley, CA: California University Press, 1997).

A. Breton, *Mad Love*, trans. M. A. Caws (Lincoln NB and London: University of Nebraska Press, 1987 [1937]).

C. Breward, *The Culture of Fashion* (Manchester: Manchester University Press, 1994).

H. Brill, 'Fin de Siècle', in *The Art Press* (London: Tate Gallery, 1976), pp. 23–31.

A. Brittan, *Masculinity and Power* (Oxford: Blackwell, 1989).

Bruce Weber, exhibition catalogue for Fahey/Klein Gallery, Los Angeles (Tokyo: Treville Co., 1991).

J. Brumberg, *Fasting Girls: The Emergence of Anorexia Nervosa as a Modern Disease* (Cambridge, MA: Harvard University Press, 1988).

V. Burgin, 'Photographic Practice and Art Theory', in V. Burgin (ed.), *Thinking Photography* (London: Macmillan, 1982), pp. 39–83.

——, 'Newton's Gravity', in C. Squiers (ed.), *The Critical Image* (Seattle: Bay Press, 1990), pp. 165–72.

R. Burton, *The Sotadic Zone* (Boston: Milford House, 1973).

J. Butler, *Gender Trouble* (London and New York: Routledge, 1990).

——, *Bodies that Matter – On The Discursive Limits of "Sex"* (London and New York: Routledge, 1993).

——, 'Melancholy Gender/Refused Identification', in M. Berger, B. Wallis and S. Watson (eds), *Constructing Masculinity* (London and New York: Routledge, 1995).

E. Carter, *The Changing World of Fashion* (London: Weidenfeld and Nicolson, 1977).

N. Caskey, 'Interpreting Anorexia Nervosa' in S. R. Suleiman (ed.), *The Female Body in Western Culture: Contemporary Perspectives* (Cambridge, MA: Harvard University Press, 1985), pp. 175–89.

W. Cather, *My Ántonia* (London: Virago, 1980).

——, *Death Comes for the Archbishop* (London: Virago, 1981).

——, *Lucy Gayheart* (London: Virago, 1985).

R. Chapman and J. Rutherford (eds), *Male Order – Unwrapping Masculinity* (London: Lawrence and Wishart, 1988).

P. Church Gibson and R. Gibson (eds), *Dirty Looks: Women, Pornography, Power* (London: BFI, 1993).

H. Cixous, 'The Laugh of the Medusa', in E. Marks and I. de Courtivron (eds), *New French Feminisms* (New York: Schocken, 1981), pp. 245–64.

W. Cobbett, *Advice to Young Men And (Incidentally) to Young Women in the Middle and Higher Ranks of Life in a Series of Letters, addressed to a Youth, a Bachelor, a Lover, a Husband, a Father, a Citizen or a Subject* (London: the author, 1829).

M. Cohen, *Lewis Carroll's Photographs of Nude Children* (Philadelphia: The Philip H. and A. S W. Rosenbach Foundation, 1978).

N. Coleridge, *The Fashion Conspiracy* (London: Mandarin, 1989).

R. W. Connell, *Masculinities* (Cambridge: Polity Press, 1995).

J. Conrad, *Under Western Eyes* (Harmondsworth: Penguin, 1989).

R. Coward, *Female Desires: How They Are Sought, Bought and Packaged* (New York: Grove, 1985).

J. Craik, *The Face of Fashion: Cultural Studies in Fashion* (London and New York: Routledge, 1994).

J. Crump, *George Platt Lynes – Photographs from the Kinsey Institute* (Boston and London: Little, Brown and Co., 1993).

J. Culler, *Structuralist Poetics; Structuralism, Linguistics and the Study of Literature* (London: Routledge, Kegan and Paul, 1975).

——, *Barthes* (London: Fontana, 1983).

A. C. Danto, *Playing with the Edge: The Photographic Achievement of Robert Mapplethorpe* (Berkeley, CA: University of California Press, 1996).

A. Davis, *Women, Race and Class* (New York: Random House, 1981).

J. Derrida, *Dissemination*, trans. B. Johnson (London: Athlone Press, 1981).

——, *Margins of Philosophy*, trans. A. Bass (Chicago: University of Chicago Press, 1982).

——, *Glas*, trans. J. P. Leavey and R. Rand (Lincoln NB: University of Nebraska Press, 1987).

——, *The Truth in Painting*, trans. G. Bennington and I. McLeod (Chicago: Chicago University Press, 1987).

J. Diamond, *The Rise and Fall of the Third Chimpanzee* (London: Radius, 1991).

J. Donald and A. Rattansi (eds), *'Race', Culture and Difference* (Buckingham: Open University Press, 1993).

T. Downing, *Olympia* (London: BFI, 1992).

K. R. Dutton, *The Perfectible Body: The Western Ideal of Physical Development* (London: Cassell, 1995).

A. Dworkin, *Pornography: Men Possessing Women* (New York: Dutton, 1979).

R. Dyer, *Stars* (London: BFI, 1979).

——, 'Getting Over the Rainbow: Identity and Pleasure in Gay Cultural Politics', in G. Bridges and R. Brunt (eds), *Silver Linings: Some Strategies for the Eighties* (London: Lawrence and Wishart, 1981), pp. 53–67.

——, *White* (London and New York: Routledge, 1997).

A. Easthope, *What A Man's Gotta Do: The Masculine Myth in Popular Culture* (London: Paladin, 1986).

A. Easthope and K. McGowan, *A Critical and Cultural Theory Reader* (Buckingham: Open University Press, 1992).

T. Edwards, *Men in the Mirror: Men's Fashion, Masculinity and Consumer Society* (London: Cassell, 1997).

A. Ellenzweig, *The Homoerotic Photograph* (New York: Columbia University Press, 1992).

C. Evans and L. Gamman, 'The Gaze Revisited, Or Reviewing Queer Viewing', in P. Burston and C. Richardson (eds), *A Queer Romance* (London and New York: Routledge, 1995).

C. Evans and M. Thornton, *Women and Fashion: A New Look* (London: Quartet Books, 1989).

W. A. Ewing, *The Photographic Art of Hoyningen Huene* (London: Thames and Hudson, 1988).

——, *The Body* (London: Thames and Hudson, 1994).

F. Fanon, *The Wretched of the Earth*, trans. C. Farrington (New York: Grove Press, 1963).

——, *Black Skin, White Masks*, trans. C. Lam Markmann (London: Pluto Press, 1986 [1952]).

Fashion Photography in the Nineties (London: Scalo, 1996).

M. Featherstone, M. Hepworth and B. S. Turner (eds), *The Body: Social Process and Cultural Theory* (London: Sage, 1991).

H. Foster, *Compulsive Beauty* (Cambridge, MA.: MIT Press, 1993).

M. Foucault, *Discipline and Punish: The Birth of the Prison*, trans. A. Sheridan (New York: Pantheon, 1977).

——, *The History of Sexuality: Vol. 3, The Care of the Self*, trans. R. Hurley (Harmondsworth: Penguin, 1986 [1984]).

——, *The History of Sexuality: Vol. 1, An Introduction*, trans. R. Hurley (Harmondsworth: Penguin, 1990).

K. Fraser (ed.), *On the Edge: Photographs from 100 Years of Vogue* (New York: Random House, 1992).

S. Freud, *The Standard Edition*, Vol. 18, edited by J. Strachey (London: Hogarth Press, 1955).

——, *The Standard Edition*, Vol. 13, ed. J. Strachey (London: Hogarth Press, 1955).

——, *The Standard Edition*, Vol. 12, ed. J. Strachey (London: Hogarth Press, 1958).

——, *The Standard Edition*, Vol. 22, ed. J. Strachey (London: Hogarth Press, 1964).

——, *On Sexuality*, trans. J. Strachey, ed. A. Richards (Harmondsworth: Penguin, 1977).

——, *On Metapsychology*, trans. J. Strachey, ed. A. Richards (Harmondsworth: Penguin, 1984).

——, *Civilization, Society and Religion*, trans. J. Strachey, ed. A. Richards (Harmondsworth: Penguin, 1985).

D. Fuss, *Identification Papers* (London and New York: Routledge, 1995).

S. W. Fussell, *Muscle: Confessions of an Unlikely Bodybuilder* (New York: Poseidon Press, 1991).

T. R. Fyvel, *The Insecure Offenders: Rebellious Youth in the Welfare State* (Harmondsworth: Pelican, 1963).

L. Gamman and M. Makinen, *Female Fetishism: A New Look* (London: Lawrence and Wishart, 1994).

M. Garber, *Vested Interests: Cross-Dressing and Cultural Anxiety* (London and New York: Routledge, 1992).

M. Gatens, *Imaginary Bodies: Ethics, Power and Corporeality* (London and New York: Routledge, 1996).

J. Genet, *Querelle of Brest*, trans. G. Streatham (London: Paladin, 1987).

C. Geist and J. Nachbar (eds), *The Popular Culture Reader* (Bowling Green, OH: Bowling Green University Popular Press, 1983).

D. Gibbs (ed.), *Nova 1965–1975 – THE Style Bible of the 60s and 70s* (London: Pavilion Books, 1993).

A. Gide, *If It Die . . .* , trans. D. Bussy (London: Secker and Warburg, 1950).

B. Glassner, 'Men and Muscles', in M. S. Kimmel and M. A. Messner (eds), *Men's Lives* (New York: Macmillan, 1989), pp. 310–20.

C. Gordon (ed.), *Power/Knowledge: Selected Interviews and Other Writings 1972–77 by Michel Foucault* (Brighton: Harvester, 1980).

E. Gross, 'The Body of Signification', in J. Fletcher and A. Benjamin (eds), *Abjection, Melancholia and Love: The Work of Julia Kristeva* (London and New York: Routledge, 1990), pp. 80–103.

M. Gross, *Model: The Ugly Business of Beautiful Women* (London and New York: Bantam Press, 1995).

N. Hall-Duncan, *The History of Fashion Photography* (New York: Alpine Book Co. Inc., 1979).

I. M. Harris, *Messages Men Hear* (London: Taylor and Francis, 1995).

M. Harrison, *Bailey: Black and White Memories* (London: J. M. Dent and Sons, 1983).

——, *Appearances – Fashion Photography Since 1945* (London: Jonathan Cape, 1991).

W. Hartshorn and M. Foresta, *Man Ray In Fashion* (New York: International Center of Photography, 1990).

D. Hebdige, *Subculture: The Meaning of Style* (London: Methuen and Co., 1979).

G. W. F. Hegel, *Philosophy of the Mind*, trans. W. Wallace (Oxford and New York: Oxford University Press, 1971).

——, *The Phenomenology of the Spirit*, trans. A. V. Miller (Oxford and New York: Oxford University Press, 1977).

D. Hill, *Designer Boys and Material Girls: Manufacturing the 80s Pop Dream* (Poole: Blandford Press, 1986).

L. Hine, *Men at Work: Photographic Studies of Modern Men and Machines* (New York: Dover, 1977).

P. Holland, 'What Is A Child?', in P. Holland, J. Spence and S. Watney (eds), *Photography/Politics Two* (London: Photography Workshop, 1986), pp. 43–56.

B. hooks, *Black Looks: Race and Representation* (Boston, MA: South End Press, 1992).

F. V. Hoover III, *Beefcake: The Muscle Magazines of America 1950–1970* (Cologne: Taschen, 1995).

T. Hopkinson, *Picture Post 1938–50* (London: Chatto and Windus, 1986).

M. Horkheimer, 'The End of Reason' [1941], in A. Arato and E. Gebhardt (eds), *The Essential Frankfurt School Reader* (Oxford: Blackwell, 1978), pp. 26–48.

P. Horne and R. Lewis (eds), *Outlooks: Lesbian and Gay Sexualities and Visual Cultures* (London and New York: Routledge, 1996).

L. Irigaray, 'The Power of Discourse and the Subordination of the Feminine', in *This Sex Which Is Not One*, trans. C. Porter (Ithaca, NY: Cornell University Press, 1985), pp. 68–85.

F. Jameson, *Postmodernism; or, the Cultural Logic of Late Capitalism* (London and New York: Verso, 1991).

P. Jobling, *Bodies of Experience: Gender and Identity in Women's Photography Since 1970* (London: Scarlet Press, 1997).

——, 'Keeping Mrs. Dawson busy: safe sex, gender and pleasure in condom advertising since 1970', in M. Nava, A. Blake, I. MacRury and B. Richards (eds), *Buy*

This Book: Studies in Advertising and Consumption (London and New York: Routledge, 1997), pp. 157–77. —

—— and D. Crowley, *Graphic Design–Reproduction and Representation Since 1800* (Manchester and New York: Manchester University Press, 1996).

A. Kaes, M. Jay and E. Dimendberg, *The Weimar Republic Sourcebook* (Berkeley, CA: University of California Press, 1994).

I. Kant, *The Critique of Judgement*, trans. J. C. Meredith (Oxford: Oxford University Press, 1952).

E. A. Kaplan, 'Is the Gaze Male?', in A. Snitow, C. Stansell and S. Thompson (eds), *Desire: The Politics of Sexuality* (London: Virago, 1983), pp. 321–32.

M. Kazmaier, *Horst – 60 Years of Photography* (London: Thames and Hudson, 1991).

R. Kinross, *Modern Typography: An Essay in Critical History* (London: Hyphen Press, 1992).

L. Kipnis, '(Male) Desire and (Female) Disgust: Reading Hustler', in L. Grossberg, C. Nelson and P. A. Treichler (eds), *Cultural Studies* (London and New York: Routledge, 1992), pp. 373–91.

A. M. Klein, *Little Big Men: Bodybuilding Subculture and Gender Construction* (Albany, NY: State University of New York Press, 1993).

W. Klein, *In and Out of Fashion* (New York: Random House, 1994).

K. Korff, 'Die illustrierte Zeitschrift', in *Fünfzig Jahre Ullstein 1877–1927* (Berlin: Ullstein, 1927), pp. 279–303.

E. Kosofsky Sedgwick, *Epistemology of the Closet* (Harmondsworth: Penguin, 1990).

R. Krauss and J. Livingstone, *L'Amour Fou: Photography and Surrealism* (London: Arts Council, 1986).

J. Kristeva, *Desire in Language: A Semiotic Approach to Literature and Art*, ed. L. S. Roudiez (New York: Columbia University Press, 1980).

——, *Powers of Horror: An Essay in Abjection*, trans. L. S. Roudiez (New York: Columbia University Press, 1982).

——, *Revolution in Poetic Language*, trans. M. Waller (New York: Columbia University Press, 1984).

A. and M. Kroker (eds), *Body Invaders: Panic Sex in America* (New York: St Martin's Press, 1987).

J. Lacan, *Écrits: A Selection*, trans. A. Sheridan (New York: Norton, 1977).

——, *The Four Fundamental Concepts of Psychoanalysis*, trans. Alan Sheridan (New York: Norton, 1978).

——, *The Seminars of Jacques Lacan, Book II: The Ego in Freud's Theory and in the Technique of Psychoanalysis, 1954–1955*, trans. S. Tomaselli (Cambridge: Cambridge University Press, 1988).

S. Lalvani, *Photography, Vision and the Production of Modern Bodies* (New York: State University of New York, 1996).

T. Laqueur, *Making Sex: Body and Gender from the Greeks to Freud* (Cambridge, MA: Harvard University Press), 1990.

H. Lee, *Willa Cather: Double Lives* (New York: Vintage, 1989).

E. Lemoine-Luccioni, *Partage des femmes* (Paris: Éditions du Seuil, 1976).

G. Lipovestsky, *The Empire of Fashion: Dressing Modern Democracy*, trans. C. Porter (Princeton, NJ: Princeton University Press, 1994).

M. Lister (ed.), *The Photographic Image in Digital Culture* (London and New York: Routledge, 1995).

Look-In Fashion Model Annual (London: Independent Television Publications Ltd, 1971).

L. Lovatt-Smith and P. Remy (eds), *Fashion: Images de Mode* (Göttingen: Steidl, 1996).

D. M. Lowe, *The Body in Late-Capitalist USA* (Durham, NC: Duke University Press, 1995).

F. Lyotard, *The Differend: Phrases in Dispute*, trans. George Van Den Abeele (Minneapolis: University of Minnesota Press, 1988).

M. MacSween, *Anorexic Bodies: A Feminist and Sociological Perspective on Anorexia Nervosa* (London and New York: Routledge, 1993).

B. Maddow, *Edward Weston, His Life and Photographs* (New York: Aperture, 1979).

Male Super Models: The Men of Boss Models (New York: Boss Models Inc., 1996).

S. Mann, *Immediate Family* (London: Phaidon, 1992).

R. Martin, *Fashion and Surrealism* (London: Thames and Hudson, 1988).

R. Martin and H. Koda, *Jocks and Nerds: Men's Style in the Twentieth Century* (New York: Rizzoli, 1989).

A. Marwick, *British Society Since 1945* (Harmondworth: Pelican, 1982).

D. Mellor and M. Harrison, *David Bailey: Black and White Memories* (London: Victoria and Albert Museum, 1983).

K. Mercer, *Welcome to the Jungle: New Positions in Black Cultural Studies* (London and New York: Routledge, 1994).

M. A. Messner and D. F. Sabo (eds), *Sport, Men and the Gender Order* (Champaign, IL: Human Kinetic Books, 1990).

R. Miles, 'Representations of "Race"', in her *Racism* (London: Routledge, Chapman and Hall, 1989), pp. 32–40.

——, *The Rites of Man: Love, Sex and Death in the Making of the Male* (London: Grafton Books, 1991).

D. A. Miller, *Bringing Out Roland Barthes* (Berkeley, CA: University of California Press, 1992).

Mintel, *Men 2000* (London: Mintel, 1993).

W. J. T. Mitchell, *Picture Theory: Essays on Verbal and Visual Representation* (Chicago: Chicago University Press, 1994).

T. Moi (ed.), *The Kristeva Reader* (Oxford: Blackwell, 1986).

P. Morrisoe, *Mapplethorpe: A Biography* (London: Papermac, 1995).

F. Mort, *Cultures of Consumption: Masculinities and Social Space in Twentieth Century Britain* (London and New York: Routledge, 1996).

L. Mulvey, *Visual and Other Pleasures* (Basingstoke: Macmillan, 1989).

National Union of Journalists, *Freelance Fees Guide* (London: NUJ, 1987).

——, *Freelance Fees Guide* (London: NUJ, 1989).

L. Nead, *The Female Nude: Art, Obscenity and Sexuality* (London and New York: Routledge, 1992).

H. Newton, *White Women* (New York: Stonehill Publishing Co., 1976).

——, *Portraits* (London: Quartet Books, 1987).

S. Nixon, *Hard Looks: Masculinities, Spectatorship and Contemporary Consumption* (London: University College London Press, 1996).

G. O'Brien, 'Pink Thoughts', in *The Idealizing Vision: The Art of Fashion Photography* (New York: Aperture, 1991).

D. O'Donahue, *Lifestyles and Psychographics* (London: Institute of Practitioners in Advertising, 1989).

Out of Fashion: Photographs by Nick Knight and Cindy Palmano (London: Photographer's Gallery, 1989).

W. Owen, *Magazine Design* (London: Lawrence King, 1991).

Plato, *Phaedrus and Letters VII and VIII*, trans. W. Hamilton (Harmondsworth: Penguin, 1973).

H. Radner, *Shopping Around – Feminine Culture and the Pursuit of Pleasure* (London and New York: Routledge, 1995).

M. Ray, *Self-Portrait: Man Ray* (London: André Deutsch, 1963).

M. Z. Rosaldo and L. Lamphere (eds), *Women, Culture and Society* (Stanford, CA: Stanford University Press, 1974).

R. Rylance, *Roland Barthes* (London: Harvester Wheatsheaf, 1994).

E. Said, *Orientalism* (Harmondsworth: Penguin, 1978).

F. de Saussure, *Course in General Linguistics*, trans. Roy Harris (Chicago and La Salle, IL: Open Court, 1986).

C. Seebohm, *The Man Who Was Vogue: The Life of Condé Nast* (New York: Viking, 1982).

L. Segal, *Slow Motion: Changing Masculinities, Changing Men* (London: Virago Press, 1990).

M. Shanahan (ed.), *Richard Avedon – Evidence 1944–1994* (London: National Portrait Gallery, 1994).

G. B. Shaw, *Plays Unpleasant* (Harmondsworth: Penguin, 1946 [1898]).

N. Shawcross, *Roland Barthes on Photography* (Gainseville, FL: University Press of Florida, 1997).

J. Shrimpton, *The Truth About Modelling* (London: W. H. Allen, 1964).

——, *An Autobiography* (London: Sphere, 1991).

K. Silverman, *Male Subjectivity at the Margins* (London and New York: Routledge, 1992).

W. Simon, *Postmodern Sexualities* (London and New York: Routledge, 1996).

M. Simpson, *Male Impersonators* (London: Cassell, 1994).

A. Sinfield, *The Wilde Century: Effeminacy, Oscar Wilde and the Queer Movement* (London: Cassell, 1994).

S. Sontag, *On Photography* (Harmondsworth: Penguin, 1977).

—— (ed.), *Barthes: Selected Writings* (London: Fontana Press, 1983).

——, 'Fascinating Fascism' in B. Taylor and W. van der Will (eds), *The Nazification of Art* (Winchester: The Winchester Press, 1990), pp. 204–18.

V. Steele, 'Erotic Allure', in *The Idealizing Vision: The Art of Fashion Photography* (New York: Aperture, 1991), pp. 80–101.

N. Strossen, *Defending Pornography: Free Speech, Sex and the Fight for Women's Rights* (London: Abacus, 1996).

J. Szarkowski, *Irving Penn* (New York: Museum of Modern Art, 1984).

Y. Tasker, *Spectacular Bodies* (London and New York: Routledge, 1993).

J. Teller, *Juergen Teller* (Cologne: Taschen Books, 1996).

The Body in Question (New York: Aperture, 1990).

The Idealizing Vision: The Art of Fashion Photography (New York: Aperture, 1991).

K. Theweleit, *Male Fantasies*, trans. S. Conway (Cambridge: Polity Press, 1987).

R. Thody, *Roland Barthes: A Conservative Estimate* (London: Macmillan, 1977).

C. Thomas, *Male Matters* (Chicago: University of Illinois Press, 1996).

B. Thompson, *Soft Core* (London: Cassell, 1994).

T. Triggs, 'Framing Masculinity', in Ash and Wilson, *Chic Thrills* (1992), pp. 25–9.

Inez Van Lamsweerde, exhibition catalogue (Zürich: Kunsthaus, Zÿrich, 1996).

P. Weiermair, *The Hidden Image: Photographs of the Male Nude in the 19th and 20th Centuries* (Cambridge, MA: MIT Press, 1988).

M. Whitford (ed.), *The Irigaray Reader* (Oxford: Blackwell, 1991).

L. Williams, *Hard Core: Power, Pleasure and the 'Frenzy of the Visible'* (Berkeley, CA: University of California Press, 1989).

E. Wilson, *Adorned in Dreams: Fashion and Modernity* (London: Virago Press, 1985).

L. Wolf (ed.), *The Essential Dracula* (New York and London: Plume, 1993).

N. Wolf, *The Beauty Myth* (London: Vintage, 1991).

V. Woolf, *To the Lighthouse* (Oxford: Oxford University Press, 1992).

W. Wordsworth, *Complete Poems* (Oxford: Oxford University Press, 1965).

J. Wozencroft, *The Graphic Language of Neville Brody* (London: Thames and Hudson, 1988).

——, *The Graphic Language of Neville Brody 2* (London: Thames and Hudson, 1994).

(iii) Magazines and Articles

D. Aaronovitch, 'Outrageous!', *Independent Section Two* (21 November 1995), pp. 2–3.

J. Adams, 'Live long and prosper', *The Observer Life* (1 December 1996), pp. 27–30.

S. Adler, 'The beauty myth', *The Observer Magazine* (13 January 1994), pp. 17–24.

L. Alford, 'Don't get your knickers in a twist over fashion', *The Observer* (30 May 1993), p. 52.

——, 'Superguys strutting into the valley of the dolls', *The Observer* (4 September 1994), p. 7.

——, 'Beauty of a certain age', *The Observer Life* (30 April 1995), pp. 40–3.

M. Amis, 'Madonna exposed', *The Observer Magazine* (11 October 1992), pp. 22–5 and 32–36.

A. Anthony, 'The girlie show-off', *The Observer Life* (1 September 1996), pp. 12–13.

——, 'The way to a woman's heart is through his stomach', *The Observer Review* (1 February 1998), p. 7.

'Are these pictures offensive?', *Independent on Sunday* (30 May 1993), p. 22.

L. Armstrong, '*Vogue*: giving the myth a little reality', *The Independent* (9 May 1991), p. 19.

——, 'Who's that girl?', *The Independent on Sunday Review* (9 August 1992), p. 37.

——, 'Come on guys, it's only me. Little Liz Tilberis', *The Independent on Sunday Review* (22 August 1992), pp. 32–3.

——, 'Booty keeps beasts on the bratwalk', *The Observer Review* (5 November 1995), p. 3.

S. Armstrong, 'Bodies of opinion', *The Guardian Media* (6 November 1995), p. 3.

G. Asaria, 'Devinez qui est derrière "Guess"?', *Vogue Hommes International Mode* (Autumn/Winter 1991/92), pp. 84–7.

L. Baker, 'London girls', *The Face* (June 1992), pp. 36–42.

——, 'A teen idoliser', *Observer Life* (16 April 1995), pp. 68–9.

M. Baker, 'Sexual shock and the emergence of New Man', *M* (February 1992), pp. 69–75.

P. Baker, 'Exposing the shape of things to come', *The Guardian* (26 May 1992), p. 4.

T. Baker, 'The work of Alan David-Tu', *The Face* (October 1987), pp. 100–01.

A. Barbieri, 'Doing the Cybercatwalk', *The Independent on Sunday Review* (4 June 1995), pp. 48–9.

R. Barthes, 'The scandal of horror photography', *Creative Camera* (July 1969).

——, 'Réponses', *Tel Quel*, 47 (1971), p. 97.

G. Bataille, 'The big toe', *Documents*, Vol.1, No.6 (1929).

G. Bataille, 'Mouth', *Documents*, Vol.2, No.5 (1930).

E. Bell, 'Oversexed, overhyped and over here', *The Observer* (17 February 1991), p. 39.

J. Bernstein, 'Survival of the fattest', *The Face* (August 1995), p. 109.

L. Bersani, 'Is the rectum a grave?', *October*, 43 (Winter 1987), pp. 197–222.

H. K. Bhabha, 'Of mimicry and man: the ambivalence of colonial discourse', *October*, 28 (Spring 1984), pp. 25–33.

A. Billen, 'No one looks at Vogue and thinks "I want to look like that". No one is that stupid', *The Observer Review Section* (4 August 1996), p. 7.

A. Billson, 'Rough diamonds', British *GQ* (August 1992), pp. 70–5.

S. Bodine and M. Dunas, 'Dr. M. F. Agha, Art Director', *AIGA Journal*, 3:3 (1985).

A. Bonnet, '"White Studies": the problems and projects of a new research agenda', *Theory, Culture and Society*, 13:2 (1996), pp. 145–55.

C. Bowen-Jones, 'Adman finds a New Woman', *The Times* (16 March 1988), p. 26.

J. Briscoe, 'Chic, worthy, sexy, successful', *The Observer Review Section* (22 August 1993), p. 1.

British *Vogue* (June 1991)–Special 75th anniversary issue.

R. Brookes, 'Double-page spread–fashion and advertising photography', *Camerawork*, No.17 (January/February 1980), pp. 1–3.

A. Brown, 'Making a Knight of it', *The Sunday Times Magazine* (9 December 1990), pp. 82–5.

'Bruce Weber redefines manhood', *International Collections For Men* (Summer 1994), pp. 47–9.

T. Brûlé, 'The gloss on the pink press', *The Guardian Media* (7 February 1994), p. 13.

S. Bucks, 'Real people', *The Independent on Sunday Review* (21 February 1993), pp. 36–7.

M. Bywater, 'If Mapplethorpe made me a pervert, then there's always Esther Rantzen to save me', *New Statesman* (20 September 1996), pp. 38–9.

R. Carroll, 'An interview with Bruce Weber', *Bomb* (Spring/Summer 1985).

L. Chambers, 'Horst on Horst', British *Vogue* (March 1991), pp. 143–7.

A. Chauduri, 'Pornspotting', *The Guardian* (6 February 1996), p. 6.

L. Chunn, 'A Wintour's tale', *The Guardian* (29 April 1991), p. 32.

——, 'A new vogue in editors', *The Guardian* (20 April 1992).

'Cindy goes to Hollywood', *International Collections* (Summer 1992), pp. 74–7 and 88.

A. K. Clark, 'The girl: a rhetoric of desire', *Cultural Studies*, 1:2 (May 1987), pp. 195–203.

N. Cohn, 'Ready, steady, gone', *The Observer Magazine* (27 August 1967), p. 12.

A. D. Coleman, 'Censorship', *European Photography*, 11:1 (January–March 1990), pp. 13–14.

J. Coles, 'The gee in GQ', *The Guardian Media* (28 September 1992), p. 23.

N. Compton, 'Likely lads', *The Face* (August 1995), pp. 40–51.

P. Conrad, 'The body perfect', *The Observer* (4 February 1990).

E. Cooper, 'The censorship debate: a British experience', *Creative Camera*, 7 (December 1990/January 1991), pp. 30–2.

R. Coward, 'Innocence made ripe for the plucking', *The Observer* (26 September 1993), p. 21.

L. Craik, 'Pixelvision', *The Face* (March 1996), pp. 116–17.

'Cross dressing', *Details* (October 1996), pp. 56–7.

J. Crump, 'The Kinsey Institute Archive: a taxonomy of erotic photography', *History of Photography*, 18:1 (Spring 1994), pp. 1–12.

S. Daly, 'Model world', *The Face* (September 1994), pp. 124–7.

H. David, 'In the pink', *The Times Saturday Review* (13 June 1992), pp. 10–11.

N. Davies, 'Dirty business', *The Guardian Weekend* (26 November 1994), pp. 12–17.

——, 'Red light for blue squad', *The Guardian* (29 November 1994), pp. 6–7.

Dazed and Confused, third anniversary fashion issue (August 1997).

J. Derrida, 'Signature, event, context', in *Glyph*, I, (Baltimore: Johns Hopkins University Press, 1977), pp. 172–97.

——, 'The parergon', *October*, 9 (1979).

K. Dieckmann, 'Immediate family', *The Village Voice Literary Supplement*, (November 1992), p. 15.

T. Douglas, 'Magazines that could explode the male myth', *The Observer* (26 April 1987), p. 37.

'Do you think I'm sexy?', *New Woman* (May 1997), pp. 64–7 .

B. D'Silva, 'Some like it Hoyt', *FHM* (September 1993), pp. 111–13.

R. Dyer, 'Don't look now–the male pin-up', *Screen*, 23:3–4 (September/October 1982), pp. 61–73.

——, 'Seen to be believed: some problems in the representation of gay people as typical', *Studies in Visual Communication*, 9:2 (Spring 1983), pp. 2–19.

D. Edgar, 'Shocking entertainment?', *The Guardian* (11 March 1997), p.3.

S. H. Edwards, 'Pretty babies: art, erotica or kiddie porn?', *History of Photography*, 18:1 (Spring 1994), pp. 38–46.

M. El-Faizy, 'The naked and the deadly', *The Guardian Media* (6 December 1993), pp. 10–11.

J. Ellis, 'Photography/Pornography/Art/Pornography', *Screen*, 21:1 (1980), pp. 81–108.

M. Etherington-Smith, 'Mad about the poise', *The Independent on Sunday* (15 September 1991), pp. 38–9.

'Exposed', *Creative Review* (September 1997), p. 55.

R. Fani-Kayode, 'Traces of Ecstasy', *Ten.8*, No. 28 (1988), pp. 36–43.

L. Farrelly, 'So you want to be a rock 'n' roll star. . .', *The Face* (October 1996), pp. 164–8.

'Fashion: a bluffer's guide', *The Face* (August 1993), pp. 32–7.

'Femme ordinaire', *The Observer Review Section* (21 January 1996), p. 3.

K. Flett, 'sex, success and the single girl . . . exposed', *Arena* (July/August 1992), pp. 88–95.

K. Flett-Flanagan, 'Defrocked', *The Observer Preview* (7–13 April 1996), pp. 6–9.

——, 'Why is this 15-year-old girl selling clothes to women twice her age?', *Observer Life* (15 September 1996), pp. 18–20.

A. Forster, 'The male nude in photography', *The Photographic Collector*, 5:3 (1986), pp. 331–44.

N. Fountain, 'Just a light facelift', *The Guardian Media Section* (1 August 1988), p. 21.

E. Francis and K. Mercer, 'Black people, culture and resistance, *Camerawork* (November 1982), pp. 6–8.

S. Frankel, 'New Model Army', *Time Out* (3–10 March 1993), pp. 26–7.

K. Fraser, 'The tender trap', *The Independent on Sunday Review* (11 October 1992), pp. 44–47.

'The furor over fashions', *Time* (3 December 1965), p. 66.

D. Fuss, 'Fashion and the homospectatorial look', *Critical Inquiry*, 18:4 (Summer 1992), pp. 713–37.

C. Gant, 'Model world', *The Face* (April 1992), pp. 72–5.

S. Garratt, 'Naomi Campbell', *The Face* (November 1992), pp. 102–5.

——, 'The making of Kate', *The Face* (March 1993), pp. 40–6.

——, interview with Nick Moss, *The Face* (August 1993), pp. 60–1.

——, 'Getting on . . . not famously', *The Guardian Media* (24 June 1996), p. 14.

——, 'Funny, useful and selling', *The Guardian Media*, 17 February 1997, pp. 6–7.

R. Gerber, 'Manipulated lady', *The Independent on Sunday* (12 July 1992), pp. 44 and 46.

N. Gerrard, 'Little girls lost', *The Observer Review* (31 August 1997), p. 5.

R. Gibson, *Chris Garnham, photographer 1958–1989*, exhibition pamphlet (London: National Portrait Gallery, 1991).

J. Godfrey, 'Man child', *The Face* (November 1992), pp. 42–51.

L. Grant, 'The old colour of money', *The Guardian G2* (15 April 1997), p. 8.

——, 'Women who buy a full monty', *The Guardian G2* (30 September 1997), p. 8.

D. Green, 'Classified subjects', *Ten. 8*, No. 14 (1984), pp. 30–7.

R. Greenslade, 'The Yank's a swank', *The Guardian Media* (8 November 1993), p. 17.

A. Gross, 'Turbeville: an interview', American *Vogue* (December 1981), pp. 248, 335–7.

M. Gross, 'Camera chameleon', *Vanity Fair* (June 1986), pp. 100–6 and 116–18.

S. Gupta, 'Homosexualities, Part One: USA', *Ten.8*, No. 31 (1989), pp. 2–6.

S. Gupta and P. Parmar, 'Homosexualities, Part Two: UK', *Ten.8*, No. 32 (1989), pp. 22–35.

S. Hall, 'The social eye of *Picture Post*', *Working Papers in Cultural Studies*, 2 (Spring 1972), CCCS, University of Birmingham, pp. 71–121.

C. Hammond, 'Thin end of the Reg', *The Guardian G2* (16 September 1997), p. 13.

C. Harrison, 'Flesh is more', *Observer Life* (8 June 1997), pp. 25–30.

M. Harrison, 'Bruce Weber', *The Sunday Correspondent* (24 September 1989), pp. 13–14.

——, 'The female eye', *The Independent on Sunday* (6 September 1992, pp. 36 and 38.

——, 'Classic camera', *The Independent on Sunday Review* (2 April 1995), pp. 48–50.

A. Heath , 'Linda Evangelista', *The Face* (August 1993), pp. 74–7.

——, 'Maximum exposure', *The Observer Life* (6 March 1994), pp. 6–7.

——, 'Sonic boom boy', *The Face* (April 1994), pp. 80–5.

——, 'Nadja', *The Face* (September 1994), pp. 36–42.

——, 'The waif escape', *The Face* (November 1994), pp. 44–51.

——, 'Profile: Helmut Newton', *The Face* (November 1994), pp. 138–9.

——, 'Super girls', *The Face* (May 1995), pp. 74–83.

S. Heath, 'Difference', *Screen*, 19:13 (1978), pp. 51–112 .

D. Hebdige, 'Towards a cartography of taste 1935–1962', *Block*, 4 , pp. 39–55.

——, 'The bottom line on Planet One–squaring up to THE FACE', *Ten.8*, 19 (1985), pp. 40–9.

Z. Heller, 'At Home with Helmie', *The Independent on Sunday Review* (3 July 1994), pp. 12–13 and 15.

G. Henry, 'Robert Mapplethorpe–collecting quality: an interview', *Print Collector's Newsletter*, 13:4 (September/October 1982), pp. 128–30.

D. Hill, 'From New Lad to Millennium Man', *The Observer* (20 October 1996), p. 14.

P. Hillmore, 'Cutting edge of haute couture', *The Observer* (19 September 1993), p. 9.

C. Hindmarch, 'Do they mean us?', *Arena* (March/April 1992), p. 31.

P. Hoare, 'I'm a wonderful thing, baby', *Arena Homme Plus* (Autumn/Winter 1994), pp. 59–64.

A. Holden, 'Any colour . . . so long as it's black', *The Guardian* (17 September 1990), p. 20.

M. Honigsbaum, 'Blitz–no time to grow up', *The Guardian Media Section* (2 September 1991), p. 23.

L. Horsburgh, 'Seize the Day', *British Journal of Photography* (8 July 1993), pp. 16–17.

R. Hughes, 'Art, morals and politics', *New York Review of Books* (23 April 1992), pp. 21–7.

B. Hugill, 'TV ads show black in the shade of white', *The Observer* (24 August 1997), p. 4.

M. Hume, 'Super power', *The Independent on Sunday Review* (7 March 1993), p. 40.

——, 'When fashion is no excuse at all', *The Independent* (26 May 1993), p. 22.

——, 'The cat in the hat', *The Independent on Sunday* (19 September 1993), pp. 18–21.

——, 'Absolutely Fabien', *The Independent on Sunday Review* (5 June 1994), pp. 45–6.

——, 'Out of Africa', *Independent on Sunday Review* (6 August 1995), p. 40.

R. Hunt, 'GQ goes for a new super model', *The Guardian Media* (18 September 1995), p. 15.

T. Imrie, 'Double page dream', *BJP Annual* (1984).

'The information', *The Observer Review* (11 August 1996), p. 16.

P. Jackson, 'Black male: advertising and the cultural politics of masculinity', *Gender, Place and Culture*, 1:1 (1994), pp. 49–59.

D. Jarman, 'In art, as life', *The Independent on Sunday* (8 November 1992), pp. 3–7.

N. Jeal, 'Gee! cue for peacocks', *The Observer* (30 October 1988), p. 36.

——, 'Black style', *The Observer Weekend* (27 November 1988), pp. 35 and 37.

——, 'Radical chic: *Vogue* but not vague', *The Observer Living* (19 July 1992), p. 53.

'Jeans ads dropped after protestors see blue', *The Guardian* (29 August 1985), pp. 1–2.

L. Jobey, 'The Big Easy', British *Vogue* (December 1988), pp. 214–17.

——, 'The major league', *The Independent on Sunday Review* (18 August 1991), pp. 27–9.

——, 'Who's zooming who?', British *Vogue* (August 1992), pp. 142–5.

——, 'Caught in his own spotlight', *The Independent on Sunday* (3 October 1993), pp. 48–9.

——, 'Helmut's second coming', *The Independent on Sunday Review* (13 November 1994), pp. 52–3 and 55.

P. Jobling, 'Who's that girl?: "Alex Eats", a case study in abjection in contemporary fashion photography', *Fashion Theory*, 2:3 (1998), pp. 209–24.

D. Jones, 'Big shots', *The Observer Magazine* (15 November 1992), pp. 30–5.

——, 'Bruce Weber', *Observer Life* (2 November 1997), pp. 14–16.

I. Julien, 'True Confessions: A discourse on images of black male sexuality', *Ten. 8*, No. 22 (1986), pp. 4–9.

R. Kee, 'The Falklands Garrison', *The Observer Magazine* (23 April 1989), pp. 23–4.

P. Keers, letter to the editor, *Campaign* (2 May 1985), p. 20.

A. M. Klein, 'Fear and loathing in Southern California: narcissism and fascism in bodybuilding subculture', *Journal of Psychoanalytic Anthropology* (Spring 1987), pp. 117–37.

'Klein of the times', *Sky* (July 1997), pp. 90–6.

S. Koch, 'Guilt, grace and Robert Mapplethorpe', *Art in America* (November 1986), pp. 145–50.

R. Koenig, 'The man who loves women', British *Vogue* (November 1988), pp. 196–7 and 282.

H. Lacey, 'The übergirl cometh', *Independent on Sunday Real Life* (26 November 1995), p. 3.

H. Lassalle, 'The sightless woman in surrealist photography', *Afterimage*, 15:5 (December 1987), pp. 4–8.

G. Lau, 'Through the lens: female power-fantasies?', *Camerawork*, 32 (Summer 1985), pp. 24–5.

C. Leggett, 'high five', *Arena Homme Plus* (Autumn/Winter 1994), pp. 14–15.

K. Leston, '1992 – review of the year', *The Face* (January 1993), pp. 54–7.

N. Logan, 'My decade', *The Sunday Correspondent* (24 September 1989), p. 8.

N. Logan and D. Jones, 'Ray Petri', *The Face* (October 1989), p. 10.

'Love, lust and phoney baloney', *The Guardian* (21 June 1990), p. 38.

A. Lycett, 'Style's in, skin's out', *The Times* (6 September 1989), p. 32.

E. McCabe, 'A Ray of light in a phoney world', *The Guardian Media* (25 February 1991), p. 33.

D. McClintock, 'Colour', *Ten.8*, 22 (1986), pp. 26–9.

S. Marquis, 'The publishing conundrum: How to reach the "New Man"', *Campaign* (26 July 1985), p. 39.

A. Maxted, 'The sizes they are a-changin", *Independent on Sunday Real Life* (20 August 1995), p. 5.

S. Maynard, 'What color is your underwear? Class, whiteness and homo-erotic advertising', *Border/Lines*, 32 (1994), pp. 4–9.

G. Melly, 'Why the tables have turned on macho males', *Campaign* (18 July 1986), pp. 40–1.

S. Menkes, 'Fashion: why you can't see the clothes for the art', *Campaign* (4 April 1986), pp. 44–5.

'Men's fashion is Logan's latest run', *Campaign* (15 August 1986), p. 18.

K. Mercer, 'Skinhead sex thing: racial difference and the homoerotic imaginary', *New Formations*, 16 (1992), pp. 1–23.

E. Mills, 'Kittens on the catwalk', *The Observer* (12 May 1996), p. 5.

S. Mower, 'Surrealism in *Vogue*', British *Vogue* (May 1988), pp. 175–7 and 225.

——, 'The reality test', British *Vogue* (March 1991), pp. 262–3.

A. Murphy, 'Tainted ladies', *Observer Life* (8 June 1997), pp. 18–19.

K. Myers, 'Fashion 'n' passion', *Screen*, 23: 3–4 (1982).

——, 'Meet Mrs. Bradshaw', *Blitz* (September 1988), pp. 78–82.

'Nan Goldin talks to Nuyoboshi Araki', *Artforum* (January 1995).

P. Naville, 'Beaux-arts', *La Révolution Surréaliste* (15 April 1925), p. 27.

A. Nayak and M. Kehily, 'Playing it straight: masculinities, homophobias and schooling', *Journal of Gender Studies*, 5:2 (1996), pp. 211–29.

New Formations, 25, 'Michel Foucault: J'Accuse' (Summer 1995).

New Internationalist (November 1989), Special issue on homosexuality.

The New Man, pamphlet (Nottingham, C. J. Welton, 1919).

'New Man – the same old story?', *The Guardian* (20 June 1990), p. 17.

S. Nixon, 'Looking for the Holy Grail: publishing and advertising strategies and contemporary men's magazines', *Cultural Studies*, 7:3 (October 1993), pp. 466–92.

P. Norman, 'The shock of the neo', *The Guardian Weekend* (30–31 May 1992), pp. 4–5.

Karen Offen, 'Depopulation, nationalism and Feminism in fin-de-siècle France', *American Historical Review*, 89 (1984).

L. O'Kelly, 'Body talk', *The Observer Life* (23 October 1994), pp. 30–3.

S. Orbach, 'The cruel fact is that most women want to change something about their bodies', *The Guardian G2* (10 February 1998), pp. 4–5.

P. Osborne and L. Segal, 'Gender as performance: an interview with Judith Butler', *Radical Philosophy*, 67 (Summer 1994), pp. 32–7.

J. Paoletti, 'Ridicule and role models as factors in American men's fashion change 1900–1910, *Costume*, 29 (1985), pp.121–34.

T. Parsons, 'David Bailey', *The Face* (December 1984), pp. 62–8.

I. Phillips, 'A revolutionary of realism', *Independent on Sunday* (17 September 1995), pp. 44–5.

J. Picardie, 'Understudies', *Independent on Sunday Review* (10 December 1995), pp. 52 and 54.

R. Picardie, 'Not quite New Man but less of a chore than sloth', *The Independent II* (25 February 1994), p. 22.

M. Pumphrey, 'Why do cowboys wear hats in the bath? Style politics and the older man', *Critical Quarterly*, 31:3 (Autumn 1989), pp. 78–100.

'Rachel Williams', *Arena* (July/August 1995), pp. 94–7.

A. Raphael, interview with Emma Balfour, *The Face* (August 1993), pp. 38–9.

C. Raven , 'Future sex', *Observer Life* (29 October 1995), pp. 32–5.

J. Riviere, 'Womanliness as masquerade', *International Journal of Psychoanalysis*, Vol. 10 (1929), pp. 303–13.

M. Roberts, 'High anxiety: The Anna Wintour story', *Independent on Sunday Review* (6 October 1991), pp. 36–7.

J. Rumbold, 'Know a man by the seat of his pants', *The Guardian Style* (9 January 1989), p. 17.

——, 'It's all spots and fat egos', *The Guardian Media* (25 February 1991), p. 33.

B. Russell, 'Wilhelm von Pluschow and Wilhelm von Gloeden: two photo essays', *Studies in Visual Communication*, 9:2 (Spring 1983), pp. 57–82.

J. Sale, 'Founding father of GQ', *The Guardian Media* (20 April 1992), p. 3.

J. Savage, 'What's so new about the new man?', *Arena* (March/April 1988), pp. 33–9.

B. E. Savedoff, 'Transforming images: photographs of representations', *The Journal of Aesthetics and Art Criticism*, 50:2 (Spring 1992), pp. 93–106.

M. Sawyer, 'What Kate did', *Observer Life* (9 April 1995), pp. 10–15.

C. Schorr, 'A pose is a pose is a pose: fashion and art and fashion', *Frieze* (March/April 1997), pp. 60–5.

W. Scobie, 'Pride and prejudice', *The Observer Magazine* (12 January 1986), pp. 14–17.

A. Sekula, 'The body and the archive', *October* (Winter 1986), pp. 3–64.

'Sell out', *Time Out* (28 February–6 March 1996), pp. 7–35.

'Shopping new man', *The Guardian* (20 January 1998), p. 14.

'Siding with Rosie', *New Statesman* (20 September 1996), p. 5.

S. Sontag, 'The Avedon eye', British *Vogue* (December 1978), pp. 104–7.

N. Spencer and D. Jones, 'Clothes Lines: the ascent of stylish man', *Arena* (July/August 1992), pp. 66–73.

R. Stengel, 'Men as sex objects', *M* (July 1992), pp. 72–9.

A. Stephen, 'Newton's principles', *The Observer Magazine* (13 November 1988), pp. 63–7.

D. W. Stowe, 'Uncoloured people: the rise of whiteness studies', *Lingua Franca* (September/October 1996), pp. 68–77.

J. Tannenbaum, 'Robert Mapplethorpe: The Philadelphia Story', *Art Journal*, 50:4 (1991), pp. 71–6 .

S. Taylor, 'Men with attitude', *The Observer* (2 April 1995), p.5.

S. Tesler, 'Ten by ten', Blitz (September 1990), pp. 84–95.

'The Face that launched a hundred', *Media Week* (22 July 1988), pp. 28–9.

'The ideal homme magazine', *Media Week* (12 February 1988), p. 43.

P. Theroux, 'Undressing women', *The Observer Magazine* (26 September 1993), p. 34.

L. Thompson, 'Shooting stars', *The Guardian Society* (29 November 1995), pp. 8–9.

J. Thrift, 'Type fashion fusion', *Eye*, 6:22 (Autumn 1996), pp. 46–53.

T. Timblick, 'Ads on the offensive', *The Observer Magazine* (7 June 1992), pp. 24–6.

'Transformers', *The Face* (September 1994), pp. 112–20.

R. Tredre, 'Whatever happened to New Man?', *The Independent on Sunday* (25 July 1993), p. 6.

——, 'The new power of male shots', *The Observer Arts* (31 October 1993), pp. 14–15.

——, 'Men at the strutting edge', *The Observer Review* (4 February 1996), p. 3.

A. Treneman, 'Body and soul', *The Independent on Saturday Magazine* (11 October 1997), pp. 24–6.

A. Tuck, 'First class males', *Time Out* (29 May–5 June 1996), pp. 27–31.

R. Tyrrel, 'The New Male Order', British *Elle* (June 1993), pp. 22–4.

L'Univers Illustré, No.1 (22 May 1858).

J. Updike, 'The American male', *The Observer Magazine* (2 January 1994), p. 24.

'Vogue Men gets set to stand on its own', *Campaign* (26 September 1986), p. 7.

K. Walton, 'Transparent pictures: on the nature of photographic realism', *Critical Inquiry*, 11 (1984), pp. 245–58 .

S. Watney, 'Sort of left out: some reflections on photography, teaching and Clause 28', *Ten.8*, No. 29 (1988), pp. 52–4.

T. Waugh, 'Musclebound underground', *Square Peg*, 19 (1988), pp. 6–8.

A. Williams, 'Re-viewing the look: photography and the female gaze', *Ten.8*, 25 (1987), pp. 4–11.

V. Williams, 'Agenda benders', *The Guardian Weekend* (4 September 1993), pp. 20–1 and 24.

J. Williamson, 'Short circuit of the New Man', *New Statesman* (20 May 1988), pp. 28–9.

——, 'Survival of the thinnest', *The Guardian Weekend* (22 March 1997), p. 8.

E. Wilson. 'Are you man enough?', *The Independent on Sunday* (29 March 1992), pp. 36–7.

J. Winship, 'Back to the future – a style for the eighties', *New Socialist* (July/August, 1987), pp. 48–9.

J. Withers and A. Fawcett, 'Expo: Photographer's Gallery', *The Face* (April 1984), pp. 58–63.

I. Wolff, 'Blokes head for the locker room', *The Observer* (13 November 1994), p. 24.

G. Wood, 'Shoot to thrill', *The Observer Review* (24 March 1996), p. 8.

——, 'Burger Queens', *The Observer Review* (11 August 1996), p. 8.

M. Woolf, 'Body Shop turns cheek to chic', *The Observer* (9 June 1996), p. 24.

C. Worthington, 'Time for the men to try it', *The Independent on Sunday* (September 1994), pp. 44–5.

R. Yates, 'Flash geezers', *The Observer Review* (1 December 1996), p. 9.

L. Young, interview with Tyra Banks, *The Face* (August 1993), pp. 92–3.

——, 'Kristen McMenamy', *The Face* (August 1993), pp. 116–19.

(iv) Official Reports

Report of the Committee on Obscenity and Film Censorship, chairman Bernard Williams (London: HMSO, 1979).

(v) Film, Radio and Television

BBC 2, 'Cindy Palmano', *The Late Show* (1989).

BBC 2, *The Look* (1992) programme 3.

BBC 2, *My Name is Albert Watson* (1994).

BBC 2, 'Fatal Exposure', *The Works* (1997).

BBC Radio 4, *The Stylographers* (29 September 1988).

Blow-Up, director Antonioni (MGM, 1966).

The Eyes of Laura Mars, director Irvin Kershner (Columbia Pictures, 1978).

Madonna, 'Vogue' (1990), directed by Herb Ritts, *Madonna: The Immaculate Collection* (Warner Music Vision, 1990).

Olympia (1938), director Leni Riefenstahl (National Film Archive, London, 1939).

Once Upon A Time In America, director Serge Leone (Warner Brothers, 1984).

Querelle, director R. Fassbinder (Planet/ Albatross/Gaumont, 1982).

Index

abjection, 109, 130–1, 133, 134, 177
Abstract Expressionism, 23
Agha, M.F., 20
AIDS – see HIV/AIDS
Allen Poe, E., 42
Andreolli, K., 44
androgyny, 23, 44, 95, 108, 111, 125, 144
   Lennox, A., 44
   Moss, N., 144
   Prince, 44, 107
see also gender
anorexia, 24, 112, 113, 126–35, 140n66
Antonioni, 121
Area, 65
Arena, 6, 7, 8, 9, 17, 18, 38, 49–57, 61, 96,
   111, 146, 149
   circulation, 50
      'Fairground Attraction', 172
      'fin de siècle', 53–4, 61, 93, 165
      'Hard Edged', 152
      'Have a Nice Day', 172
      'high tension', 158
      'Idle Kitsch', 120
      'Kid Gloves', 118
      'NYC – Urban Cowboy', 150
      'On and Off the Road', 154
      'once upon a time', 53, 54–6, 61, 93,
         152, 158
      'South of the Border', 172
      'Throwback', 151
      'Wide Boys Awake', 154
Arena Homme Plus 7, 53
   'Close Encounters', 4, 150, 173–7
Armani, G., 49
Armstrong, L., 119
Armstrong-Jones, A, 21
Art Nouveau, 19
Arts, A., 135

see also *The Face*, 'Alex Eats' and 'Alex
   Works'
Arts and Crafts, 19,
Ashworth, P, 36, 37
Asio, 152
Aurell, A., 179
Avedon, R., 5

Badulescu, E., 52
Bailey, D., 21, 22, 31n11
Bakhtin, M., 91, 129
Baker, C., 108
Balfour, E., 111, 113
Barthes, R.,
   Essais Critiques, 80
   Elements of Semiology, 81n9
   The Fashion System, 1, 9, 62, 66–103,
      135, 171
   class, 75–6, 87
   'commutation test', 86
   fashionability, 85–6
   gender, 66, 79, 94–7, 101
   image-clothing, 10, 66, 73–4, 84, 86,
      93
   OVS matrix, 74, 81n8, 93
   photography, 74, 88–90, 93
   poetics of clothing, 26, 77, 101, 102n1,
      114, 152, 177
   reason of Fashion, 77, 79–80, 101
   rhetorical system, 71–2, 74, 84–7
   shifters, 71–2
   terminological system, 71–2, 74, 84–6
   technological/real system, 71–2, 74, 84,
      86
   time, 70, 80–1
   vesteme, 74
   work, 79, 158
   worldly signified, 77–9, 101

written clothing, 10, 66, 72–4, 76, 84, 86, 88, 93, 98n16, 101
  Image/Music/Text, 94
  Le Plaisir du Texte, 102, 103n6
  'Myth Today', 18, 59–61, 76, 146
    inoculation, 146, 168
  'The Photographic Message', 89, 115
  Roland Barthes, 107, 179
Bataille, G., 131, 156
  bassesse, 131
Baudrillard, J, 5, 45, 83
  hyperreality, 5, 18, 30, 40–1, 56, 65, 99n28
BAZAAR, 161
Beatles, The, 37, 114
Beckford, T., 152
Berkin, D., 53, 151, 154
Bettles, A., 162
Beukers, A., 38
Bhabha, H.K., 155, 156
Blahnik, M., 26
Blame, J., 44, 125
Blitz, 17, 35, 96, 143
Blow-Up, 121–2, 138n39
body, the, 107–86, 128
  body double, 109
  body fascism, 12, 147, 170, 181n23
  female body, 112–35
    the 'girl', 111–12, 126
    ectomorphism, 126–35
  phallic body, 109–79
    female, 158–65, 184n66
    non-white, 152–8, 164
Bolan, M., 144
Borch-Jakobsen, M, 157
Bordo, S., 127
see also anorexia
Bourdin, G., 11, 22,
Bowles, H., 108
Brading, M., 36, 38, 52, 53, 108, 154
Bradshaw, Dò, 38, 53, 152, 158, 172
Brassa, 161
Breton, A., 159–60, 162
  Mad Love (L'Amour Fou), 160–61
Brody, N., 7, 35, 37, 42, 50, 148
Brooks, R., 152
Bulger, J., 117
  Robert Thompson, 117

  Jon Venables, 117
bulimia
  see anorexia
Burton, R., 156
Butler, J., 10, 12, 94, 109, 163, 165, 170–3, 178, 179
see also performativity

Callaghan, G., 158
Callaghan, S., 178
camp, 179
Campbell, N., 152
cannibalism, 131
Caputi, J., 127
Carroll, L., 116
Carter, E., 22
Cather, W., 9, 23, 26–8, 45, 56, 61
censorship, 109, 115–17, 118
  Advertising Standards Authority, 116
  Feminists Against Censorship, 116, 137n20
  Jesse Helms, 137n18
  Obscene Publications Act, 115
  Protection of Children Act, 115
  Williams Report, 116, 137n20
Chanel, C., 126, 159, 170
Chapman, R., 51–2
Charity, R., 38
Chatelain, A., 23
Cixous, H., 143
Clark, A.K., 112
Clinton, W.J., 3
Cobbett, W., 146, 180n14
computer systems, 179
  Barco, 179
  Paintbox, 179
  Quantel, 197
Condé Nast, T., 19, 30n4
Conrad, J., 28
Cooper, G., 115
Cosmopolitan, 17, 31n11, 50, 113
  Cosmo Man, 50
Coward, R., 123, 143
Crolla, S., 42, 43
Crozier, M., 70, 81n4
Culler, J., 83–5

Dal', S., 160

dandy, the, 158, 180n7, 184n65
d'Argy-Smith, M., 113
David-Tu, A., 162
Davies, G., 49
Day, C., 2, 6, 8, 11, 24, 36, 38, 66, 96, 112
see also The Face, 'borneo' and 'England's
   Dreaming'; Vogue (British), 'Under
   Exposure'
Dazed and Confused, 17
deconstruction, 87–8, 166
   supplementarity, 166–7
Demarchelier, P., 22, 114
Derrida, J., 88, 162
   parergon, 87, 166
   pharmakos, 92
Dolce e Gabbana, 54, 168
Donovan, T., 21, 31n11
Don't Tell It, 17
Dourdan, G., 152
Duffy, B., 21, 31n11
Dunaway, F., 121
Dyer, R., 97, 151, 157

Edwards, S., 118
Elle, 17
Elle (French) 67n5, 70, 76, 80, 81n8, 87,
   97n7, 102
   'Amoureuse', 10, 21, 66, 72–4, 77–9, 80,
   90–4, 144
Erdman, R., 108
erotic, the 25, 115–16, 135, 158
   homoerotic, 144, 149–51, 154
The Eyes of Laura Mars, 121–22

Fabulous, 7, 37
The Face, 6, 9, 17, 18, 35–47, 50–3, 61, 96,
   102, 107, 111, 143, 146, 168
   circulation, 45–6, 113
   'Alex Eats', 7, 11, 112–13, 115,
   126–35, 145
   'Alex Wo⁻rks', 119
   'Another Country', 108
   'Apparitions', 9, 42–4, 61, 111
   'Army Dreamers', 179
   'The Baby Sitter', 118
   'Back to the Future', 8,
   'Beached Bums', 135
   'borneo', 66, 78, 82n13, 114

'Brute 33', 179
'Cherry Drops and Jelly Babes', 127
'Crimes of Passion', 111
'The Daisy Age', 114
'England's Dreaming', 115–16
'Fashion Vampires', 125
'Flesh', 31n11, 145
'Forever Leather', 164
'For Your Pleasure', 124–5
'grease monkeys', 145, 148–9
'Guys N Dolls', 3–5, 173
'Heavy Metal', 96–7
'Hotel Motel, Holiday In', 111, 165
'London – March 88', 162
'Malcolm X', 153, 155
'Oh You Pretty Thing', 111
'Performance', 179
'Punk', 155–6
'Role over and enjoy it', 108
'Simplex Concordia', 179
'Suit Yourself', 108
'Trade', 178
'Veiled Threats', 9, 43–4, 47n34, 54, 61,
   94, 111
'Wet', 172
'Who's Shooting Who?', 66–7, 101–02,
   103n2, 158
'Yard Times', 127
Faithfull, M., 4, 37
Fanon, F., 154, 155
fascism, 147, 186n112
fashion models, 7, 21, 24, 31n11, 96, 108,
   115, 127, 135, 144, 152
Fassbinder, W.M., 173
fetishism, 119, 121, 157, 161
FHM, 17, 49, 50, 146
Foale M., 22
For Him – *see FHM*
For Women, 167
Foster, R., 152
Foucault, M., 5, 108, 127, 169
Foxton, S., 38, 53, 173
see also Arena Homme Plus, 'Close
   Encounters'
Frecker, P., 53
Freud, S., 10, 125, 160, 162, 172, 186n112
   cannibalism, 131–2
   fort/da, 126, 139n56

homosexuality, 169
infantile sexuality, 161
'Oedipus complex', 131, 133, 157,
   164–5, 170
penis envy, 126, 139n59, 161, 170
Fuss, D., 11, 125, 126
Fussell, S., 169

Galliano, J., 43
Garner, K., 172
Garratt, S., 36
Gaultier, J.P., 31n11, 43, 49, 114
gaze, the, 123–6, 135, 151, 156, 163, 165,
   174–5, 179
vampiric, 125, 139n56
gay, 10, 11, 12, 22, 23, 25, 51, 56n10,
   96–7, 107, 11–77, 118, 122, 123–5, 126,
   139n56, 144–5, 147–51, 154, 155, 164,
   165, 167, 168–9, 172–9
see also gender; erotic, homoerotic;
   performativity
gender, 10, 12, 66, 94, 107, 170–9
femininity 92, 94–5, 117–35
masculinity, 10, 12, 79, 95–6, 143–89
see also the body; gay; performativity
Genet, J.
Querelle de Brest, 4, 173–7
see also gay
Gestrich, M., 111
Gide, A., 139n56
Gill, J., 111
Glassner, B., 169
Gordon, A., 11, 119
see also The Face, 'Alex Eats' and 'Alex
   Works'
GQ, 7, 8, 17, 49, 50, 56n1, 93, 96, 147
Grieve, A., 42
Griffiths, C., 38, 158, 172
grunge, 114
Jerome, 144
Martin, K., 144
gym culture, 97, 147, 149, 158, 168–70,
   182n27

Haddi, M., 36, 39, 52, 53, 60, 118, 144,
   151, 154
half-tone, 19
Hall, S., 156

Hall-Duncan, N., 1, 5
Hamnett, K., 49
Harpers and Queen, 17, 25
Harper's Bazaar, 114
Harrison, M., 5, 21, 98n16
Heartfield, J., 50
Hebdige, D., 9, 18, 30, 114, 128, 155, 169
   The Face, 39–42, 45
see also incorporation
Hegel, 40, 88, 90
Heidegger, 83
heroin chic, 2–3, 113, 115–16
Heseltine, M, 49
Hill, D., 37, 44
Hine, L., 55, 56
historicism, 25–30, 43, 44, 47n34, 53–6, 59
HIV/AIDS, 51, 155, 170
Holland, P., 117
homosexuality
see gay
Horkheimer, M., 170
Horst P. Horst, 5, 20, 21, 53, 144
Horvat, F., 95
Howell, M., 27
Hoyningen-Huene, G., 20, 53
Hugell, A., 118
Hume, M., 112, 114, 122

i-D, 8, 17, 35, 38, 96, 143
incorporation, 113–14, 119, 136n9, 155,
   169
inoculation, 146, 168
intertextuality
see word and image
intratextuality
see word and image
Irigaray, L., 11, 92, 120, 123–4, 126, 163,
   164
see also gay; mimicry

Jakobson, R., 71
Jameson, F., 30
Jardin des Modes, 67n5, 70, 76, 7–9, 80,
   87, 97n7
'Monsieur J.M.', 79, 95, 98n35
Jenkins, L., 162
Jones, D., 8, 38
Jones, E., 67

see also The Face, 'Who's Shooting Who?'

Kant, I., 166
Karl and Derick, 39, 153, 172
Kasterine, C., 112
see also Vogue, 'Under Exposure'
Keers, P., 49
Kehily, M., 172
Kersher, I., 121
Kidscape, 115
Kilpatrick, J., 115, 136n14
Klein, A., 147, 149
Klein, C., 25, 49, 114, 115, 144, 154
    American Family Association, 115
Klein, S., 179
Klein, W., 21
Knight, N., 6, 8, 36, 38, 52, 53, 97, 144,
    155, 173
see also Arena Homme Plus, 'Close
    Encounters'
Kohn, M., 108
Korff, K., 20
Kracauer, S., 45
Kristeva, J., 11, 123, 126, 130–1, 132, 133,
    134, 143, 177
    homosexual maternal, 123–4, 126,
    138n48
    chora, 126
see also abjection

Labovitch, C., 49
Lacan, J., 10, 126, 160, 162, 167, 171,
    183n60, 184n65, 186n116
    'The Mirror Stage', 108, 110n10, 134,
    145, 162–3
    the gaze, 123, 165
    the Symbolic, 130, 133, 157
see also phallogocentrism
La Mode Pratique, 20
Lapape, P., 83
Lauren, R., 54, 152
Lavender, A., 127, 128
see also The Face, 'Alex Eats'
Lebon, M., 38, 164
L'Echo de la Mode, 70, 75
Lee, S., 153
Leone, S., 54, 55, 56, 61
lesbianism

see gay
Levi jeans, 49, 51
Lewis, R., 123, 125
Liberman, A., 21, 25
Linard, S., 37
Loaded, 50
Logan, N., 7, 35, 36, 38, 50, 52, 167
logocentrism, 9, 40, 66
see also phallogocentrism
Lowe, D., 128
Luchford, G., 36, 125
L'Univers Illustré, 20
Lush, K., 112
see also The Face, 'Alex Eats'
Lyotard, J., 120–21
    differend, 120–21

McCabe, E., 1
McCann-Erickson, 51
MacKinnon, C., 117
Macpherson, A., 36, 42, 52, 61
MacSween, M., 128
see also anorexia
Madonna, 31n11, 114
Maddow, B., 29
Mainman, D., 152
Man About Town, 49, 143
Mann, S., 116
ManStudy Report, 51, 180n13
Mapplethorpe, R., 116, 154, 155, 156
Marie Claire, 17
Marignac, B., 118
Martin, J., 152
Mason, D., 108, 164
Maxim, 50
Maxwell, O., 67
see also The Face, 'Who's Shooting Who?'
Maynard, S., 154
melancholia, 134, 165
Men Only, 49
Mercer, K., 78, 153
Mesdon, R., 38, 53, 55, 61
Miller, D.A., 149
Milne, D., 179
mimicry, 109, 117, 120, 121, 150, 155, 156,
    164, 184n66
Mintel, 146, 181, n20
Mizer, B., 150

Mondino, J.B., 44, 53, 162, 170
money shot, 134, 141n89
Monheim, A., 179
Morgan, J., 38, 66, 96, 144
see also Petri, R, Buffalo Boy; *The Face*
   'Heavy Metal'
Moss, K., 24, 78, 96, 112, 114, 115, 127,
   129, 135
see also The Face 'borneo'; *Vogue* (British),
   'Under Exposure'
Mulvey, L., 123

narcissism, 134, 144, 147, 158, 168
   primary, 124, 126
Nayak, A., 172
Neue Sachlichkeit
see New Objectivity
Newburn, T., 118
Newhall, N., 29
new man, 9, 51–2, 96, 145–47, 168,
   180n14, 181n15
see also gay; gender
New Musical Express, 35
New Objectivity, 20, 53–4
Newton, H., 5, 8, 11, 22, 24, 36, 119, 120,
   121, 122, 124
New Woman, 168
Next for Men, 49
Nikos, 96
Nocella, C., 172
nostalgia
see historicism
Nova, 22, 133

Obadia, J., 50
O'Callaghan, D., 168
O'Polo, M., 26
Orbach, S., 113, 115, 122
Other the, 7–8, 108–09, 130, 133, 156,
   158, 163, 170, 179

paedophilia, 10, 113, 116–18, 122, 127, 135
Paradis, V., 126
Penn, I., 5, 21, 22,
performativity, 9, 12, 87, 94, 109, 145, 164,
   170–9, 186n116
see also Arena Homme Plus, 'Close
   Encounters'; the body; gay; gender

Per Lui, 49
   'Album. Phototour', 150–51
Petri, R., 38, 66, 96, 144, 150, 154, 172
   Buffalo Boy, 38, 96
see also The Face, 'Heavy Metal'
phallogocentrism, 122, 157–8, 167
phallus, 153–5, 158, 165, 183n60, 184n66
photography
   photographers' gender, 112, 119, 120
   photographic fees, 36, 46n6
   realism, 115, 136n6
Physique Pictorial, 150
Pictorialism, 53
Picture Post, 41
plaisir/pleasure, 92, 96, 103n6, 108, 167,
   168, 178
see also spectatorship
Plato, 98n12, 126
Platt-Lynes, G., 25
pornography, 22, 107, 109, 112, 114–18,
   120, 121, 127, 135
Postmodernism, 40, 41, 45, 128, 162
   metanarrative, 55, 59
   simulation, 53, 59, 128, 151
prostitution, 134
Punk, 155

Quant, M., 22
Queen, 22

race, 55, 78, 107, 109, 152–7, 163, 179
see also the body, female; non-white
Radner, H., 18, 23, 102
Ray, Man, 4, 5, 159, 161, 162
readerships, 38, 45–6, 50, 51, 113, 114,
   122–23, 148, 150, 167–8
see also spectatorship
Richards, H., 144
Richmond/Cornejo, 43
Riefenstahl, L., 25, 147
Ritts, H., 6, 22, 23, 31n11, 36, 144, 147,
   148, 170
Riviere, J., 96
Robot, 37
Rock, S., 36, 37
Rodway, K., 144
Roger, M., 162
Rohde, N., 179

Rolley, K., 123, 125
Rosza, J., 149, 150
Roversi, P., 23, 38

St Laurent, Y., 23
Sander A., 25
Santoro, 21, 66
see also *Elle* (French), 'Amoureuse'
Saussure de F., 69–70, 84
Schatzberg, J., 21
Schoerner, 36
Scott, V., 39, 111
Sednaoui, S., 53, 162
semiology, 69–70, 71, 76
sexuality
see androgyny; the body; gay; gender;
    performativity
Shadee Perez, D., 53
Shelley, I., 152
Shrimpton, J., 21,22
Shulman, A., 119
Sieff, J., 22, 133
Sims, D., 36, 111
Smash Hits, 35
Smith, G., 36
Smith, P., 26, 49
Smith, R., 65
Sontag, S., 134, 147
Sopp, R., 51
Sorrenti, D., 2–3
'Sotadic Zone', 156
spectatorship, 96, 101–02, 108–09, 112,
    115–17, 121, 122–6, 135, 150, 167–9,
    178–9
see also readerships
Sprouse, S., 148
Steichen, E., 5, 20, 53
Stember, J., 119
Stoker, B., 125
structuralism, 69
Sturges, J., 116
stylist, 38–9
see also Petri, R. and Appendix 1
Surrealism, 4, 7, 12, 20, 53, 54, 131,
    159–62
    automatism, 159
    convulsive beauty, 159–62, 184n79
    trouvaille, 160

Teller, J., 36, 39, 52
Templer, K., 178
Ten, 8, 39, 40
Testino, M., 23
Thatcher, M., 43
Theweleit, K., 164
Thody, P., 84
Time, 24
Tomlinson, M., 44
Tuffin, S., 22
Turbeville, D., 10, 22, 23, 24
typography, 42, 54, 148
see also word and image

Unique, 7, 17, 50, 96, 146
  'High Noon', 149

van Lamsweerde, I., 39, 124, 179
Versace, G., 170
Vinoodh Matadin, 39, 125
Virilio, P., 40, 46n21
Vogue (American), 2, 5, 10, 19, 20, 22, 23,
    53, 102
Vogue (British), 6, 7, 8, 17, 18, 19–33,
    32n28, 35, 36, 39, 50, 53, 54, 56, 61,
    66, 77, 126, 129, 133, 143
  circulation, 113, 122
  'Bodyline', 120
  'New Morning Nebraska', 9, 26–8, 55,
    61, 94, 122
  'Soft Understatements', 119
  'Sri Lanka – Fashion in the Sun and
    Serendip', 66, 77–8
  'Under Exposure', 7,8, 11, 93, 96,
    112–26, 127, 145
  'Under Weston Eyes', 9, 26, 28–29, 55,
    61, 94
Vogue (French), 10, 22, 53, 70
Vogue Pour Hommes, 49
von Unwerth, E., 6, 53, 120, 121, 172
von Wangenheim, C., 11, 22

Ward, M., 38, 66
Watson, N., 6, 22, 38, 39, 53, 96, 150, 172
Weber, B., 6, 8, 9, 22, 23, 24, 25–30, 37,
    42, 44–5, 54, 55, 56, 61, 144, 147,
    150–51
see also *Vogue*, 'New Morning Nebraska'

and 'Under Weston Eyes'; Per Lui,
   'Album. Phototour'
Welton, C.J., 146
West, J., 144
Weston, E., 9, 26, 28–9, 45, 56, 61
Westwood, V., 164
Wicke, J., 117
Williams, V., 113
Williamson, J., 39, 146
Wilson, E., 21, 107, 113, 170
Winship, J., 47, n34
Wintour, A., 19, 24
Woman's Own, 17

Woolf, V., 143
Woolman, E., 19
word and image, 5, 9, 26–9, 39–45, 47n36,
   54–6, 59–62, 65–6, 72–5, 86–94, 98n27,
   101–02, 109, 117, 125, 127, 148–51,
   153, 155, 165, 173–9
Wordsworth, W., 47n36

Yamamoto, Y., 54
York, P., 146
Yuppies, 50

Za-Zuza, 37